OPERATIVE TECHNIQUES

spine

surgery

OPERATIVETECHNIQUES

spine
surgery

Alexander R. Vaccaro, MD, FACS
Professor
Department of Orthopaedics and
Neurosurgery
Co-Director of the Delaware Valley Regional
Spinal Cord Injury Service
Co-Chief of Spine Surgery
Thomas Jefferson University and
The Rothman Institute
Philadelphia, Pennsylvania

Eli M. Baron, MD
Attending Spine Surgeon
Attending Neurosurgeon
Cedars-Sinai Institute for Spinal Disorders
Los Angeles, California

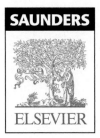

SAUNDERS

ELSEVIER

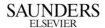

SAUNDERS
ELSEVIER

1600 John F. Kennedy Blvd.
Ste 1800
Philadelphia, PA 19103-2899

OPERATIVE TECHNIQUES: SPINE SURGERY   ISBN: 978-1-4160-3279-3

Notice

Knowledge and best practice in this field are constantly changing. As new research and experience broaden our knowledge, changes in practice, treatment and drug therapy may become necessary or appropriate. Readers are advised to check the most current information provided (i) on procedures featured or (ii) by the manufacturer of each product to be administered, to verify the recommended dose or formula, the method and duration of administration, and contraindications. It is the responsibility of the practitioner, relying on their own experience and knowledge of the patient, to make diagnoses, to determine dosages and the best treatment for each individual patient, and to take all appropriate safety precautions. To the fullest extent of the law, neither the Publisher nor the Editor assumes any liability for any injury and/or damage to persons or property arising out or related to any use of the material contained in this book.

The Publisher

Library of Congress Cataloging-in-Publication Data
Operative techniques : spine surgery/[edited by] Alexander R. Vaccaro, Eli M. Baron.—1st ed.
    p. ; cm.
Includes bibliographical references and index.
ISBN 978-1-4160-3279-3
1. Spine—Surgery—Atlases. I. Vaccaro, Alexander R. II. Baron, Eli M. III. Title: Spine surgery.
[DNLM: 1. Spine—surgery. 2. Orthopedic Procedures—methods. WE 725 O613 2007]
RD768.O68 2007
617.5'6059—dc22   2007025412

Acquisitions Editor: Kimberly Murphy
Design Direction: Steven Stave

Printed in China

Last digit is the print number: 9 8 7 6 5 4 3 2

I dedicate the effort behind this book to my wife Midge and three children Max, Alex and Juliana for their tolerance and support in allowing me the time and effort needed to complete this undertaking.

Alexander R. Vaccaro

I dedicate this book to my neurosurgical and orthopaedic instructors and students who have enabled me to gain a better grasp of the art and science of spine surgery. I also dedicate the book to my parents for their tireless support of me and my endeavors.

Eli M. Baron

CONTRIBUTORS

Kuniyoshi Abumi, MD
Professor of Orthopaedic Surgery, Hokkaido
    University, Sapporo, Japan
    Cervical Pedicle Screw Fixation

Todd J. Albert, MD
Professor of Orthopaedic Surgery and Neurosurgery,
    Jefferson Medical College of Thomas Jefferson
    University; Chairman of Orthopaedic Surgery
    Department, Thomas Jefferson University Hospital
    and The Rothman Institute, Philadelphia,
    Pennsylvania
    Posterior Far Lateral Disk Herniation

Howard S. An, MD
The Morton International Professor of Orthopaedic
    Surgery, and Director of Division of Spine Surgery
    and Spine Fellowship, Department of Orthopaedic
    Surgery, Rush University Medical Center, Chicago,
    Illinois
    Halo Placement in the Pediatric and Adult Patient

Neel Anand, MD
Co-Director, Institute for Spinal Disorders, Cedars-
    Sinai Medical Center, Los Angeles, California
    Posterior Cervical Osteotomy Techniques

David T. Anderson, MD
Resident, Orthopaedic Surgery, Thomas Jefferson
    University Hospital, Philadelphia, Pennsylvania
    Anterior Cervical Corpectomy/Diskectomy

D. Greg Anderson, MD, PhD
Associate Professor, Department of Orthopaedics,
    Thomas Jefferson University Hospital and The
    Rothman Institute, Philadelphia, Pennsylvania
    Posterior Far Lateral Disk Herniation; Minimally
        Invasive Exposure Techniques of the Lumbar Spine

Paul A. Anderson, MD
Associate Professor of Orthopedic Surgery,
    Department of Orthopedic Surgery and
    Rehabilitation, University of Wisconsin, Madison,
    Wisconsin
    Anterior Cervical Disk Arthroplasty

Ronald I. Apfelbaum, MD
Professor, and Attending Physician in Neurosurgery,
    Department of Neurosurgery, University of Utah,
    Salt Lake City, Utah
    Odontoid Screw Fixation

Eli M. Baron, MD
Attending Spine Surgeon and Attending
    Neurosurgeon, Cedars-Sinai Institute for Spinal
    Disorders, Los Angeles, California
    Anterior Odontoid Resection: The Transoral
        Approach; Anterior C1–C2 Arthrodesis: Lateral
        Approach of Barbour and Whitesides

Mohan Belthur, MD
Clinical Fellow, Department of Orthopaedics, Alfred
    I. duPont Hospital for Children, Nemours
    Children's Clinic, Wilmington, Delaware
    Thoracoplasty for Rib Deformity

Edward C. Benzel, MD
Professor of Surgery, Cleveland Clinic Lerner College
    of Medicine of Case Western Reserve University;
    Director, Center for Spine Health, Cleveland Clinic,
    Cleveland, Ohio
    The Lateral Extracavitary Approach for
        Vertebrectomy

John Birkness, MD
Chief Neurosurgical Resident, Jefferson Medical
    College of Thomas Jefferson University,
    Philadelphia, Pennsylvania
    Resection of Intradural Intramedullary or
        Extramedullary Spinal Tumors

Scott L. Blumenthal, MD
Orthopedic Surgeon, Texas Back Institute, Plano,
    Texas
    Lumbar Spine Arthroplasty: Charité Total Disk
        Replacement

Oheneba Boachie-Adjei, MD
Chief of the Scoliosis Service, Hospital for Special
    Surgery, New York, New York
    Hemivertebrae Resection

Keith H. Bridwell, MD
Asa C. and Dorothy W. Jones Professor of
Orthopedics, and Professor of Neurological
Surgery, Washington University in St. Louis; Chief,
Adult/Pediatric Spine Surgery, Washington
University in St. Louis, Barnes Hospital, and St.
Louis Children's Hospital, St. Louis, Missouri
Osteotomy Techniques (Smith-Petersen and Pedicle
Subtraction) for Fixed Sagittal Imbalance

Christopher Brown, MD
Spine Fellow, Emory University, Atlanta, Georgia
Cervical Laminoplasty

Jacob M. Buchowski, MD, MS
Assistant Professor of Orthopaedic Surgery and
Neurological Surgery, Washington University;
Surgeon, Barnes-Jewish Hospital, St. Louis,
Missouri
Transforaminal Lumbar Interbody Fusion

Robert M. Campbell, Jr., MD
Professor of Orthopaedics, The President's Council/
Dielmann Chair in Pediatric Orthopaedics,
University of Texas Health Science Center at San
Antonio; Director, The Thoracic Institute,
CHRISTUS Santa Rosa Children's Hospital, San
Antonio, Texas
VEPTR Opening Wedge Thoracostomy for
Congenital Spinal Deformities

David Choi, MA, MB, ChB, FRCS(SN), PhD
Consultant Neurosurgeon, The National Hospital for
Neurology and Neurosurgery, Queen Square,
London, United Kingdom
Anterior Odontoid Resection: The Transoral
Approach

David H. Clements, MD
Associate Professor of Orthopedic Surgery, Cooper
Bone and Joint Institute, Robert Wood Johnson
School of Medicine, Camden, New Jersey; Director
of Spinal Surgery, Cooper University Hospital,
Camden, New Jersey; Attending Surgeon, Shriner's
Hospital for Children, Philadelphia, Pennsylvania
Reduction of High-Grade Spondylolisthesis

H. Alan Crockard, DSc, FRCS, FRCS(Ed), FDS, RCS(Eng)
Consultant Neurosurgeon, The National Hospital for
Neurology and Neurosurgery, Queen Square,
London, United Kingdom
Anterior Odontoid Resection: The Transoral
Approach

Tapan Daftari, MD
Orthopaedic Spine Fellow, William Beaumont
Hospital, Royal Oak, Michigan
Sacropelvic Fixation

Michael D. Daubs, MD
Assistant Professor, Department of Orthopaedic
Surgery, and Surgeon, University of Utah Medical
Center; Surgeon, Primary Children's Medical
Center, Salt Lake City, Utah
Anterior Lumbar Interbody Fusion; Transforaminal
Lumbar Interbody Fusion

Gregory D. Dikos, MD
Resident, Department of Orthopaedic Surgery,
Indiana University School of Medicine,
Indianapolis, Indiana
Complete Vertebral Resection for Primary Spinal
Tumors

Thomas J. Errico, MD
Associate Professor of Orthopedic and Neurological
Surgery, New York University School of Medicine;
Chief, Division of Spine Surgery, New York
University Hospital for Joint Diseases, New York,
New York
Operative Management of Scheuermann's Kyphosis

Daniel R. Fassett, MD, MBA
Resident, Department of Neurosurgery, University of
Utah, Salt Lake City, Utah
Odontoid Screw Fixation

Michael A. Finn, MD
Resident, Department of Neurosurgery, University of
Utah, Salt Lake City, Utah
Odontoid Screw Fixation

Jeff Fischgrund, MD
Spine Surgeon, William Beaumont Hospital, Royal
Oak, Michigan
Sacropelvic Fixation

Charles Fisher, MD, FRCSC
Spine Surgeon, Vancouver, British Columbia, Canada
Interspinous Process Motion-Sparing Implant

Ernest Found, MD
Associate Professor of Orthopaedics, The University
of Iowa, Iowa City, Iowa
Spondylolysis Repair

Kyle Fox, PA-C
Private Practice, Milwaukee Neurological Institute,
Milwaukee, Wisconsin
Anterior Thoracic Diskectomy and Corpectomy

Peter G. Gabos, MD
Assistant Professor, Jefferson Medical College of
Thomas Jefferson University, Philadelphia,
Pennsylvania; Co-Director, Division of Scoliosis and
Spine Surgery, Alfred I. duPont Hospital for
Children, Wilmington, Delaware
Anterior Thoracolumbar Spinal Fusion with Single-
or Dual-Rod Instrumentation via Open Approach
for Idiopathic Scoliosis

John A. Handal, MD
Chairman, Department of Orthopaedic Surgery,
Albert Einstein Medical Center, Philadelphia,
Pennsylvania
Posterior C1–C2 Fusion Techniques: Harms
Technique and Magerl Technique

Colin Harris, MD
Resident, Department of Orthopaedics, University of
Medicine and Dentistry-New Jersey Medical
School, Newark, New Jersey
Closed Cervical Skeletal Tong Placement and
Reduction Techniques

James S. Harrop, MD
Assistant Professor of Neurosurgery and
Orthopaedics, Thomas Jefferson University,
Philadelphia, Pennsylvania
Anterior Odontoid Resection: The Transoral
Approach; Resection of Intradural Intramedullary
or Extramedullary Spinal Tumors

Alan S. Hilibrand, MD
Associate Professor of Orthopaedic Surgery and
Neurosurgery, and Director of Medical Education,
Jefferson Medical College of Thomas Jefferson
University/The Rothman Institute, Thomas
Jefferson University Hospital, Philadelphia,
Pennsylvania
Anterior Cervical Corpectomy/Diskectomy

Jack I. Jallo, MD, PhD
Associate Professor, Temple University School of
Medicine, Philadelphia, Pennsylvania
Occipital-Cervical Fusion

J. Patrick Johnson, MD
Director, Academic Research and Fellowship
Programs, Cedars-Sinai Institute for Spinal
Disorders; Director, California Institute of
Neurological Surgeons, Los Angeles, California
Endoscopic Thoracic Diskectomy

Stepan Kasimian, MD
Attending Spine Surgeon, University of Southern
California, Los Angeles, and Saint John's Health
Center, Santa Monica, California
Endoscopic Thoracic Diskectomy

Daniel H. Kim, MD
Neurosurgeon, Ochsner Clinic, New Orleans,
Louisiana
Anterior Thoracic Diskectomy and Corpectomy

Timothy R. Kuklo, MD, JD
Professor of Orthopaedic Surgery, and Associate
Professor, Washington University School of
Medicine, St. Louis, Missouri
Posterior Thoracolumbar Fusion Techniques for
Scoliosis—Lenke Classification

Joon Y. Lee, MD
Assistant Professor of Orthopaedic Surgery,
University of Pittsburgh Medical Center, University
of Pittsburgh, Pittsburgh, Pennsylvania
Posterior C1–C2 Fusion Techniques: Harms
Technique and Magerl Technique; Cervical Pedicle
Screw Fixation

Max C. Lee, MD
Private Practice, Milwaukee Neurological Institute,
Milwaukee, Wisconsin
Anterior Thoracic Diskectomy and Corpectomy

Howard B. Levene, MD, PhD
Adjunct Assistant Professor, Temple University
College of Engineering; Chief Resident,
Neurosurgery, Temple University Hospital,
Philadelphia, Pennsylvania
Occipital-Cervical Fusion

Isador H. Lieberman, MD, MBA, FRCS(C)
Professor of Surgery, Cleveland Clinic Spine Institute;
Director, Minimally Invasive Surgery Center, and
Director, Center for Advanced Skills Training, The
Cleveland Clinic Foundation, Cleveland, Ohio
Kyphoplasty

Moe R. Lim, MD
Assistant Professor of Orthopaedic Surgery,
University of North Carolina at Chapel Hill, Chapel
Hill, North Carolina
Cervical Pedicle Screw Fixation

Jason E. Lowenstein, MD
Orthopaedic Spine Surgeon, Spine Austin, Austin,
Texas
Cervical Laminoplasty

Neil A. Manson, MD, FRCSC
Lecturer, Dalhousie University, Halifax, Nova Scotia;
Active Staff Physician, Department of Orthopaedic
Surgery, Atlantic Health Sciences Centre, Saint
John, New Brunswick, Canada
Halo Placement in the Pediatric and Adult Patient

Ralph J. Mobbs, BSc, MB, BS, MS, FRACS
Department of Surgery, University of New South
Wales; Consultant Neurosurgeon, Spinal Surgery
and Neurosurgery, Prince of Wales Hospital,
Sydney, Australia
Interspinous Process Motion-Sparing Implant

Donna D. Ohnmeiss, MD
Associate Director of Clinical Research, Texas Back
Institute Research Foundation, Plano, Texas
**Lumbar Spine Arthroplasty: Charité Total Disk
Replacement**

F.C. Öner, MD, PhD
Associate Professor, Orthopaedic Surgery, and Head,
Spine Unit, University Medical Center Utrecht,
Utrecht, The Netherlands
**Balloon-Assisted End Plate Reduction (BAER)
Techniques**

Alpesh A. Patel, MD
Spine Fellow, Department of Orthopaedic Surgery,
Thomas Jefferson University, Philadelphia,
Pennsylvania
**Anterior Resection of Ossification of the Posterior
Longitudinal Ligament**

Brian Perri, DO
Associate Director, Institute for Spinal Disorders,
Cedars-Sinai Medical Center, Los Angeles,
California
Posterior Cervical Osteotomy Techniques

Matías G. Petracchi, MD
Spine Fellow, Hospital for Special Surgery, New York,
New York
Hemivertebrae Resection

Kornelis A. Poelstra, MD, PhD
Assistant Professor of Orthopaedics, Department of
Orthopaedic Surgery, University of Maryland
Spine Program, Baltimore, Maryland
**Minimally Invasive Exposure Techniques of the
Lumbar Spine**

John Ratliff, MD
Assistant Professor of Neurosurgery, Jefferson
Medical College of Thomas Jefferson University,
Philadelphia, Pennsylvania
**Resection of Intradural Intramedullary or
Extramedullary Spinal Tumors**

Minn Saing, MD
Resident, Department of Orthopaedic Surgery,
Albert Einstein Medical Center, Philadelphia,
Pennsylvania
**Posterior C1–C2 Fusion Techniques: Harms
Technique and Magerl Technique**

Rick C. Sasso, MD
Assistant Professor, Clinical Orthopaedic Surgery,
Indiana University School of Medicine;
Orthopaedic Spine Surgeon, Indiana Spine Group,
Indianapolis, Indiana
**Anterior Cervical Disk Arthroplasty; Complete
Vertebral Resection for Primary Spinal Tumors**

Teresa M. Schroeder, MBA
Director, Clinical Affairs, Musculoskeletal Clinical
Regulatory Advisors, LLC, Washington, DC
**Posterior Thoracolumbar Fusion Techniques for
Scoliosis—Lenke Classification**

Suken A. Shah, MD
Assistant Professor of Orthopaedic Surgery, Jefferson
Medical College of Thomas Jefferson University,
Philadelphia, Pennsylvania; Co-Director, Division of
Scoliosis and Spine Surgery, and Attending
Pediatric Orthopaedic Surgeon, Alfred I. duPont
Hospital for Children, Nemours Children's Clinic,
Wilmington, Delaware
Thoracoplasty for Rib Deformity

Alok D. Sharan, MD
Assistant Professor of Orthopaedic Surgery,
Montefiore Medical Center, Albert Einstein College
of Medicine; Chief, Orthopedic Spine Service,
Montefiore Medical Center, Bronx, New York
Operative Management of Scheuermann's Kyphosis

Ashwini Sharan, MD
Assistant Professor, Neurosurgery and Neurology,
Jefferson Medical College of Thomas Jefferson
University, Philadelphia, Pennsylvania
**Resection of Intradural Intramedullary or
Extramedullary Spinal Tumors**

Daniel Shedid, MD, MSc, FRCS(C)
Assistant Professor, Division of Neurosurgery, Spine
Surgery Unit, University of Montreal; Assistant
Professor, Notre Dame Hospital, Centre Hospitalier
de l'Université de Montreal, Montreal, Quebec,
Canada
Kyphoplasty

Kern Singh, MD
Assistant Professor, Department of Orthopaedic
  Surgery, Rush University Medical Center, Chicago,
  Illinois
  Anterior Resection of Ossification of the Posterior
    Longitudinal Ligament; Cervical Spine: Lateral
    Mass Screw Fixation; Lumbar Spine Arthroplasty:
    Charité Total Disk Replacement

Swetha Srinivisan, MD
Medical Student, Department of Orthopaedics,
  Thomas Jefferson University, Philadelphia,
  Pennsylvania
  Minimally Invasive Exposure Techniques of the
    Lumbar Spine

Chadi Tannoury, MD
Orthopaedic Resident, Thomas Jefferson University
  Hospital and The Rothman Institute, Philadelphia,
  Pennsylvania
  Posterior Far Lateral Disk Herniation; Minimally
    Invasive Exposure Techniques of the Lumbar Spine

Vincent C. Traynelis, MD
Professor of Neurosurgery, The University of Iowa,
  Iowa City, Iowa
  Spondylolysis Repair

Rachana Tyagi, MD
Spine Surgery Fellow, Department of Orthopedics,
  Shriners Hospitals for Children, Philadelphia,
  Pennsylvania
  Reduction of High-Grade Spondylolisthesis

Kene T. Ugokwe, MD
Neurosurgery Resident, Cleveland Clinic, Cleveland,
  Ohio
  The Lateral Extracavitary Approach for
    Vertebrectomy

Alexander R. Vaccaro, MD, FACS
Professor, Department of Orthopaedics and
  Neurosurgery, Co-Director of the Delaware Valley
  Regional Spinal Cord Injury Service, and Co-Chief
  of Spine Surgery, Thomas Jefferson University and
  The Rothman Institute, Philadelphia, Pennsylvania
  Anterior Odontoid Resection: The Transoral
    Approach; Anterior C1–C2 Arthrodesis: Lateral
    Approach of Barbour and Whitesides; Anterior
    Resection of Ossification of the Posterior
    Longitudinal Ligament; Posterior C1–C2 Fusion
    Techniques: Harms Technique and Magerl
    Technique; Cervical Spine: Lateral Mass Screw
    Fixation; Sacropelvic Fixation; Posterior Far Lateral
    Disk Herniation; Lumbar Spine Arthroplasty:
    Charité Total Disk Replacement

J.J. Verlaan, MD, PhD
Resident, Orthopaedic Surgery, University Medical
  Center Utrecht, Utrecht, The Netherlands
  Balloon-Assisted End Plate Reduction (BAER)
    Techniques

Michael J. Vives, MD
Associate Professor, Department of Orthopaedics,
  University of Medicine and Dentistry-New Jersey
  Medical School, Newark, New Jersey
  Closed Cervical Skeletal Tong Placement and
    Reduction Techniques

Brian Walsh, MD
Assistant Professor of Neurosurgery, University of
  Wisconsin, Madison, Wisconsin
  Spondylolysis Repair

Bart Wojewnik, BS
Medical Student, Chicago Medical School, Chicago,
  Illinois
  Lumbar Spine Arthroplasty: Charité Total Disk
    Replacement

Demian M. Yakel, DO
Fellow, Texas Back Institute, Plano, Texas
  Lumbar Spine Arthroplasty: Charité Total Disk
    Replacement

S. Tim Yoon, MD, PhD
Assistant Professor, Department of Orthopaedic
  Surgery, Emory University; Chief of Orthopaedic
  Surgery, Atlanta VA Medical Center, Atlanta,
  Georgia
  Cervical Laminoplasty

Joseph M. Zavatsky, MD
Resident, Department of Orthopaedic Surgery,
  Albert Einstein Medical Center, Philadelphia,
  Pennsylvania
  Posterior C1–C2 Fusion Techniques: Harms
    Technique and Magerl Technique

PREFACE

Today, there are a plethora of textbooks written on spinal surgery. Most are an overview of the general science of spinal care or represent a reference text for specific spinal procedures. These may include the background on a particular topic, its clinical presentation, treatment options and outcomes, or a review of the nuances of a pathologic condition with a discussion of the non-operative and operative treatments with case examples.

This book was written to serve a much different purpose. While some atlases of spine surgery do exist, none are truly meant to serve as an operating room companion. We envisioned writing this text to serve and function as an indispensable tool for a spinal surgeon who wants to accent their knowledge and exposure to interesting and commonly performed surgical procedures encountered in daily practice. Thirty-seven of the most commonly performed spinal procedures are presented by highly experienced practitioners. Each chapter includes step-by-step illustrations of particular spinal procedures along with practical expert advice. Many pearls of wisdom are conveyed by the authors in order to assist in the learning curve and avoid the commonly experienced pitfalls encountered by many practitioners.

We feel that this text will represent a source of information that will be used over and over again by the busy spinal clinician. The surgeon will find that they will want to consult with this text routinely before embarking on a particular procedure in order to feel comfortable and confident regarding their chosen techniques. A DVD is included which illustrates master practitioners performing their trademark surgical procedures as they counsel and guide the surgeon through each surgical step. This addition wonderfully complements the overall appeal of this learning aid.

We hope this text serves as a valuable resource to not only orthopedic surgeons, neurosurgeons, and surgical trainees such as residents and fellows, but also physician assistants, nursing staff personnel and anyone else involved in the operative care of patients undergoing spinal surgery.

Alexander R. Vaccaro, MD
Eli M. Baron, MD

FOREWORD

It seems fair to say that the development of spine surgery over the last 50 years has been nothing short of breathtaking. Advances in mechanical engineering and biomaterials as well as increasing anatomic sophistication have led to a surge of surgical treatment options for patients with spinal disorders. During this time period, the care of spinal disorders has matured from a peripheral possibility requiring some improvisational management skills to a highly diversified specialty in its own right. On the publications side there has been a similar increase in the number of textbooks and journals dealing with spinal disorders. Several of the classic textbooks on the spine have blossomed to multivolume tomes containing highly differentiated discussions on the many complex issues surrounding this subject. The result, borrowing the words of Thomas De Quincey [1785–1859], is that *"Worlds of fine thinking lie buried in the vast abyss . . . , never to be disentombed or restored to human admiration."* (from Coleridge's "Reminisces of the English Lake Poets"). Indeed, the somewhat overwhelming plethora of spine publications has led to frequently heard inquiries to the tune of "What should I read first?" and "Where can I find a quick description of . . . ?" by many involved in spine care.

It certainly is a privilege to have been asked to provide introductory words to a refreshingly novel, yet thorough approach towards presenting this increasingly large body of knowledge in the world of spinal surgery to a widely differing audience. The editors, of *Operative Techniques: Spine Surgery*, Alexander Vaccaro and Eli Baron draw from a extensive clinical background across surgical specialty lines and have a near unparalleled research background, as any Medline search will readily demonstrate. The editors have taken the challenge of information overflow head-on by providing a meaningful condensation of the myriad surgical techniques available and presenting it in a well-structured and meaningful fashion. The reader will find quite helpful the organization of each procedure into sections on Surgical Anatomy, Positioning, Portals and Exposures, and step-by-step surgical plans, accompanied by subsections on Pearls and Pitfalls. The open-ended questions of spine surgery are addressed in straightforward fashion in the subsections on Controversies. The latter will pique the interest of even seasoned spine surgeons as they invite thought-provoking deliberations on how to further develop the field of spine surgery. Key references are listed in an evidence-based bibliography, with brief synopses of some of the most relevant publications given. The quality of the state-of-the-art illustrations are in a way emblematic of this book, with their concise yet eminently detailed depictions of anatomy providing meaningful assistance for a brief review of a specific area of interest.

Undoubtedly this book will be an asset to a wide array of health providers associated with spine care for the eminently approachable and resource-rich material that it provides.

Jens R. Chapman
Professor
HansJörg Wyss Endowed Chair
Chief of Spine Service
Departments of Orthopaedic and
Neurologic Surgery
University of Washington School of Medicine
Seattle, Washington

CONTENTS

Contents

CERVICAL SPINE
Immobilization Techniques

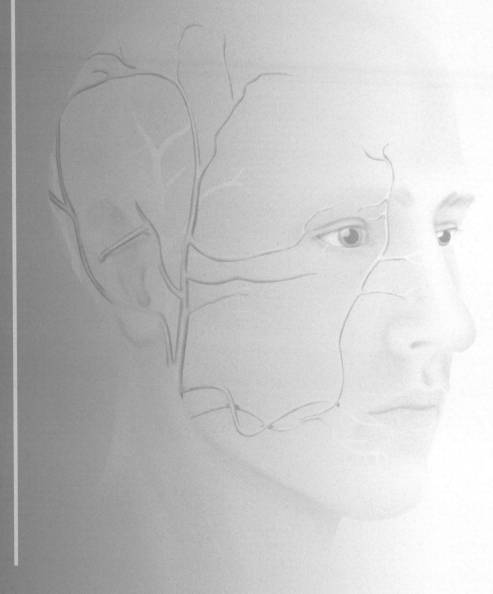

Closed Cervical Skeletal Tong Placement and Reduction Techniques

Michael J. Vives and Colin Harris

Controversies

- Magnetic resonance imaging (MRI) prior to closed reduction of dislocated facets, to exclude an associated disk herniation, is advocated by some.
- For awake, alert patients, closed reduction may be attempted without MRI. If closed reduction fails, MRI should be obtained prior to operative reduction under general anesthesia.

Treatment Options

- Open reduction by anterior or posterior approach
- Anterior (or combined anterior-posterior) approach is commonly recommended if MRI shows large associated disk herniation at the level of the dislocation.

Indications

- Subaxial cervical fractures with malalignment
- Unilateral and bilateral subaxial cervical facet dislocations
- Displaced odontoid fractures, selected types of hangman's fractures, and C1-2 rotary subluxations

Examination/Imaging

- A thorough neurologic examination should be documented prior to procedure.
- High-quality imaging of the cervical spine (including visualization of the occipital-cervical and cervical-thoracic junctions) should be obtained prior to reduction attempts (Fig. 1).

Surgical Anatomy

- Correct pin placement site is 1 cm above the pinna, in line with the external auditory meatus and below the equator of the skull (Figs. 2 and 3).
- The temporalis muscle and superficial temporal artery and vein are at risk if pins are placed too anterior.

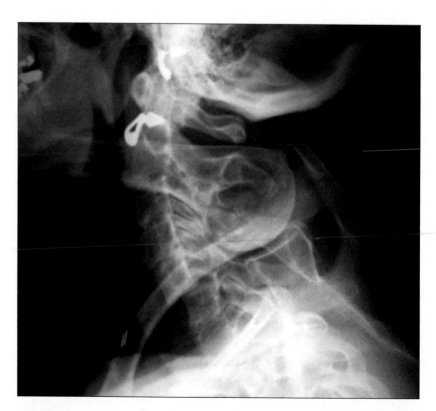

FIGURE 1

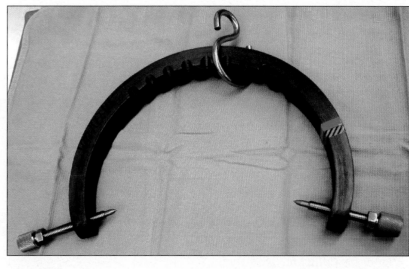

FIGURE 2

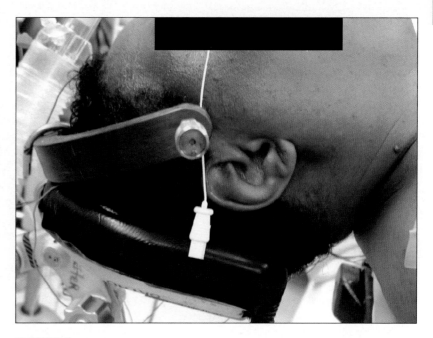

FIGURE 3

Positioning

- The patient is positioned supine on the operative table, Stryker table, or Roto-Rest bed.

Portals/Exposures

- The skin is prepped with a povidone-iodine solution.
- Shaving or skin incisions are not necessary with the use of tapered Gardner-Wells pins.
- Local anesthetic is used to infiltrate the skin and down to the skull periosteum.

Equipment

- MRI-compatible graphite tongs and titanium pins have lower failure loads due to deformation. Stainless steel tongs are therefore recommended if greater than 50 lbs of traction are anticipated.

Procedure

STEP 1

- The pins are angled upward slightly and simultaneously tightened until the spring-loaded force indicator (found on one of the two pins) protrudes 1 mm above the flat surface of the pinhead (Fig. 4).

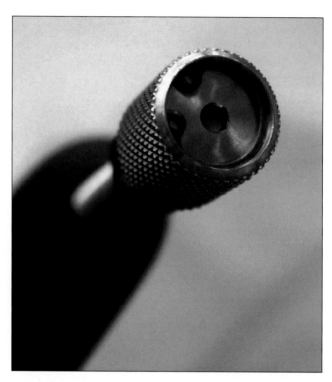

FIGURE 4

STEP 2

- An initial weight of 10 lbs is applied.
- The neurologic examination is repeated and a lateral radiograph is taken.

STEP 3

- Weights are increased at 5- to 10-lb increments at intervals of 20-30 minutes to overcome muscle spasm and to obtain a soft tissue creep effect.
- Serial neurologic examinations and radiographs are obtained after each increase in weight.

Equipment

- In general, the amount of weight required depends on the level of the injury (5 kg per level).
- More weight is generally required to reduce a unilateral facet dislocation than a bilateral facet dislocation.

Controversies

- Some authors have recommended weight limits of 66-70 lbs. Other authors have reported use of up to 140 lbs.

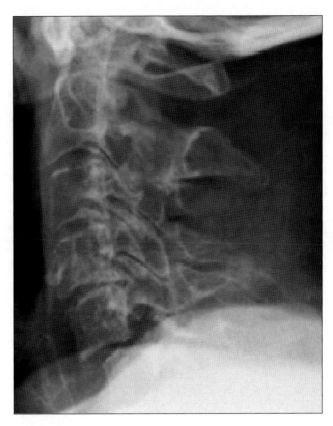

FIGURE 5

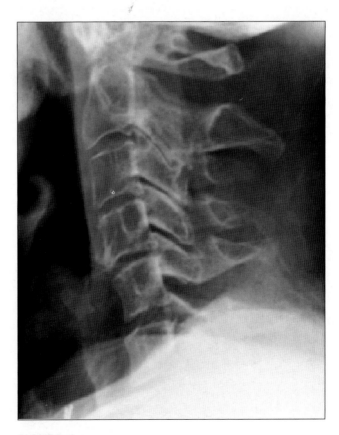

FIGURE 6

PEARLS

• *Facets should be distracted to a perched position prior to attempting manipulative reduction.*

STEP 4: REDUCTION OF UNILATERAL FACET DISLOCATION

- Manipulation may assist in the final reduction of dislocated facets.
- An axial load is applied to the normal facet while the head is rotated 30-40 degrees past midline in the direction of the dislocated facet (Fig. 7).
- Stop the reduction once resistance is felt, and verify the reduction radiographically.

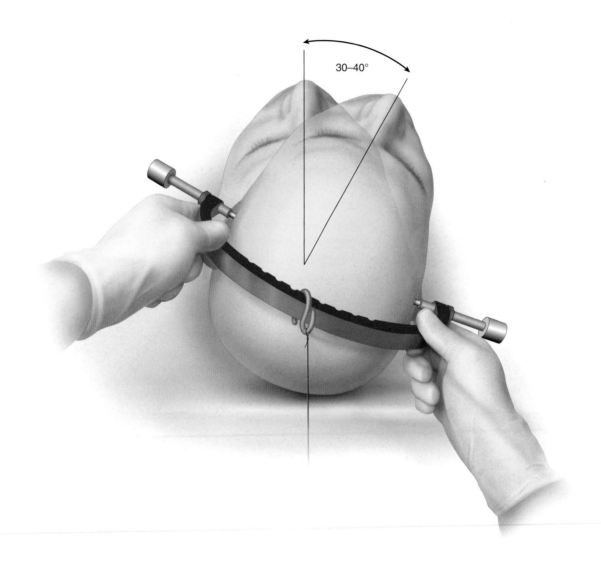

30–40°

FIGURE 7

• *Facets should be distracted to a perched position prior to attempting manipulative reduction.*

PITFALLS

• *An irreducible bilateral facet dislocation is unstable and should be treated with urgent open reduction (after MRI evaluation is performed).*

PEARLS

• *A Rota-Rest bed can be useful at this stage while the patient awaits definitive treatment.*

PITFALLS

• *Tongs should be retightened 24 hours after initial application until the indicator again protrudes 1 mm from the flat surface of the pinhead.*

STEP 5: REDUCTION OF BILATERAL FACET DISLOCATION

■ An anteriorly directed force is applied just caudal to the level of the dislocation, which is usually palpable as a stepoff in the spinous processes (Fig. 8).
■ The head is rotated 30-40 degrees beyond midline toward one side, then the maneuver is repeated toward the opposite side if successful.

Postoperative Care and Expected Outcomes

■ After reduction is achieved, traction weight typically can be reduced to about 10-20 lbs.

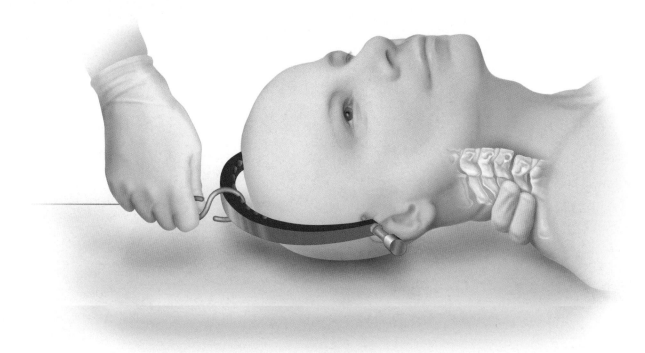

FIGURE 8

Evidence

Cotler HB, Miller LS, DeLucia FA, Cotler JM, Davne SH. Closed reduction of cervical spine dislocations. Clin Orthop Rel Res. 1987;214:185-99.

A cadaver study was performed to delineate the anatomy of pin placement, in addition to a review of 24 patients with cervical facet dislocations treated with closed reduction and traction. Ninety percent of patients improved at least one Frankel grade, and 71% were treated successfully with closed reduction.

Cotler JM, Herbison GJ, Nasuti JF, Ditunno JF Jr, An H, Wolff BE. Closed reduction of traumatic cervical spine dislocation using traction weights up to 140 pounds. Spine. 1993;18:386-90.

This review of 24 cases demonstrates that traction weights of up to 140 lbs can be used safely in the reduction of facet dislocations without associated fractures. Seventeen patients in this series required over 50 lbs for successful reduction, with total time to successful reduction ranging from 8 to 187 minutes. None of the patients had worsening neurologic status during or after the procedure.

Littleton K, Curcin A, Novak V, Belkoff S. Insertion force measurement of cervical traction tongs: a biomechanical study. J Orthop Trauma. 2000;14:505-8.

Biomechanical study on cadaver specimens that demonstrated that overtightening of pins can result in substantial increases in force exceeding that needed to penetrate the skull. In addition, the possible complications of tong placement are discussed.

Vaccaro AR, Falatyn SP, Flanders AE, Balderston RA, Northrup BE, Cotler JM. Magnetic resonance evaluation of the intervertebral disc, spinal ligaments, and spinal cord before and after closed traction reduction of cervical spine dislocations. Spine 1998; 24:1210-7.

Prospective study utilizing MRI to evaluate the incidence of intervertebral disk herniations and ligamentous injuries before and after closed traction reduction of facet dislocations. Of 11 patients in the study, 9 had successful closed reduction, 2 had disk herniations on pretraction MRI, and 5 had disk herniations on post-traction MRI. None of the patients who sustained disk herniations during the reduction developed neurologic deficits.

Vital J, Gille O, Sénégas J, Pointillart V. Reduction technique for uni- and biarticular dislocations of the lower cervical spine. Spine 1998;23:949-54.

This is a review of 168 consecutive cases of lower cervical facet dislocations treated with gradual traction, followed by closed reduction under anesthesia and finally open reduction when necessary. Fifty-nine percent of unilateral dislocations and 73% of bilateral dislocations were treated successfully with closed reduction techniques or traction alone.

Halo Placement in the Pediatric and Adult Patient

Neil A. Manson and Howard S. An

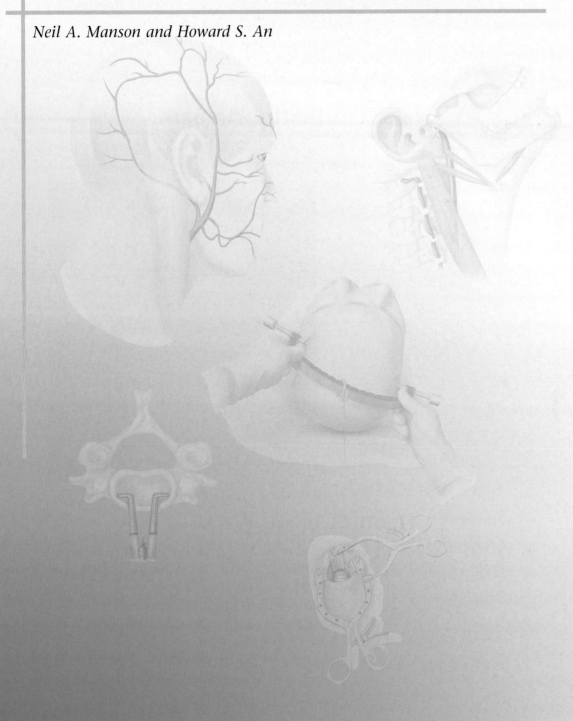

Treatment Options

• Consider rigid collar immobilization in a compliant, young, healthy patient with a minimally displaced, stable fracture.
• Consider surgical intervention in an elderly or noncompliant patient with an unstable or displaced fracture, a fracture of high nonunion potential, ligamentous injury, or associated injury.
• Move to surgical intervention for failure of halo fixation: loss of fracture alignment, symptomatic nonunion, neurologic deterioration.

Indications

■ Jefferson fracture
■ Odontoid fracture: type III or specific type II
■ Hangman's fracture: type II
■ One-column bony cervical spine fracture
■ Fracture in ankylosing spondylitis
■ Preoperative traction or stabilization
■ Postoperative stabilization of arthrodesis, infection, tumor resection

Examination/Imaging

■ Radiographs should be taken to determine the specific fracture type (Fig. 1).

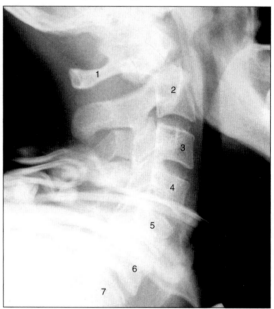

FIGURE 1 Courtesy of Howard S. An, MB.

Surgical Anatomy

■ Relevant anatomy pertains to pin placement. Correct placement prevents direct neural or vascular injury, inner calvarial plate penetration, and pin migration, while providing adequate strength of fixation.
■ Anterior pins
  • Safe zone of placement: anterolateral skull, 1 cm superior to the orbital rim (eyebrow), above the lateral two thirds of the orbit, and below the greatest circumference of the skull.
  • Structures to avoid (medial to lateral): frontal sinus, supratrochlear nerve, supraorbital nerve, zygomaticotemporal nerve, temporal artery, temporalis muscle (Kang, Vives, Vaccaro, 2003) (Fig. 2).

- *It is preferrable if the patient is awake and responsive to report any progression of pain or neurologic loss. Light sedation (midazolam) may be provided for comfort.*

- *Crash-cart access should be assured during halo application.*

Equipment

- Assure that all necessary equipment is available prior to halo application (adapted from Botte et al., 1995):
  - Sterile halo ring/crown in preselected size
  - Sterile halo pins
  - Halo torque screwdrivers or breakaway wrenches
  - Halo pin locknuts
  - Halo vest in preselected size
  - Halo upright post and connecting rods
  - Headboard
  - Spanners or ratchet wrenches
  - Iodine solution
  - Iodine ointment
  - Sterile gloves
  - Syringes
  - Needles
  - Lidocaine for injection
  - Crash cart (including airway supplies, endotracheal tube)
- Three people are recommended during application.
- Measure head and chest circumference and obtain appropriate size halo and vest prior to halo application.

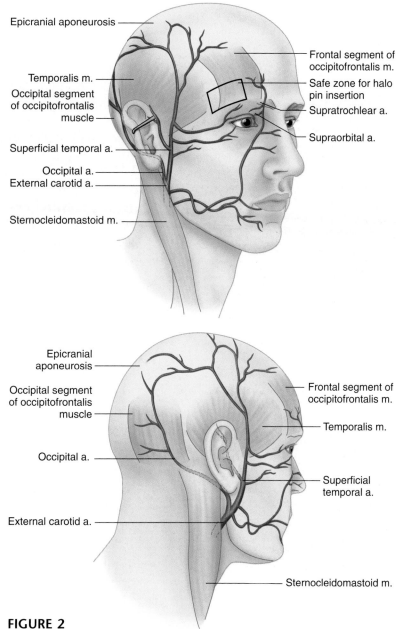

FIGURE 2

- Posterior pins
  - Placement: posterolateral skull, at 4 and 8 o'clock positions or approximately diagonal to the corresponding contralateral anterior pins, below the greatest circumference of the skull and above the upper helix of the ear.
  - No specific structures to avoid.

Positioning

- Typical halo application is performed in the supine position utilizing in-line cervical stabilization by a knowledgeable care provider while two providers apply the apparatus.

PEARLS

- *Prior to supine halo application, consider positioning the vest's posterior shell under the patient to minimize movements during the application process. This could take place, for example, when transferring the patient to an operating room table for the application process.*

PITFALLS

- *The patient's eyelids should be closed and relaxed during application. Pin malposition or sliding during insertion may tent the periorbital tissues and limit eyelid closure. This should be avoided.*

Controversies

- The traditional construct utilizes four pins of 8 inch-pounds torque each. Cadaver and clinical studies have demonstrated improved stability and decreased pin site complications with six- and eight-pin contructs.

- For stable fractures or nonfracture treatment, halo application in the upright position is prefered to optimize cranial-cervical-thoracic alignment and patient comfort.
- A cervical collar can provide additional stability until the halo construct is completed.

Procedure: Halo Application

STEP 1: CROWN AND PIN PLACEMENT

- Identify proper crown size: small for 48- to 58-cm head circumference, large for 58- to 66-cm head circumference. Choose the smallest crown size that allows at least 1 cm of space between head and crown.
- Identify proper pin sites as previously described under Surgical Anatomy.
- Shave hair at posterior sites and cleanse skin at all sites with Betadine or alcohol preparation.
- Instruct patient to keep eyes closed and face musculature relaxed.
- Utilize positioning pins to align and maintain halo position: 1 cm above eyebrow and top of ear and below largest circumference of the head.
- Inject 1% lidocaine with epinephrine at the intended pin sites. Pass the needle through the pin holes of the halo ring to optimize anesthetic positioning. Inject from skin though to periosteum for patient comfort during pin placement.
- Traditionally, four pins provide halo fixation.
- Initial skin incision at the pin sites is not necessary and does not influence scar formation.
- Placement of all pins should occur simultaneously to maintain halo position and balance pin forces. Simultaneous advancement to the skin, through the soft tissue, and to the skull should occur, with final security achieved with release of the breakaway torque-limiting caps (Fig. 3) (see the Depuy Spine Bremer Halo Systems technical monograph).
- Confirm torque to 8 inch-pounds utilizing a torque wrench.
- With pins secure to the skull, tighten the locking nuts to secure the pins to the halo ring.
- Areas of tethered or tented skin surrounding the pins can be released using a scalpel as needed.

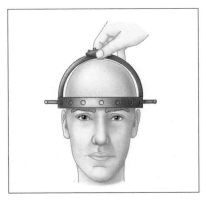

1. Position Halo crown on patient's head.

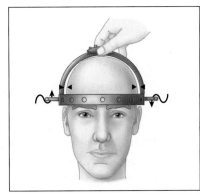

2. Adjust Halo crown and positioning pads, ensuring 1 cm separation between the crown and the head at the pin sites.

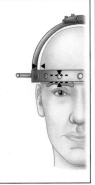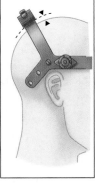

3. Ensure, with the aid of the positioning pads that the Halo crown position and alignment are correct.
   The crown should be
   a. 1cm from the skin at the pin sites
   b. 1cm above the eyebrows
   c. Not in contact with the ears
   d. The posterior pin should be below the equator of the skull
   e. If there is a capital arch it should not touch the top of the head

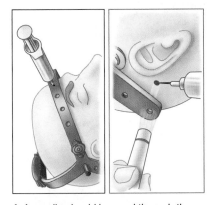

4. A needle should be used through the selected pinholes to provide local anesthetic to the periostium and skin. Make sure the eyes are closed while injecting through the anterior pin sites.

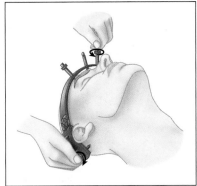

5. Insert the skull pins in selected holes, tightening opposing pins till they penetrate the skin. The patient's eyes should remain closed and the Halo crown should be maintained in position by another person holding the crown. If the crown becomes mispositioned, the pins should be backed out and the crown should be repositioned.

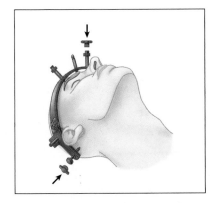

6. Either a torque wrench preset to 8 pounds or manufacturer supplied torque limiting cap should be used to tighten opposing pins 2 turns at a time.

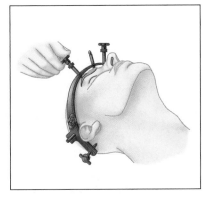

7. For sets with torque limiting caps, this should be done till the caps break off.

FIGURE 3

PITFALLS

- *Patient obesity may necessitate custom vest sizing or preclude halo management altogether.*

STEP 2: VEST APPLICATION

- Identify proper vest size based on chest circumference 5 cm below the xiphoid process and patient height: short vest for circumference of 70-97 cm and height less than 170 cm, large vest for circumference up to 112 cm and height greater than 170 cm.
- In-line cervical stabilization is maintained as required.
- Logrolling or trunk elevation allows placement of the posterior shell of the vest (Magnum and Sunderland, 1993) (Fig. 4).
- The anterior shell is positioned and secured to the posterior shell.
- The vertical bars are secured on the vest and positioned for fixation to the crown.

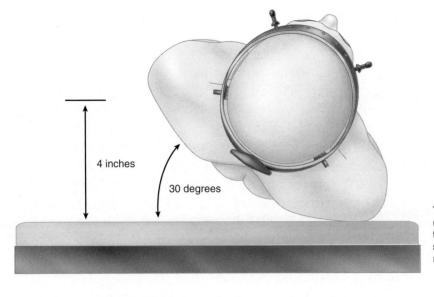

4 inches

30 degrees

The patient should be log rolled 30 degrees (or roughly 4 inches off the mattress) while the posterior vest is put in place. Great care should be taken to ensure the head and neck remains in proper alignment.

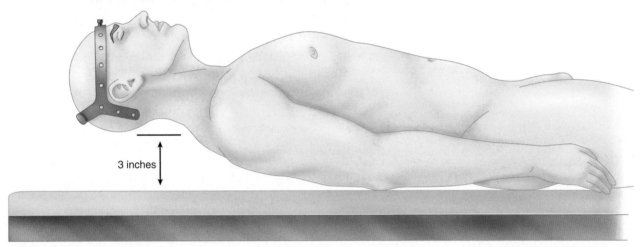

3 inches

Alternatively the patient may be lifted 3 inches (as a maximum) so the posterior shell of the vest can be slipped under the patient.

FIGURE 4

Step 3: Construct Alignment

■ Each posterior vertical bar is attached to its ipsilateral anterior bar by the horizontal crown connector. Loosen all joints within the construct to allow appropriate alignment of the bars relative to the crown.

■ Time spent in optimizing bar position prior to attachment to the crown will minimize patient discomfort and risk of loss of cervical alignment, which can occur when adjustments are made with the construct secured to the crown (Magnum and Sunderland, 1993) (Fig. 5).

■ Assure symmetry between left and right bar constructs.

■ Final tightening of all joints of the crown and vest construct should provide security with no concern for loosening.

■ Only when final stability is obtained may the rigid collar be removed and in-line stabilization released.

■ Final cranial-cervical-thoracic alignment is crucial to (1) maintain fracture alignment, (2) provide patient comfort, and (3) optimize patient function, specifically concerning normal vision and swallowing ability.

Step 4: Follow-up

■ Immediate Follow-up

• Imaging is required to confirm cervical alignment and/or fracture alignment. Lateral radiograph is standard.

• If possible, sit patient upright to assess cervical alignment, construct security, and patient comfort.

■ Short-Term Follow-up

• Further imaging (radiographs or computed tomography) is obtained as needed.

• Retightening of pins is performed at 24 hours after halo application. Locking nuts are first loosened and each pin is retightened to 8 inch-pounds utilizing the torque wrench. Locking nuts are retightened. All joints of the crown-vest construct are retightened.

PEARLS

• *Application tools should be kept at the bedside or taped to the vest in case emergency removal of the vest is required.*

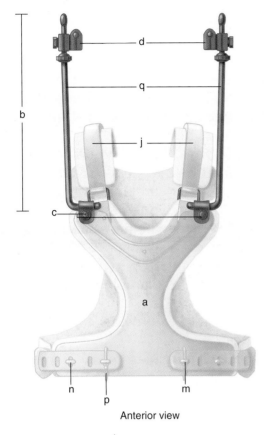

Anterior view

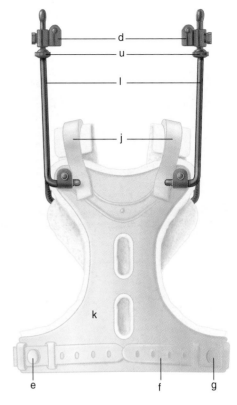

Posterior view

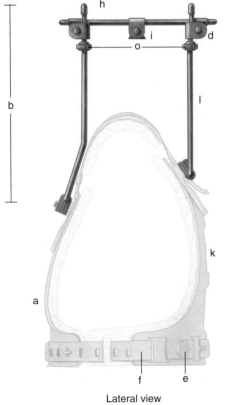

Lateral view

FIGURE 5

a. anterior vest shell
b. superstructure
c. vest joints
d. universal joints
e. posterior locking knobs
f. thoracic bands
g. threaded hole
h. transverse bar
i. halo clamps

j. Velcro shoulder straps
k. posterior vest shell
l. posterior upright
m. medial hold
n. locking post
o. black traction knob
p. plastic cable tie
q. anterior upright

Procedure: Halo Application in the Child or Infant

- Relevant differences in halo application in the pediatric population pertain to skull thickness, skull hardness, and the presence of open cranial sutures. Cranial penetration must be avoided.
- Consider general anesthesia depending on age and diagnosis. While an anesthetized patient cannot provide feedback regarding neurologic status, this may be irrelevant in the very young child or infant.
- A custom crown and vest may be necessary, although pediatric sizes are available.
- Consider preapplication computed tomography to identify cranial sutures and plan pin placement (Mubarak et al., 1989) (Fig. 6).
- Eight to 10 pins are utilized to provide stable fixation at lower torque forces.
- Torque to 2 inch-pounds utilizing a torque wrench. Consider torquing to finger tightness only in the very young child or infant.

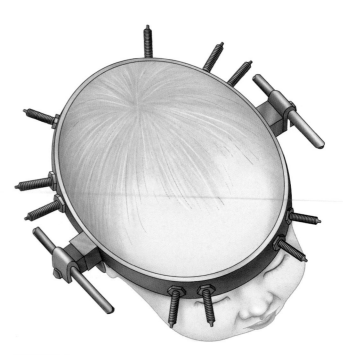

FIGURE 6

Postoperative Care and Expected Outcomes

- Long-Term Follow-up
  - Pin retightening at 1 week after halo application
  - Pin site care twice daily:
    - Inspection for crusting, drainage, redness, or swelling
    - Cleansing using hydrogen peroxide (full or half strength)
    - Reporting any changes to the care team
  - Patient education regarding self-care and independence: Magnum and Sunderland (1993) provides valuable information.
  - Complications are high but manageable through meticulous care and awareness.
- Final Care
  - One third of patients regard their pin scars as severe. During removal of the halo, the pin sites should be massaged with peroxide-saturated gauze to loosen adhesions between skin and bone. The patient should move the skin over the pin holes for several days to prevent reattachment of adhesions and thus minimize scarring.

Evidence

Botte MJ, Byrne TP, Abrams RA, Garfin SR. The halo skeletal fixator: current concepts of application and maintenance. Orthopedics. 1995;18:463-71.

Kang M, Vives MJ, Vaccaro AR. The halo vest: principles of application and management of complications. J Spinal Cord Med. 2003;26:186-92.

Letts M, Girouard L, Yeadon A. Mechanical evaluation of four versus eight-pin halo fixation. J Pediatr Orthop. 1997;17:121-4.

Magnum S, Sunderland PM. A comprehensive guide to the halo brace. AORN J. 1993;58:534-46.

Manthey DE. Halo traction device. Emerg Med Clin North Am. 1994;12:771-8.

Morishima N, Ohota K, Miura Y. The influence of halo-vest fixation and cervical hyperextension on swallowing in healthy volunteers. Spine. 2005;30:e179-82.

Mubarak SJ, Camp JF, Vuletich W, Wenger DR, Garfin SR. Halo application in the infant. J Pediatr Orthop. 1989;9:612-4.

Nemeth JA, Mattingly LG. Six-pin halo fixation and the resulting prevalence of pin-site complications. J Bone Joint Surg Am. 2001;83:377-82.

Polin RS, Szabo T, Bogaev CA, Replogle RE, Jane JA. Nonoperative management of types II and III odontoid fractures: the Philadelphia collar versus the halo vest. Neurosurgery. 1996;38:450-7.

Product monograph. Bremer Halo Crown Traction Set. Bremer Halo Systems, Raynham, MA. 2003.

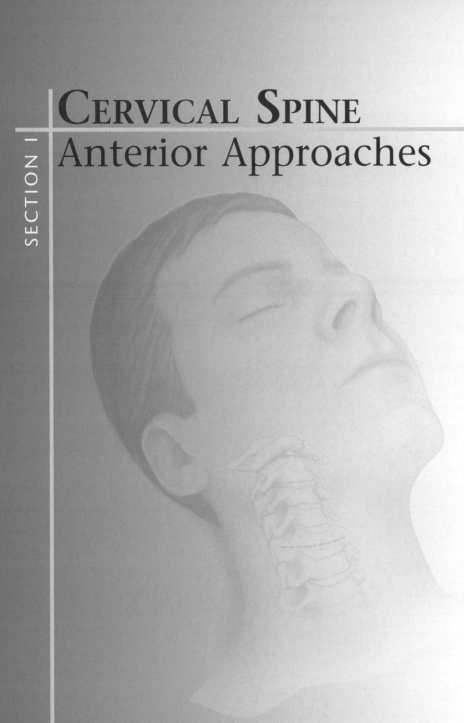

CERVICAL SPINE
Anterior Approaches

Anterior Odontoid Resection: The Transoral Approach

Eli M. Baron, David Choi, James S. Harrop, Alexander R. Vaccaro, and H. Alan Crockard

Indications

- For ventral extradural, midline pathology from the lower clivus to the C2/3 disk. Anticipated dissection should not extend laterally more than 11 mm on either side of the midline as this may result in damage to the eustachian tubes, hypoglossal nerves, or vertebral arteries.
- Commonly used to decompress neural elements, typically in patients with rheumatoid arthritis. Cervicomedullary neural compression may be due to
  - craniovertebral settling due to rheumatoid or degenerative disease
  - pseudotumor or rheumatoid pannus
  - extradural primary bone or soft tissue tumors
  - congenital basilar invagination
  - irreducible chronic nonunion of a fractured odontoid process causing neural compression
- As part of a staged procedure, may be used to excise a chordoma or other midline extradural tumor at the craniocervical junction
- May very occasionally be used for midline intradural pathology such as meningiomas and schwannomas, usually as part of a staged procedure.

Treatment Options

- Anterior odontoid resection through the transoral approach
- Combined anterior odontoid resection through the transoral approach, followed by posterior stabilization with possible decompression
- Stand-alone posterior stabilization with possible decompression
- Adjunctive traction reduction (in setting of reducible basilar invagination or atlantoaxial subluxation), followed by posterior stabilization

Examination/Imaging

- Neurologic and musculoskeletal examination.
- Rotary subluxation is a relative contraindication to this procedure, as is irreducible torticollis.
- Careful examination of the oral and pharyngeal region:
  - The relationship of the hard palate to the pathology must be studied: a hard palate located above the level of pathology allows for good access.
  - The mouth should be able to opened more than 25 mm. This is required to obtain adequate visualization of the pathology, and provide adequate access for surgical instruments.
  - Close attention must be paid to the patient's teeth: root abscesses and periodontal sepsis may be significant risk factors for postoperative infection. Any irregularities in dentition should be noted, as they may make retractor placement difficult.
  - A gum guard can be fashioned prior to surgery, which fits both the irregular dentition and the retractors.

- • Temporomandibular pathology should be taken into consideration as this may limit mouth opening and hinder a transoral approach.
- Good neck extension is required. Fixed flexion deformities of the neck can prevent sufficient mouth opening, and limit surgical access.
- A preoperative otorhinolaryngologic assessment should be performed to rule out any lower cranial nerve dysfunction. If there is vocal cord, pharyngeal, or brainstem dysfunction, then a preoperative tracheostomy should be considered.
- Preoperative imaging should include multiplanar radiographs of the cervical spine, computed tomography (CT) with sagittal and coronal reformatting, and magnetic resonance imaging (MRI) to clearly define any soft tissue pathology and the degree of neural compression (Fig. 1A and 1B).
- CT reformatted images provide detailed information about the bony elements and can be beneficial in planning posterior instrumentation procedures.
- Image guidance has been used as an adjunct for anterior odontoid resection, including frameless stereotaxy and intraoperative MRI. However, frameless stereotaxy may be inaccurate due to the mobility of the craniocervical junction.
- Magnetic resonance angiography (MRA) may be beneficial in defining the vascular anatomy and relationship of the vertebral arteries to the midline, as well as dominance of one vessel.

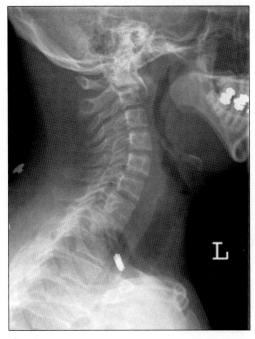 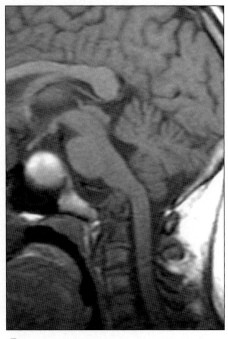

FIGURE 1A-B   A   B

Surgical Anatomy

- Below the foramen magnum, the oropharynx is separated from the prevertebral fascia by a well-defined areolar plane (Fig. 2A–2C). The oropharyngeal mucosa heals remarkably well after surgical incision and repair.

- The most important bony anatomic landmarks for the transoral approach are the midline structures: rostrally, the septal attachment to the sphenoid, the pharyngeal tubercle on the clivus, and caudally the anterior tubercle of the C1 arch. The longus coli muscles flank the dens on each side and, more laterally, the longus capitis muscles.

- The anterior longitudinal ligament extends caudally in the midline.

- Knowledge of the location of the vertebral arteries is requisite before performing a transoral procedure.
  - The vertebral arteries are located 24 mm laterally from the midline at the level of the arch of C1, and approximately 11 mm from the midline at the C2-3 disk space as well as the level of the foramen magnum.
  - Pathology such as atlantoaxial rotary subluxation can significantly distort the relationship of the vertebral arteries to the midline.
  - Visually, the anatomic midline can be accurately defined by examining the symmetry of the anterior longitudinal ligament and the longus colli muscles.

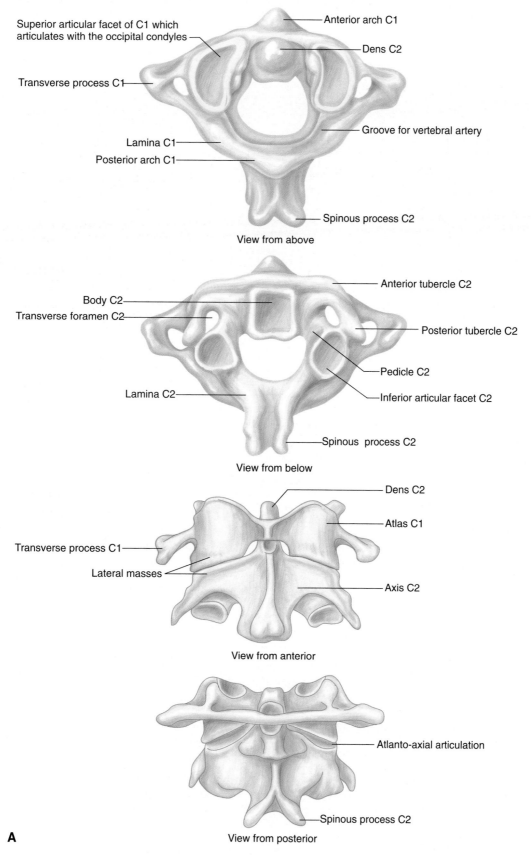

Superior articular facet of C1 which
articulates with the occipital condyles

Anterior arch C1

Dens C2

Transverse process C1

Groove for vertebral artery

Lamina C1

Posterior arch C1

Spinous process C2

View from above

Anterior tubercle C2

Body C2

Transverse foramen C2

Posterior tubercle C2

Pedicle C2

Inferior articular facet C2

Lamina C2

Spinous process C2

View from below

Dens C2

Atlas C1

Transverse process C1

Lateral masses

Axis C2

View from anterior

Atlanto-axial articulation

Spinous process C2

View from posterior

A

FIGURE 2A

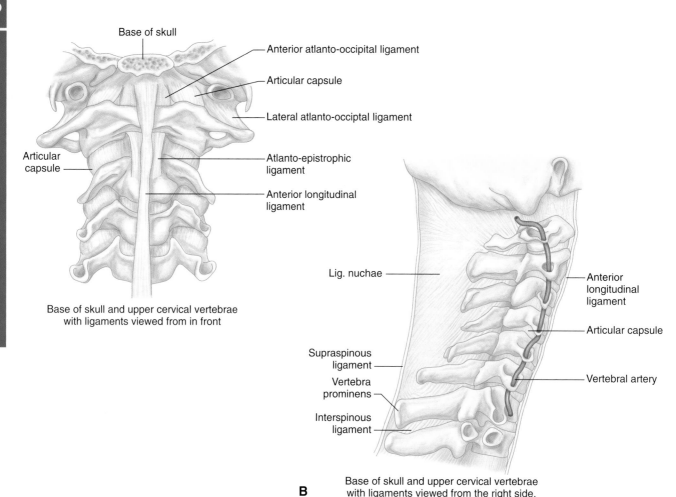

Base of skull

Anterior atlanto-occipital ligament

Articular capsule

Lateral atlanto-occiptal ligament

Articular capsule

Atlanto-epistrophic ligament

Anterior longitudinal ligament

Base of skull and upper cervical vertebrae with ligaments viewed from in front

Lig. nuchae

Anterior longitudinal ligament

Articular capsule

Vertebral artery

Supraspinous ligament

Vertebra prominens

Interspinous ligament

Base of skull and upper cervical vertebrae with ligaments viewed from the right side.

B

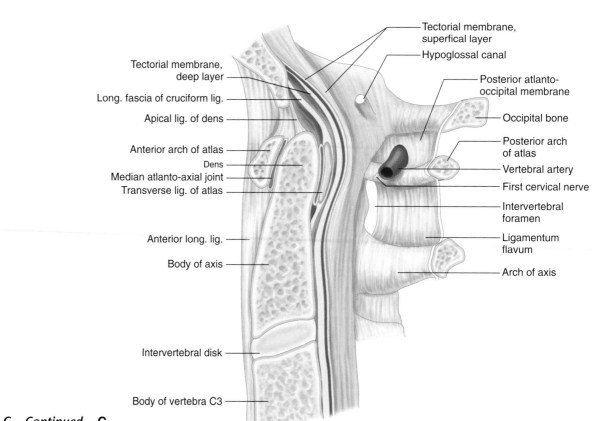

Tectorial membrane, superfical layer

Hypoglossal canal

Tectorial membrane, deep layer

Posterior atlanto-occipital membrane

Long. fascia of cruciform lig.

Apical lig. of dens

Occipital bone

Anterior arch of atlas

Posterior arch of atlas

Dens

Vertebral artery

Median atlanto-axial joint

First cervical nerve

Transverse lig. of atlas

Intervertebral foramen

Anterior long. lig.

Ligamentum flavum

Body of axis

Arch of axis

Intervertebral disk

Body of vertebra C3

FIGURE 2B,C *Continued* **C**

Positioning

- Neurophysiologic monitoring electrodes for somatosensory evoked potential and transcranial motor evoked potential monitoring are placed first.
- Fiberoptic nasotracheal intubation is then performed.
- A nasogastric tube should also be placed for intraoperative gastric drainage and postoperative feeding.
- The patient's head can be fixed in a three-pin fixation system with slight extension. Alternatively, a horseshoe with Gardner-Wells traction or the head resting on a circular headrest can be used.
- Extension should not be used in patients with fixed cervical kyphosis. Rather, they should be placed in slight Trendelenburg position to assist in the rostral extent of the dissection.
- Alternatively, patients may be positioned laterally in a Mayfield clamp (Fig. 3). The advantages of this position are that blood and washings drain out of the operative field. The head is placed in slight extension, which improves exposure. The table may

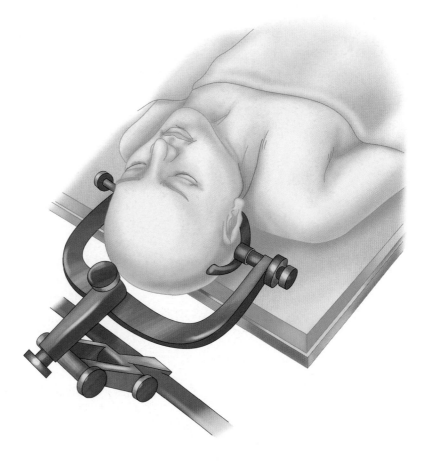

FIGURE 3

be tilted laterally, allowing optimal positioning for the patient and surgeon. After the initial procedure, a posterior stabilization can be performed after reversing the lateral tilt.

■ A fluoroscopy unit is then brought in following positioning to confirm adequate positioning and spinal alignment.

Portals/Exposures

■ Oral swabs can be obtained for culture to identify bacterial colonization prior to preparation of the mouth and oropharynx with 1% Betadine or Cetrimide.

■ The upper esophagus should be packed with a collagen sponge or gauze to minimize the ingestion of saline and blood.

■ The midlines of the oropharyngeal mucosa and soft palate are infiltrated with 1% lidocaine with epinephrine. A Crockard transoral retractor system (Codman, Raynham, MA) is used to maintain adequate exposure of the posterior oral cavity and to keep the nasotracheal and nasogastric tubes to one side, out of the surgeon's way (Figs. 4 and 5).

■ A tongue blade and soft palate retractors maximize the exposure.

■ After incision of the posterior pharyngeal wall, a Crockard toothed self-retaining retractor is inserted for lateral retraction to expose the underlying anterior longitudinal ligament and longus colli muscles.

■ Alternative techniques
  • Another technique is to use endotracheal intubation with the Spetzler-Sonntag retractor system (Aesculap, San Francisco, CA). This system protects and retracts the endotracheal tube and tongue, whereas the Crockard system displaces the nasotracheal tube out of the way.
  • The soft palate may also be retracted using sutures through the soft palate, which are brought out via the nares after they are secured to vessel loops that were passed through the nostrils into the nasopharynx (Spetzler). Alternatively the soft palate may be divided in the midline (offset to avoid the uvula) and retracted with sutures hanging out of the mouth (Crockard).

PEARLS

• *If there is doubt as to one's location during the procedure, or there is difficulty resecting the odontoid or epidural mass, fluoroscopy should be used for orientation with or without placement of radiopaque dye in the decompression defect. The midline can be estimated by determining the midpoint between the attachments of the longus colli muscles. It is important to understand the location of the vertebral arteries at the craniocervical junction. MRA may be useful to clarify the course of the arteries.*

Instrumentation

• Circumoral halo Crockard retractor
• Toothed angled retractors
• Tongue blade and palatal retractors
• Alternative: McIvor three-ring retractor system

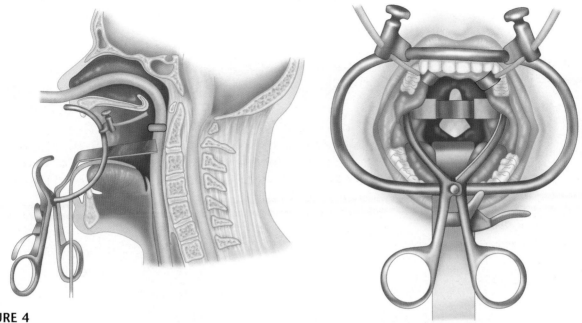

FIGURE 4

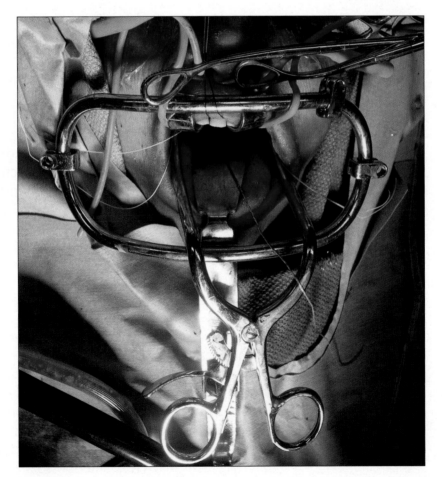

FIGURE 5

Instrumentation/ Implantation

- Though the procedure can be performed using loupes alone, the operating microscope provides enhanced visualization and illumination. Recently, the procedure has been performed endoscopically.

Procedure

STEP 1

- The anterior ridge or tubercle of the atlas is palpated. At this point, a confirmatory lateral localizing image may be taken. An operating microscope can then be used, or a surgeon may choose loupe magnification with directed illumination.
- A vertical incision is made extending approximately 2.5 cm superiorly and 2.5-3.0 cm inferiorly along the midline of the posterior oropharynx (Fig. 6).

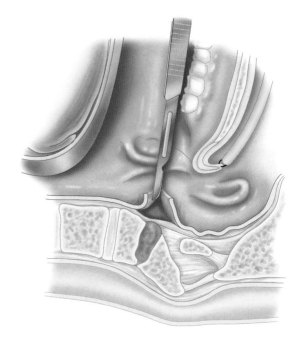

FIGURE 6

Dissection is taken through the posterior pharyngeal mucosa, the superior constrictor muscles of the pharynx, and the anterior longitudinal ligament. Incising the soft (and sometimes hard) palate can provide additional visualization of the lower clivus if needed.

- Using periosteal elevators and electrocautery, a subperiosteal dissection exposes the arch of C1. In the presence of instability, there may be a large amount of granulation tissue at the level of the inferior margin of the atlas and its junction with the anterior odontoid peg. Toothed retractor blades are then used to retract the dissected soft tissues laterally. This allows excellent visualization of the midline inferior clivus, the atlas, and the axis.

STEP 2

- A match-head burr is used to remove the anterior arch of the atlas out laterally approximately 1 cm

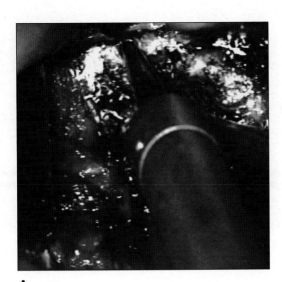

A

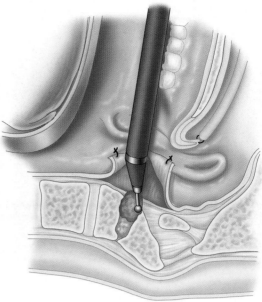

B

FIGURE 7A-B

to each side of the midline (about two thirds of the arch, exposing the shoulder of the dens bilaterally) (Fig. 7A and 7B). The odontoid mass and pannus (if present) are then resected in a rostrocaudal direction (starting at the top of the odontoid process) using a combination of drilling and curetting.

■ Alternatively, the odontoid process may be initially drilled at its base and disarticulated from the C2 body. The odontoid peg is hollowed out gradually with a 3-mm cutting burr down to the cortical bone, which is then thinned and removed with a match-head or diamond burr. The alar and apical ligaments are sharply divided, taking care not to cause a CSF leak. The proximal peg is then removed after circumferentially elevating off all soft tissue attachments. This is facilitated by grasping the odontoid peg with special forceps and pulling it down from the foramen magnum while elevating the dura off it. This allows complete removal of the dens. This technique has a greater potential for durotomy, particularly in the pediatric population, in whom the odontoid process may have a hook at its apex that can tear the dura during peg removal.

■ The posterior longitudinal ligament is seen behind the dens, which has now been removed. The fibers of the transverse ligament are also visualized at the level of the removed C1 anterior arch. With

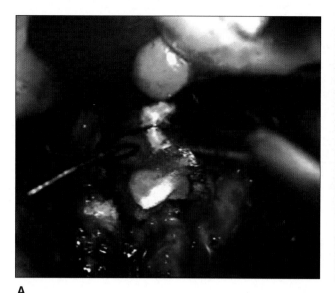

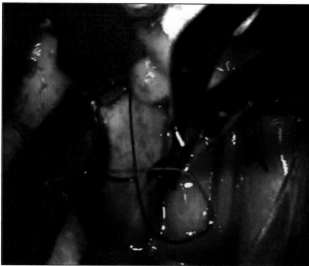

A

B

FIGURE 8A-B

division of these ligaments, the dura should be clearly seen. Ligament and soft tissue removal can be accomplished with a series of small angled curettes, transsphenoidal punches, and transoral bayoneted forceps. Typically a gap exists between the ligaments and dura. Decompression is considered adequate when the dura pulsates freely and the lateral curvature of the dura is seen bilaterally. Fluoroscopy may be used to confirm adequate decompression.

■ Any venous bleeding can be controlled with Surgicel and fibrin glue (Fig. 8A).

STEP 3

■ The posterior pharyngeal wall is then closed with a two-layered closure using 3-0 Vicryl sutures (Fig. 8B).

■ Despite the presence of bacterial flora in the oral cavity, a low infection rate of less than 3% is to be expected if the dura is not breeched. In the presence of a durotomy, great efforts should be made to close the dura in a watertight manner. This may be aided with the application of fat, fascia, dermal fat graft, and fibrin glue. Additionally, a lumbar drain should be used for about 5 days with regular drainage of CSF (10-15 ml/hr).

Postoperative Care and Expected Outcomes

■ Postoperative Care
   • Postoperatively, the nasotracheal tube is left in place for 24-48 hours. It should only be removed if

PEARLS

• *Control venous bleeding with Gelfoam, Surgicel, and fibrin glue and head-up positioning.*

• *Bending the suturing needle into a J shape may facilitate easier pharyngeal closure. To avoid dead space, the pharyngeal wall should be closed in two layers. When repairing the soft palate, a two-layer closure should be performed.*

Controversies

- Necessity and timing of a stabilization procedure is controversial. While early stabilization results in immediate fixation, it can make the investigation of a potential postoperative infection confusing, cause theoretical cross-contamination, and requires a longer anesthetic time. If the anterior and posterior stages are not performed on the same day, the occipitocervical junction should be immobilized until posterior stabilization is performed.

there is no evidence of significant labial or lingual swelling.
- The patient should be left in a halo vest, Minerva jacket, rigid collar, or traction if a posterior stabilization has not been performed at the initial procedure.
- The patient should be encouraged to sit up and to ambulate if possible, in order to minimize saliva pooling in the pharynx and the potential for breakdown of the incision.
- The patient should take nothing by mouth for 5 days after the operation. Nasogastric feeding may commence after 5 hours.
- Hydrocortisone ointment should be applied to the tongue and mucosa for the first 48 hours.
- In the event of a durotomy, lumbar drainage should be maintained for 5-10 days. Prophylactic antibiotic therapy directed against gram-positive, gram-negative, and anaerobic oral flora may be administered by some surgeons. For example, Menezes (1991) recommended CSF cultures for the initial 5 days, at which point, if the cultures remain negative, antibiotics may be stopped. Occasionally a lumbar-peritoneal shunt may be required for persistent CSF leakage.

- Complications
  - Airway complications are always a concern with the transoral approach. It is the practice of the senior author to leave the endotracheal tube in place for a minimum of 24 hours following surgery. If after this time there is evidence of swelling of the tongue or oral cavity, the endotracheal tube is left in situ until the swelling subsides. The occurrence of lingual swelling may be minimized by intermittent intraoperative release of the retractor, and ensuring the tongue is not trapped between the retractor blade and the lower teeth.
  - Delayed complications may include tongue swelling, meningitis, palatal/pharyngeal dehiscence, neurologic deterioration, retropharyngeal abscess, late pharyngeal bleeding, and velopalatine incompetence. Pharyngeal dehiscence may occur either early or late. Early dehiscence (during the first 7 days after surgery) is typically due to inadequate closure or starting oral feeding too early. This can be minimized by encouraging the patient to sit up and walk as soon

as possible to prevent pooling of saliva at the apex or weakest point of the pharyngeal incision. If early dehiscence occurs, closure should be attempted (with the assistance of head and neck colleagues if required) followed by hyperalimentation and intravenous antibiotics. In cases of late dehiscence, infection needs to be ruled out. The differential diagnosis of late dehiscence includes osteomyelitis, retropharyngeal abscess, and poor nutrition. Management of retropharyngeal abscess includes lateral drainage (rather than transoral), followed by appropriate intravenous antibiotics, hyperalimentation via a nasogastric feeding tube, and neck immobilization.

- Neurologic deterioration after transoral odontoid resection is most likely to be due to craniocervical instability. The vast majority of patients who undergo this procedure require a posterior stabilization procedure.

- In patients with altered mental status following the transoral approach, meningitis must be kept at the forefront of the differential diagnosis. This is particularly true in the elderly population with rheumatoid arthritis, in whom this diagnosis may be overlooked since confusion in this age group can be common in the critical care setting.

- Late retropharyngeal bleeding may indicate an underlying infection. Osteomyelitis and pseudoaneurysm of the vertebral artery must also be ruled out. MRI/MRA evaluation of the craniovertebral junction should be performed in addition to angiography to rule out vascular involvement. This diagnostic process also allows for potential therapeutic endovascular treatment in cases of vertebral artery compromise.

- Velopalatine incompetence (incorrect closure of the soft palate muscle during speech resulting in a nasal voice) occurs more commonly in children than in adults. It typically occurs 4-6 months after the transoral procedure and probably occurs secondary to contracture of the soft palate and nasopharynx. This requires otorhinolaryngologic evaluation. Usually it is treated with pharyngeal retraining, but a palatal prosthesis or a pharyngeal flap may also be used.

- Outcome
  - The main predictor of outcome is the degree of preoperative neurologic impairment. Rheumatoid patients who are unable to walk due to myelopathy (Ranawat classification IIIb) have a much higher mortality.

Evidence

- Although little evidence exists as to the long-term efficacy of anterior odontoid resection, with proper indications, diligent planning, and an understanding of the anatomy of the craniovertebral junction, the procedure appears to be a highly effective and safe method of addressing anterior compressive pathology at the craniocervical junction. A few small studies support the different steps outlined in this technique.

Apuzzo ML, Weiss MH, Heiden JS. Transoral exposure of the atlantoaxial region. Neurosurgery. 1978;3:201-7.

This paper reviews the positioning, surgical technique, and postoperative care related to transoral odontoid resection. (Level V evidence [expert opinion])

Crockard HA. Transoral surgery: some lessons learned. Br J Neurosurg. 1995;9:283-93.

Reviews the author's experience with the transoral approach and discusses its use in relation to different pathologies. Reviews technical pearls of preoperative patient evaluation and selection, intraoperative techniques, and postoperative management. (Level V evidence)

Crockard HA, Calder I, Ransford AO. One-stage transoral decompression and posterior fixation in rheumatoid atlanto-axial subluxation. J Bone Joint Surg Br. 1990;72:682-5.

Illustrates how the lateral position can be used for anterior odontoid resection and for posterior stabilization in the same setting. (Level IV evidence [Case series]: retrospective series of 68 patients undergoing a combined procedure)

Crockard HA, Sen CN. The transoral approach for the management of intradural lesions at the craniovertebral junction: review of 7 cases. Neurosurgery. 1991;28:88-97; discussion 97-8.

A study examining the transoral approach for intradural pathology, including meningiomas and schwannomas. Reviews the advantages and disadvantages of this approach in this clinical setting. (Level IV evidence)

Fang HSY, Ong GB. Direct anterior approach to the upper cervical spine. J Bone Joint Surg Am. 1962;44:1588-1604.

Fang and Ong published a series of patients who underwent transoral decompression of the spinal cord and brainstem for irreducible compressive atlantoaxial pathology. The high complication rate with this approach tempered their enthusiasm for the procedure. (Level IV evidence)

Frempong-Boadu AK, Faunce WA, Fessler RG. Endoscopically assisted transoral-transpharyngeal approach to the craniovertebral junction. Neurosurgery. 2002;51(5 Suppl):S60-6.

A review of the endoscopic transoral approach. (Level IV evidence [case series of 7 patients])

Hadley MN, Martin NA, Spetzler RF, Sonntag VK, Johnson PC. Comparative transoral dural closure techniques: a canine model. Neurosurgery. 1988;22:392-7.

This animal study demonstrated the superiority of a fibrin glue augmented dural closure over other methods. (Level I study: prospective study)

Kaibara T, Hurlbert RJ, Sutherland GR. Transoral resection of axial lesions augmented by intraoperative magnetic resonance imaging: report of three cases. J Neurosurg Spine. 2001;95:239-42.

Small case study supporting alternative intraoperative imaging in addition to fluoroscopy. (Level IV evidence)

Menezes AH. Complications of surgery at the craniovertebral junction—avoidance and management. Pediatr Neurosurg. 1991;17:254-66.

This article presents a detailed review of complications of the transoral approach, with specific reference to the pediatric population, and their management. (Level IV evidence as recommendations are based on author's case series)

Pollack IF, Welch W, Jacobs GB, Janecka IP. Frameless stereotactic guidance: an intraoperative adjunct in the transoral approach for ventral cervicomedullary junction decompression. Spine. 1995;20:216-20.

Small case study supporting alternative intraoperative imaging in addition to fluoroscopy. (Level V evidence)

Odontoid Screw Fixation

Michael A. Finn, Daniel R. Fassett, and Ronald I. Apfelbaum

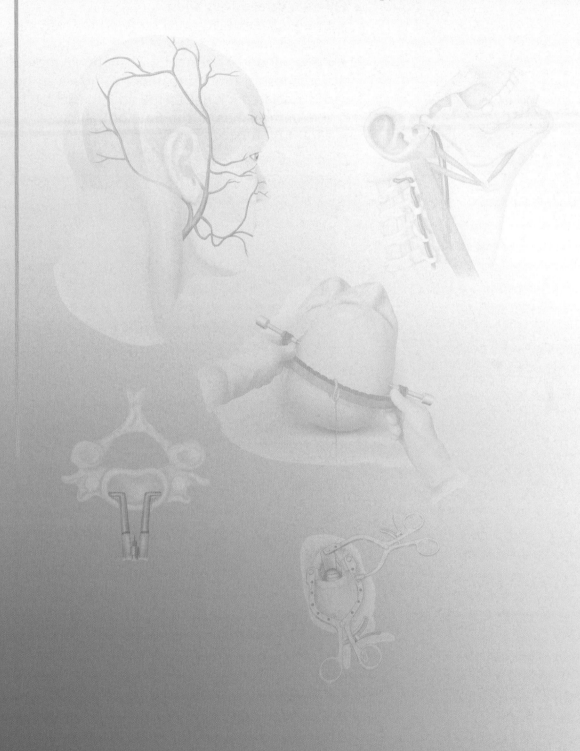

PITFALLS

- *Contraindications*

    - *Inability to achieve an appropriate screw trajectory because of chest obstructing trajectory for instruments used to place odontoid screw*

        - *Short neck*
        - *Barrel chest*
        - *Straight or kyphotic cervical alignment*
        - *Inability to extend the neck*

    - *Type III fractures with significant vertebral body involvement because of poor proximal screw fixation*

    - *Transverse ligament disruption (atlantodental interval [ADI] > 3 mm). Although magnetic resonance imaging (MRI) has been recommended by some for evaluation of transverse ligament rupture, we do not recommend this modality unless neurologic deficits or increased ADI are identified. In our experience, transverse ligament rupture in the setting of odontoid fracture is very rare.*

    - *Chronic nonunion. Fractures older than 6 months or fractures with sclerotic margins have a much lower fusion rate and should be treated by posterior atlantoaxial arthrodesis.*

    - *Nonreducible canal compromise. Intraoperative reduction has been considered more feasible by a posterior approach in combination with atlantoaxial arthrodesis; however, the guide tube system to be described allows realignment intraoperatively before placement of an odontoid screw. In our experience, almost all acute fractures are reducible with traction or intraoperatively.*

Indications

- For surgical fixation of recent (<6 months old) type II and some high type III odontoid fractures (Fig. 1A and 1B)
- Offers several advantages:
    - Immediate stability with no need for external orthosis in most cases
    - Preservation of normal C1-2 rotational motion. Some loss of motion may occur, however, because of associated injuries to the atlantoaxial lateral mass articulation at the time of trauma.
    - High fusion rate

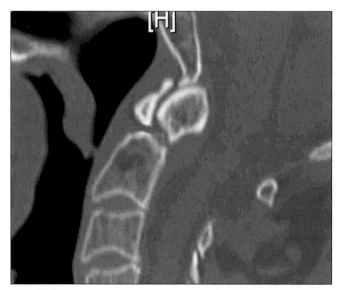

A

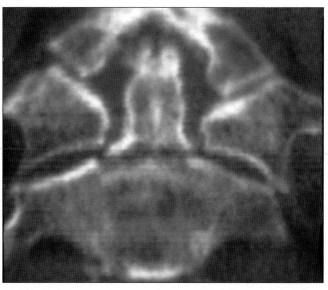

B

FIGURE 1A-B

■ *Anterior oblique fractures (posterior superior to anterior inferior) can be difficult to reduce and maintain in good alignment with odontoid screw fixation (Fig. 2A). Because the screw crosses the fracture line at an angle and thus tends to pull the odontoid anteriorly, these fractures have lower fusion rates. In our previously reported series, we found that patients with anterior oblique fractures had an approximately twofold greater risk of nonunion after odontoid screw fixation than did those with horizontal or posterior oblique fractures (anterior superior to posterior inferior) (Fig. 2B). By fixing these fractures with the odontoid positioned in a slightly posterior position and using a hard collar type of external orthosis, we have usually been able to achieve successful fixation and healing in these patients.*

Controversies

- Type III fractures (Fig. 2C)
  - Some surgeons advocate odontoid screw fixation for high type III fractures, but odontoid screw fixation is contraindicated for type III fractures when there is additional vertebral body involvement because of poor proximal screw fixation.
  - Careful study of reformatted computed tomography (CT) scans can help in identification of patients with fractures in the body of C2.
- Chronic nonunion. Although it has been reported that chronic nonunion can be treated with curettage and odontoid screw fixation, the fusion rates are very low and this fracture is probably better treated with posterior C1-2 fusion.

- Most cost-effective alternative
  - A single odontoid screw is less expensive than posterior atlantoaxial arthrodesis instrumentation alternatives.
  - Patients have earlier return to work and activity than with external orthosis.
- Procedure suited for patients of all ages, including elderly

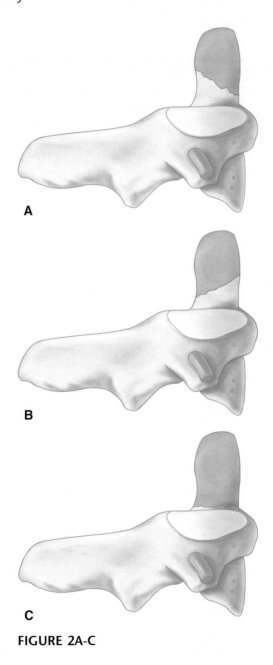

A

B

C

FIGURE 2A-C

Controversies—Cont'd

- Treatment of the elderly. In our experience, this procedure is well tolerated in older patients and allows for early mobilization with fewer general medical complications. The incidence of temporary postoperative dysphagia is greater in this group.

Treatment Options

- Nontreatment may be considered for severely debilitated elderly patients.
- External orthoses
  - Cervical collar: provides least amount of motion restriction
  - Cervical orthosis with thoracic extension (Minerva and SOMI braces) is not recommended because cervical orthoses using an under-the-chin support have been shown to increase upper cervical spine motion with talking and eating.
  - Halo vest
    - Complications include pin site infection, intracranial pin penetration or infection, loosening of hardware, and respiratory compromise.
    - The overall success rate is about 70%.
    - Halo vests are not tolerated well in elderly patients, in whom the success rate is much lower.
  - External orthoses have poor fusion rates except in younger patients. The worst fusion rates occur in older patients, patients with fractures with large gaps or subluxations, and those with comminuted fractures.
  - Treatment with all forms of external orthosis requires close follow-up and 3-6 months of significant activity restrictions.
- Posterior C1-2 arthrodesis
  - Options include transarticular screw fixation, polyaxial C1 and C2 screws with rods, and bone grafting with wiring constructs.
  - Results in loss of atlantoaxial motion (approximately 50% of normal axial rotation of the head and 10% of cervical flexion/extension occurs at this joint)

Examination/Imaging

- Neurologic and musculoskeletal examination
- Anteroposterior (AP), lateral, and open-mouth cervical spine radiographs to assess alignment and other fractures. Note that plain films alone are only 65-95% sensitive for axis fractures.
- Computed tomography (CT)
  - Greater sensitivity than plain films
  - Horizontally oriented fractures may be missed if one is relying on axial images alone; thus sagittal and coronal reconstructions should be evaluated (Fig. 3A and 3B).
  - Useful for operative planning if fracture is obliquely oriented
  - Helps exclude patients with concomitant body fractures
- Magnetic resonance imaging (MRI)
  - Should be performed in all cases in which a neurologic deficit is present
  - May be used to evaluate integrity of transverse ligament rupture. However, unless suspicion is high (ADI > 3 mm), we do not routinely perform MRI.

Treatment Options—Cont'd

- Greater surgical morbidity
- Longer postoperative recovery
- If noninstrumented atlantoaxial arthrodesis procedures are done, they should be supplemented with a rigid external orthosis until fusion is documented.

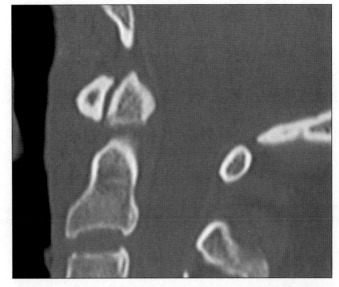

A

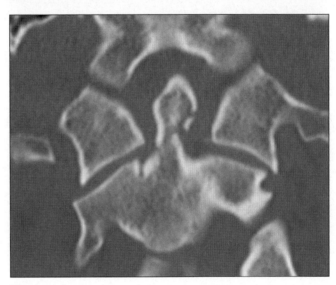

B

FIGURE 3A-B

Surgical Anatomy

- Knowledge of the neck anatomy is imperative
  - Platysma
  - Sternocleidomastoid fascia
  - Carotid sheath contents
  - Trachea and esophagus
  - Longus colli
  - C2 vertebral body

Positioning

- Awake nasotracheal or fiberoptic intubation is used if there is instability in extension.
  - Traditional laryngoscopic intubation is safe if the fracture reduces in extension.
- The patient is placed in the supine position with the head immobilized in 10 lbs of halter traction (see Fig. 4C).

Equipment

- Two C-arms
- Halter traction
- Bite block
- Shoulder bump

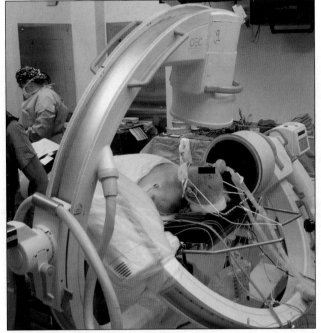

A

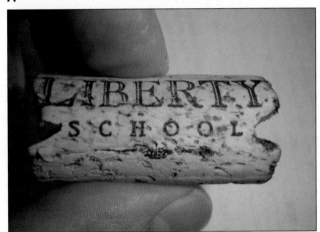

B

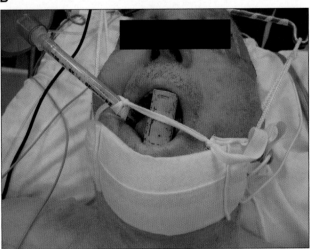

C

FIGURE 4A-C

Instrumentation

- Caspar sharp-toothed cervical retractor blades
- Modified Caspar retractor blade holder
- Superior angled retractor blade (comes in six sizes to fit patient's anatomy)

Portals/Exposures

- The initial approach is a standard Cloward or Smith-Robinson approach to the C5-6 level.
- A small unilateral skin incision is made along the natural skin crease at approximately C5. Either side can be approached, but the right side is often preferred by right-handed surgeons.
- The platysma muscle is divided horizontally.
- The sternocleidomastoid muscle is identified and the fascia along the medial border of this muscle is opened sharply.
- The carotid artery is palpated to assure that the approach is continued medial to this structure.
- Blunt dissection of natural tissue planes provides easy access to the prevertebral space. The trachea and esophagus are retracted medially.
- The prevertebral fascia is incised in the midline at the C5-6 level and the longus colli muscles are elevated to allow retractor placement.
- Caspar sharp-toothed retractor blades are inserted under the longus colli bilaterally at approximately C5 and attached to a modified retractor blade holder (Fig. 5).
- Blunt dissection with a Kittner dissector in the prevertebral fascial plane is carried out to C1 and confirmed on lateral fluoroscopy.

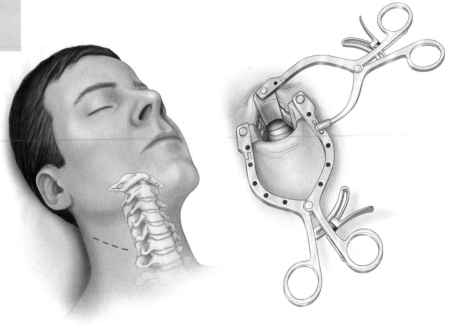

FIGURE 5

Instrumentation/ Implantation

- 2-mm K-wire
- 7-mm hollow-core hand-twist drill
- Inner and outer drill guide tubes

■ A superior angled retractor blade is inserted to retract the pharyngeal tissues off the anterior upper cervical spine and protect them (see Fig. 5). This superior retractor is secured to the modified Caspar retractor (Apfelbaum odontoid retractor system).

Procedure

STEP 1

- ■ An entry site on the anterior inferior edge of C2 is chosen and confirmed on AP and lateral fluoroscopy.
  - One midline site for one screw
  - Two paramedian sites ~2-3 mm from the midline for two screws
- ■ A 2-mm Kirschner wire (K-wire) is impacted 3-5 mm into the desired entry site (Fig. 6A).
- ■ A 7-mm hollow-core hand-twist drill is passed over the K-wire. A groove to accommodate the drill guide is drilled into the anterior face of C3 and the anulus of C2-3 (Fig. 6B-6D).

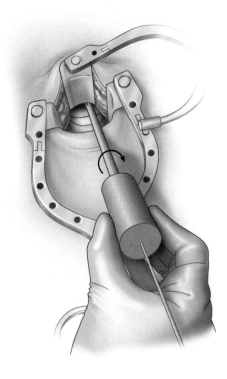

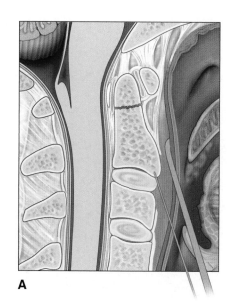

A

FIGURE 6A

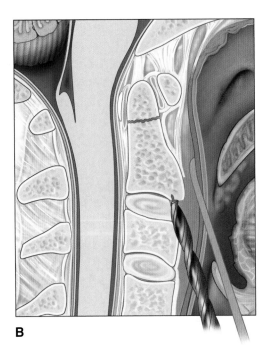

B

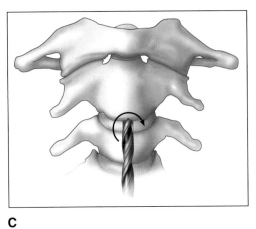

C

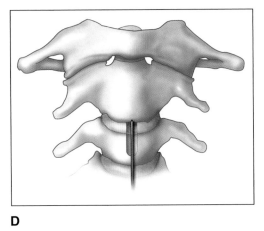

D

FIGURE 6B-D

- The inner and outer drill guides are mated and placed over the K-wire.
- The outer guide has forward-projecting spikes that are walked up the vertebral column, under live fluoroscopy, to overlie the C3 body.
  - The K-wire is trimmed so that no more than 1 cm protrudes from beyond the inner guide tube.
  - A plastic impactor is placed over the inner guide tube and a mallet is used to drive the spikes into the C3 body, securing the apparatus (Fig. 7). These spikes in C3 allow for reduction maneuvers with the guide tube to align C2-3 with the odontoid-C1 complex. They then are used for maintenance of alignment during drilling, tapping, and placement of the screw, establishing the trajectory to reach the tip of the odontoid.
- The inner guide tube is then advanced in the previously created groove (see Fig. 7, *wide arrow*) up to the bottom of C2 (see Fig. 7, *fine arrow*). At this stage, the K-wire can be removed.

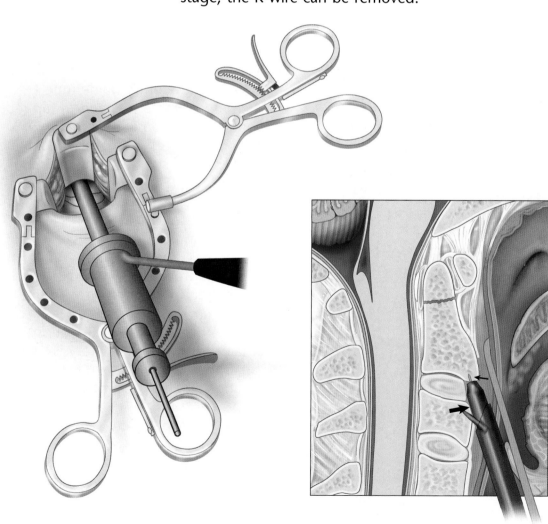

FIGURE 7

Instrumentation/ Implantation

- Calibrated drill
- A right-angled drill driver (Elan-E or Microspeed) is helpful in barrel-chested patients, but a straight drill is adequate in most cases.
- A 4-mm titanium lag screw and a 4-mm titanium fully threaded screw (if two screws are used)

Controversies

- The use of one versus two screws has not been demonstrated to result in any difference in outcome or complication rate, but the use of two screws does provide the theoretical advantage of eliminating the possibility of rotation of the odontoid about the screw.

STEP 2

- A pilot hole is drilled through the body of C2, across the fracture gap, and into the odontoid fragment using a calibrated drill bit, with attention to drill the distal cortex of the odontoid (Fig. 8A).
  - The odontoid fragment is realigned by depressing or lifting the guide tube that has been securely fixed to C3.
    - Further extension of the neck, which may improve screw trajectory, can be accomplished by removing padding from behind the head while keeping the odontoid and C2 aligned with the guide tube system.
  - The apical cortex of the odontoid should be penetrated.
  - A 3-mm drill is used for the 4-mm cortical screws as these screws have a 2.9-mm minor (core) diameter. The drill has excellent directional stability, allowing corrections to be made to the trajectory if needed.
  - The depth of the drilling is noted on the calibrated drill shaft. Adjustments in length are made for any gap between the fractured odontoid and C2.
- The inner guide is removed and the calibrated tap is inserted into the outer guide tube.
  - The tap is rotated by hand to tap (cut threads) along the previously drilled pathway.
  - The entire length of the pilot hole, including the apical cortex, should be tapped prior to placement of the screw (Fig. 8B).
- A 4-mm, buttress-threaded cortical titanium lag screw (threaded distally only) is inserted into the guide tube and the tapped hole.
  - A lag screw is placed across the fracture into the distal odontoid cortex to pull the fractured dens into better approximation with the body of C2 (Fig. 9, *arrows*). Care must be taken to ensure that the distal cortex of the odontoid is engaged. Because the screw trajectory is tangential to the canal, the dura is not endangered if the screw is advanced several millimeters beyond the odontoid tip.
  - The head of the screw should be recessed into the C2-3 anulus or the C2 body.
  - Traction should be removed from the patient's head as the screw is tightened.
- A second screw can placed in the same fashion if anatomy allows.

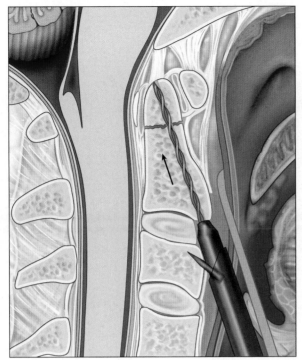 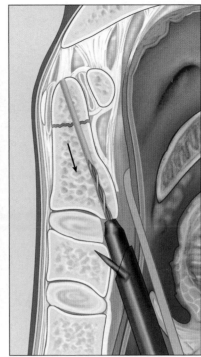

A

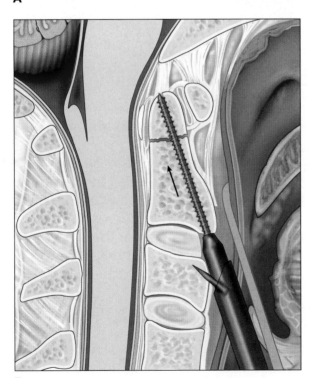

B

FIGURE 8A-B

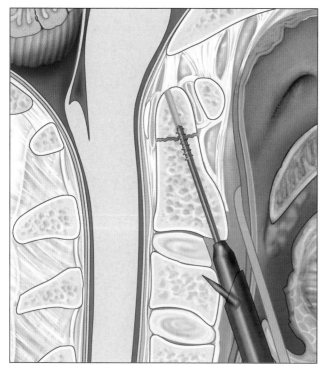 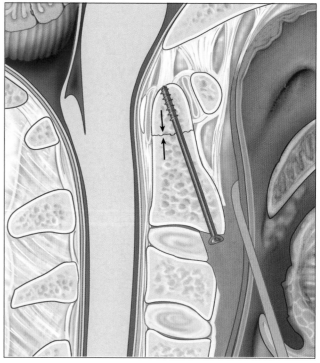

A   **B**

FIGURE 9A-B

- • Biomechanical and clinical studies have suggested there is no benefit of a second screw in most type II fractures.
- • A fully threaded screw may be used because no further lag effect is needed in the reduced fracture.
- ■ Stability can be confirmed by flexing and extending the patient's neck under fluoroscopy.
- ■ The retractors are removed, the wound is irrigated, hemostasis is ensured, and the wound is closed in layers.

Postoperative Care and Expected Outcomes

- ■ We observe all patients in a monitored setting overnight for acute complications, including hematoma development and respiratory compromise.
- ■ We do not use external orthoses in most cases. We recommend the use of a rigid collar in the case of an anterior oblique fracture (posterior superior to anterior inferior) and in patients who are very osteoporotic.

- AP and lateral plain radiographs are sufficient, but CT scanning should be considered if any concern exists about screw placement.
- Early ambulation is critical, especially in elderly patients.
- Fusion rates of 85-95% have been demonstrated in numerous studies.
  - Age, sex, and degree and direction of displacement have no effect on fusion.
  - Anterior oblique fracture orientation (anterior inferior to posterior superior) decreases the rate of fusion: 50% fuse in anatomic position, 25% fuse in nonanatomic position, and 25% fail to fuse.
- Full range of cervical motion was present in 83% of patients after fusion.

Evidence

- Although no prospective randomized trials have examined the efficacy of odontoid screw fixation, a multitude of retrospective studies have demonstrated consistent fusion rates in the 80-90% range when it is used to treat acute fractures. Additionally, preserved motion at the C1-2 joint and the minimal associated morbidity make odontoid screw fixation the treatment of choice for acute odontoid fractures.

Apfelbaum RI, Kriskovich MD, Haller JR. On the incidence, cause and prevention of recurrent laryngeal nerve palsies during anterior cervical spine surgery. Spine. 2000;25:2906-12.

The authors describe a maneuver of deflating and reinflating the endotracheal (ET) tube cuff after placement of cervical retractors to allow the ET tube to centralize within the larynx to prevent recurrent laryngeal nerve injury (RLN). With this maneuver, they reduced the rate of RLN injury from 6.4% to 1.7%. (Level IV evidence [case series]: a retrospective review of the incidence of RLN injury associated with anterior cervical spine surgery in 900 consecutive patients)

Apfelbaum RI, Lonser RR, Veres R, Casey A. Direct anterior screw fixation for recent and remote odontoid fractures. J Neurosurg. 2000;93(2 Suppl):227-36.

This study examines the optimum timing and results of odontoid screw surgery. Surgery performed within 6 months of injury and a fracture oriented in a horizontal or posterior oblique plane (anterior superior to posterior inferior) resulted in significantly higher fusion rates than fractures treated more than 18 months after injury and those oriented in an anterior oblique fashion (anterior inferior to posterior superior). (Class IV evidence: retrospective review of 147 patients)

Fountas KN, Kapsalaki EZ, Karampelas I, Feltes CH, Dimopoulos VG, Machinis TG, Nikolakakos LG, Boev AN 3rd, Choudhri H, Smisson HF, Robinson JS. Results of long-term follow-up in patients undergoing anterior screw fixation for type II and rostral type III odontoid fractures. Spine. 2005;30:661-9.

The authors report on the high fusion rate of odontoid screw fixation with a mean follow-up time of 58.4 months, confirming the long-term success of the procedure. (Class IV evidence: retrospective review of 31 patients)

Greene KA, Dickman CA, Marciano FF, Drabier JB, Hadley MN, Sonntag VKH. Acute axis fractures: analysis of management and outcome of 340 consecutive cases. Spine. 1997;22:1843-52.

Report on treatment of type II fractures with halo immobilization with a 26% overall nonunion rate, but a 67% nonunion rate in fractures displaced greater than 6 mm. (Class IV evidence [case series]: retrospective review of 340 axis fractures with 119 type II odontoid fractures in the case series)

Jenkins JD, Coric D, Branch CL Jr. A clinical comparison of one- and two-screw odontoid fixation. J Neurosurg. 1998;89:366-70.

The study demonstrated no difference in fusion rate with the use of one or two screws. A good discussion of this controversial topic is provided. (Class IV evidence: retrospective review of 42 patients)

Majercik S, Tashjian RZ, Biffl WL, Harrington DT, Cioffi WG. Halo vest immobilization in the elderly: a death sentence? J Trauma. 2005;59:350-7.

The authors report on the use of halo vest immobilization in the elderly and increased morbidity associated with this treatment. (Class IV [case series]: retrospective review of 456 consecutive cervical spine fractures)

Montesano PX, Anderson PA, Schlehr F, Thalgott JS, Lowrey G. Odontoid fractures treated by anterior odontoid screw fixation. Spine. 1991;16(3 Suppl):S33-7.

The authors report on their results with this treatment and comment on its usefulness in polytrauma patients. (Class IV evidence [case series]: retrospective review of 14 patients)

Sasso R, Doherty BJ, Crawford MJ, Heggeness MH. Biomechanics of odontoid fracture fixation: comparison of the one- and two-screw technique. Spine. 1993;18:1950-3.

This study found that odontoid screw fixation provides 50% of the stability of the unfractured odontoid and that two screws offer slightly more stiffness in extension loading only. (Cadaveric study)

Subach BR, Morone MA, Haid RW Jr, McLaughlin MR, Rodts GR, Comey CH. Management of acute odontoid fractures with single-screw anterior fixation. Neurosurgery. 1999;45:812-9; discussion 819-20.

The authors report a 96% fusion rate in 26 patients with acute fractures treated with odontoid screw surgery. (Class IV evidence: retrospective review of 26 patients)

Anterior C1–C2 Arthrodesis: Lateral Approach of Barbour and Whitesides

Eli M. Baron and Alexander R. Vaccaro

Treatment Options

- C1–C2 posterior arthrodesis
- Occipitocervical fusion

Indications

- Instability at C1-2 requiring anterior fixation or where an anterior approach is required for a diagnosis.
- Instability at C1-2 with the presence of incompetent posterior elements
- Salvage technique following a failed posterior C1–C2 arthrodesis.

Examination/Imaging

- Computed tomography (CT) scan to delineate bony anatomy of C1-2; measurements should also be made off the CT scan to estimate screw length.
- Magnetic resonance angiography or CT angiography to evaluate course of vertebral arteries
- Plain radiographs

Surgical Anatomy

- The facial nerve courses through the parotid gland. The posterior belly of the digastric muscle lies posterior to the parotid gland and runs downward to lie medial to the gland.
- The spinal accessory nerve exits the skull through the jugular foramen and then courses posteriorly and downward to enter the deep surface of the sternocleidomastoid. While it usually turns through the muscle, sometimes it runs deep to it. After supplying the sternocleidomastoid, the nerve runs downward and laterally through the posterior triangle of the neck to supply the trapezius muscle.
- The vertebral artery courses cephalad within the foramen transversarium, usually starting at C6, and winds around the surface of the lateral mass and posterior arch of the atlas before entering the foramen magnum through the posterior atlanto-occipital membrane.
- The cervical sympathetic trunk passes upward on the anterior surface of the longus colli and longus capitus muscles. It is easily injured if anterior cervical dissections are performed to far lateral or in a non-subperiostal manner in this region, potentially resulting in Horner syndrome.

Positioning

- Consider preoperative halo immobilization.
- Nasal fiberoptic intubation is preferably done opposite to the side of the approach.

- If not contraindicated, the neck should be turned to the opposite side and extended as much as possible.
- Postoperative prophylactic tracheostomy should be considered in cases in which there is significant or prolonged retropharyngeal dissection. It is usually more convenient to do this after the procedure.
- Intraoperative neurophysiologic monitoring should be used, including somatosensory evoked potentials, transcranial motor evoked potentials, and cranial nerve/electromyography (EMG) monitoring.

Portals/Exposures

- Biplanar fluoroscopy should be used to assist in this procedure. Alternatively, a single C-arm may be used in conjunction with frameless stereotaxy. If using frameless stereotaxy, consider obtaining preoperative imaging while the patient is in a halo vest to minimize shift of C1 on C2, thus reducing registration error.

Procedure

STEP 1

- A hockey stick–shaped incision is made from the tip of the mastoid process and taken distally along the anterior border of the sternocleidomastoid muscle (Fig. 1).

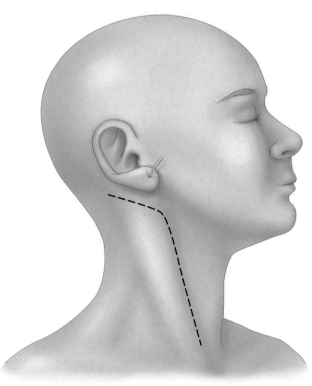

FIGURE 1

PITFALLS

- *Avoid the parotid gland, which may be seen superficially at the cranial end of the incision. Dissection into the gland may result in injury to the facial nerve or a parotid fistula.*

- *Deep at the cephalad end of the incision is the posterior belly of the digastric muscle. Avoid retraction against this muscle to minimize risk to the facial nerve, which courses between the digastric and the base of the skull.*

- *Excessive medial retraction on the nasopharynx may cause mucosal laceration and result in contamination of the field.*

- *Excessive retraction may contribute to postoperative dysphagia and possible cranial nerve injury, including the hypoglossal and superior laryngeal nerve.*

- *Excessive retraction on the spinal accessory nerve should be avoided to minimize risk of sternocleidomastoid and/or trapezius weakness.*

- The greater auricular nerve is identified as it crosses the sternocleidomastoid muscle and dissected proximally and distally to increase its laxity, facilitating retraction. If necessary, it may be divided, with a resultant small sensory deficit around the ear.
- The external jugular vein is also ligated and divided.

Step 2

- The platysma is divided parallel with the prior incision, followed by division of the deep cervical fascia investing the sternocleidomastoid.
- The sternocleidomastoid muscle is detached from the mastoid process. This is done by incising it transversely as it inserts onto the mastoid process, and then everting it, creating a corridor of entry to the retropharyngeal space (Fig. 2).
- The spinal accessory nerve is then identified, about 3 cm from the tip of the mastoid process. The nerve should then be protected with a vessel loop. Triggered EMG monitoring may facilitate its identification.

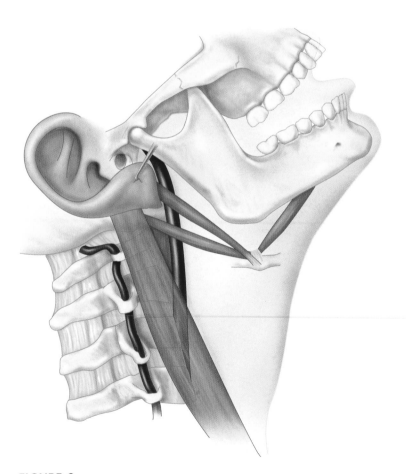

FIGURE 2

- The internal jugular vein is located in the carotid sheath and dissected from the spinal accessory nerve, for greater mobilization.
- The sternomastoid branch of the occipital artery is identified next, distal to the spinal accessory nerve, and is ligated.
- Both the spinal accessory nerves and the internal jugular veins are dissected proximally to the digastric muscle. The dissection continues posterior and lateral to the carotid sheath and medial to the spinal accessory nerve and sternocleidomastoid muscles (Fig. 3, *arrow*).

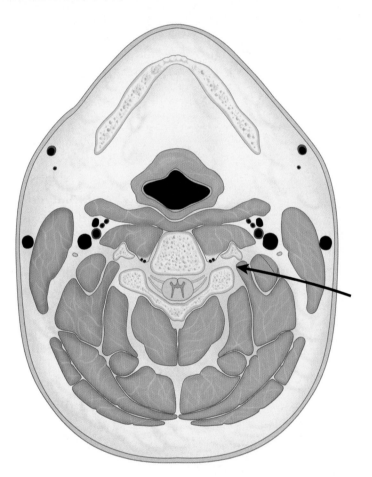

FIGURE 3

STEP 3

- Dissection continues transversely along the anterior border of the transverse processes.
- Sharpey fibers (which attach the midline viscera to the prevertebral fascia and muscles) are divided to enter the retropharyngeal space.
- Blunt dissection with a peanut is used to clear the prevertebral fascia.

■ The C1 arch is easily located by palpating its prominent transversely oriented anterior arch. C2 can also be located by palpation, as it has a prominent vertical ridge at its base.

■ A subperiostal dissection of C1 and C2 is then performed wherein the longus colli and longus capitus muscles are stripped laterally.

■ The longus colli muscle may be detached from its origin on the anterior surface of C1-2 to maximize exposure. The intertransverse membrane at C1-2 should not be violated.

■ The approach and dissection are then repeated on the contralateral side.

■ The facets are then exposed through blunt dissection. A small cutting burr and cervical curettes are used to denude the cartilaginous C1-2 articulation, and the joint space is packed with autogenous iliac crest bone graft.

STEP 4

■ Screw fixation is now performed

■ A 2-mm guidewire is placed at the anterior base of the C1 transverse process, aiming 25° from superolateral to inferomedial in the coronal plane and 10° posteriorly in the sagittal plane. At the starting point, the guidewire should be in line with the ipsilateral mastoid process.

■ Biplanar fluoroscopy should confirm wire placement.

■ Drilling is then performed with a cannulated drill, first using a 2.7-mm cannulated drill bit over the guidewire, followed by a 3.5-mm cannulated drill bit that is taken through only the C1 lateral mass for a lag technique. Alternately, a lag screw may be used.

■ The procedure is then repeated on the opposite side. A 3.5-mm tap is used, followed by a 3.5-mm × 26-mm cannulated screw, in the average adult. (Fig. 4; note screw trajectory).

STEP 5

■ Meticulous hemostasis is obtained, followed by reapproximation of the sternocleidomastoid muscle to the periosteum overlying the mastoid process.

■ A drain should then be placed, followed by customary closure of the platysma and skin.

PITFALLS

- *Dysphagia or cranial nerve injury may result from excessive traction.*

- *Cerebrospinal fluid leak and/or neural injury may occur via penetration of instrumentation into the spinal canal.*

- *The spinal accessory nerve should be identified early and protected with a rubber vessel loop. This may be facilitated using intraoperative EMG stimulation. Injury to the spinal accessory nerve during dissection may cause ipsilateral trazpezius or sternocleidomastoid weakness.*

- *Horner syndrome may result from excessive lateral dissection, especially if a strictly subperiostal plane is not maintained.*

- *Facial nerve palsy may arise secondary to injury to the parotid gland or belly of the digastric muscle.*

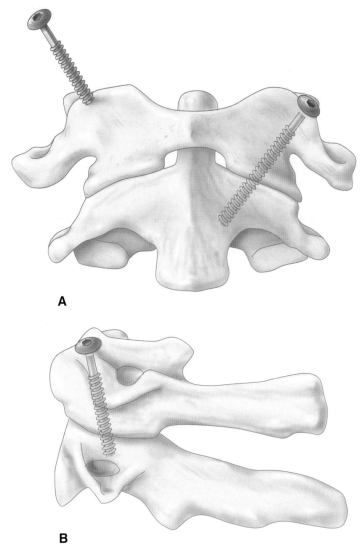

A

B

FIGURE 4A-B

Postoperative Care and Expected Outcomes

■ Postoperatively, the patient should be maintained in a Philadelphia collar for 2-3 months on average.

Evidence

Vaccaro AR, Ring D, Lee RS, Scuderi G, Garfin SR. Salvage anterior C1–C2 screw fixation and arthrodesis through the lateral approach in a patient with a symptomatic pseudoarthrosis. Am J Orthop. 1997;26:349-53.

Reviews the technique and literature of the anterolateral approach to the upper cervical spine, stressing its clinical utility. (Grade IV case report)

Whitesides TE. Lateral retropharyngeal approach to the upper cervical spine. In Sherk HH, Dunn EJ, Eismont FJ, Fielding JW, Long DM, Ono K, Penning L, Raynor R (eds). The Cervical Spine, ed 2. Philadelphia: JB Lippincott, 1989:796-804.

Reports on the author's own experience with this approach on 26 patients. Excellent technical description of the operation. (Grade IV case series)

Anterior Cervical Corpectomy/Diskectomy

David T. Anderson and Alan S. Hilibrand

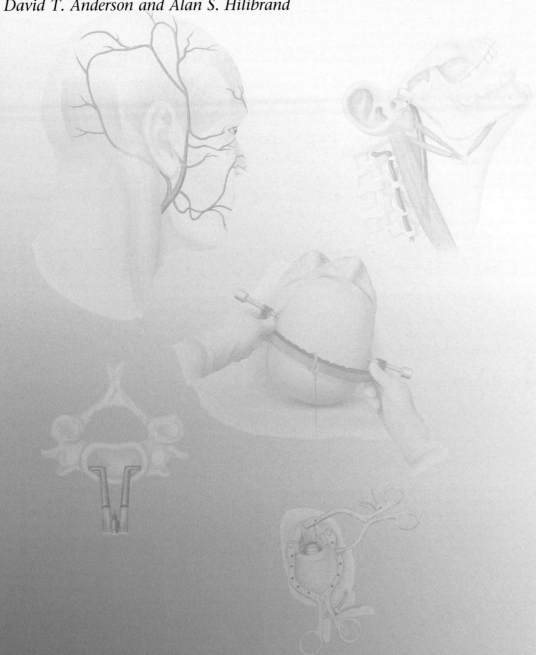

Controversies

• Some patients with arm pain due to a lateral disk herniation may also be treated with posterior foraminotomy.

Indications

■ Refractory symptoms of cervical radiculopathy, cervical myelopathy, or increasing neurologic deficit due to nerve root or spinal cord compression.

■ Additional indications include specific types of cervical trauma, tumor, or infection (Ozgen et al., 2004).

Examination/Imaging

■ Plain radiographs (lateral, flexion, and extension) assess spinal instability and overall sagittal alignment (lordosis, neutral, or kyphosis).

■ Magnetic resonance imaging (MRI) (sagittal, transaxial) is the most common study for radiographic diagnosis (Figs. 1 and 2).

■ Computed tomographic myelography is an invasive procedure requiring a spinal tap in the lumbar or cervical spine.

■ Electromyography may be indicated to confirm radiculopathy when MRI is inconclusive.

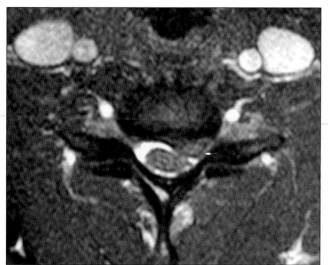

FIGURE 1

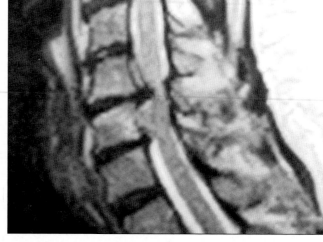

FIGURE 2

Treatment Options

- Nonsurgical management
  - Anti-inflammatory medications
  - Physical therapy
  - Cervical traction
- Operative management
  - Posterior foraminotomy (radiculopathy)
  - Laminectomy/laminoplasty ± fusion (myelopathy)

PITFALLS

- *Failure to adequately retract the shoulders may limit the ability to obtain localizing lateral radiographs.*

- *Excessive hyperextension may increase spinal cord compression and cause iatrogenic spinal cord injury.*

- *Excessive shoulder traction may cause a C5 nerve root injury or brachial plexopathy.*

Equipment

- For corpectomy and strut grafting procedures, we prefer the use of cranial tongs and traction with the head resting on a Mayfield horseshoe.
- An inflatable intravenous pressure bag is used to "dial up" cervical extension, and can be undone after graft placement for graft preloading prior to plate placement.

Surgical Anatomy

- The ventral approach is performed through a plane between the sternocleidomastoid (SCM) muscle and carotid sheath laterally and the strap muscles and tracheoesophageal viscera medially.
- At-risk structures during dissection of the platysma and opening of the cervical fascia include the external jugular vein. The 11th cranial nerve is at risk during the retraction of the SCM.
- Once the plane is established between the SCM laterally and the strap muscles medially, structures at risk include the larynx and trachea, esophagus and pharynx, laryngeal nerves, and carotid sheath (Fig. 3).

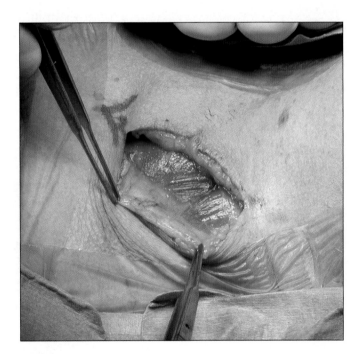

FIGURE 3

Positioning

- The patient is placed supine, and the neck is mildly extended to achieve a normal lordotic curvature. This is done by placing an inflatable bag under the shoulder blades.
- The patient's head and neck should be supported to reduce intraoperative motion.
- The patient's shoulders should be pulled down with tape to facilitate intraoperative lateral radiography, and the arms should be tucked at the sides to improve access to the patient.

Instrumentation

- Hand-held appendiceal retractors or self-retaining blade retractors may be used.

Controversies

- Right- or left-sided approaches may be chosen based upon surgeon preference, although some authors have noted a higher incidence of recurrent laryngeal nerve injury from the right side.
- Once retractor blades are placed, the endotracheal tube cuff may be deflated and then reinflated to reduce pressure on the trachea, esophagus, and laryngeal nerves.

Portals/Exposures

- A transverse incision made 2-8 cm above the clavicle from just across midline to the SCM laterally allows adequate exposure of two to three levels (Fig. 4).
- When greater exposure is needed, a longitudinal incision along the medial border of the SCM can be used.
- The SCM muscle and carotid sheath are retracted laterally, and the strap muscles and tracheoesophageal viscera are retracted medially.
- Identification of the anterior longitudinal ligament will help in finding the midline and disk.
- A spinal needle should be placed in the anticipated operative disk space to confirm location with a lateral radiograph or fluoroscopy.
- Longus colli muscles are elevated and freed from their vertebral attachments for a distance of half a vertebral body above and below the desired area of planned disk and bone resection. Retractors are used beneath the muscle edges to gain medial/lateral exposure.

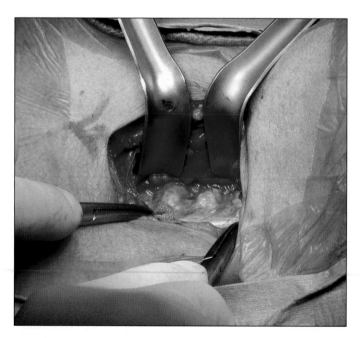

FIGURE 4

Procedure

STEP 1: DISK EXCISION

- Annuli of the C5/6 and C6/7 disks are incised, and the disks are dissected out of their respective spaces down to the posterior longitudinal ligament, removing all disk material as well as the cartilaginous end plates (Fig. 5).
- The uncovertebral joint should be identified laterally on both sides and at both levels. Drilling too far beyond the lateral aspect of this joint may result in injury to the vertebral artery.

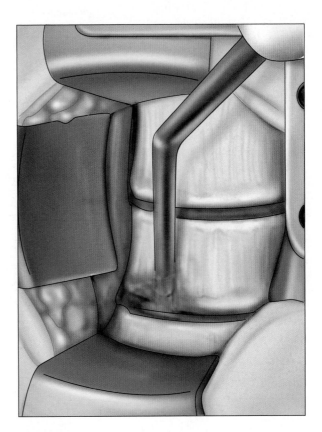

FIGURE 5

Instrumentation/ Implantion

- Higher speed burrs may be used through the vertebral bone and against the PLL without injury to the underlying dura mater.

STEP 2: DECOMPRESSION

- A trough is created symmetrically between the uncovertebral joints using a small rongeur and completed using a high-speed burr under irrigation.
- A trough measuring 16 mm is created within the corpectomized vertebral body to allow complete decompression of the width of the spinal cord.
- The trough is widened at the uncovertebral joint and deepened to the posterior longitudinal ligament (PLL), removing the posterior cortex of the vertebral body, and thus completing the decompression (Fig. 6).
- Once decompression has been the completed, hemostasis may be obtained with Gelfoam or a powdered Gelfoam-thrombin solution.

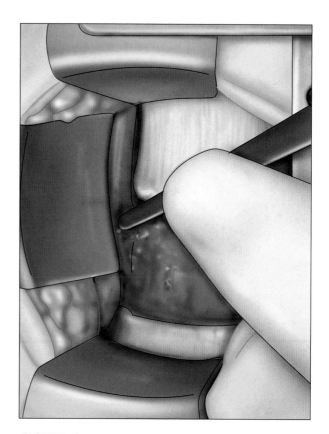

FIGURE 6

Controversies

- Removal of the PLL is controversial. Removal may allow greater spinal cord decompression but may also increase the risk of stretch injury to the C5 nerve root(s). It should be removed in the setting of disk herniation and in patients with ossification of the PLL undergoing an anterior decompression.

STEP 3: STRUT GRAFT PREPARATION AND PLACEMENT

- Using the burr, the superior and inferior end plates are decorticated to expose bleeding cancellous bone with posterior lips to prevent the graft from displacing against the spinal cord.
- A depth gauge is used to assist in shaping the graft to the appropriate depth.
- Iliac crest bone graft is harvested, or allograft bone may be selected. Grafts must be trimmed and shaped to match the vertebral recipient site (Fig. 7).
- If cranial tongs are used, an additional 20 lbs of traction is applied prior to measuring the required length of strut graft. With this additional traction maintained, the graft is carefully tamped into position.
- The graft may require modifications to optimize an ideal fit within the decompression trough.

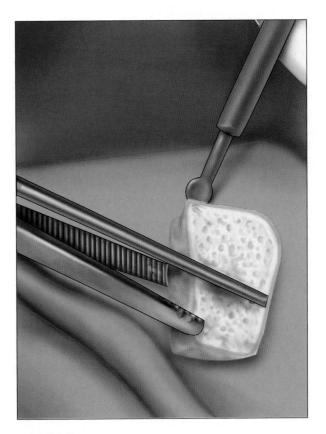

FIGURE 7

STEP 4: INTERNAL FIXATION

- Anterior cervical plates may create a rigid construct with fixed screws, a semirigid construct with variable screws allowing for partial load sharing via screw rotation, or a dynamic construct with a slotted or collapsing plate via screw/body translation.
- Holes are drilled through a guide and screws are typically used to fix the plate to the vertebral body (Fig. 8).
- Anteroposterior and lateral radiographs or fluoroscopy is used to ensure correct plate and screw placement (Figs. 9 and 10).

Postoperative Care and Expected Outcomes

- Retropharyngeal hematoma or edema can possibly lead to respiratory compromise or spinal cord compression. Patients undergoing multilevel corpectomies and certain anterior-posterior procedures are potentially at higher risk and may be kept intubated overnight.
- The patient is kept immobilized in a hard cervical collar for 4-6 weeks.
- When performing anterior cervical diskectomy and arthrodesis with autogenous strut grafting for radiculopathy, Bohlman et al. (1993) reported that 93% of patients experienced relief of arm pain.
- When performing anterior decompression and arthrodesis with autogenous bone strut grafting for cervical myelopathy, Emery et al. (1998) reported that 87% of patients with previous gait abnormality experienced improvement.

PEARLS

- *An external bone stimulator using either capacitive coupling or a pulsed electromagnetic field may increase the rapidity of bone graft consolidation following anterior cervical fusion.*

Controversies

- Anterior cervical plating may help to prevent graft dislodgement and enhance union rates. It may also minimize the need for or duration of severe postoperative immobilization.

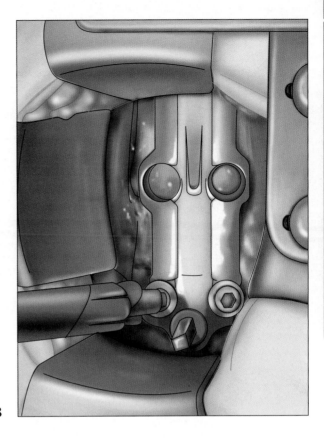

FIGURE 8

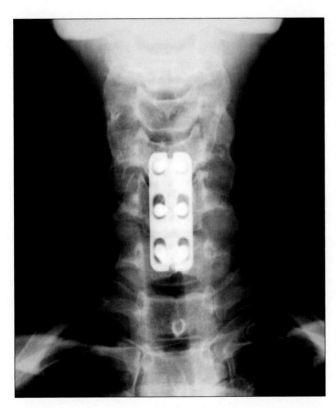

FIGURE 9

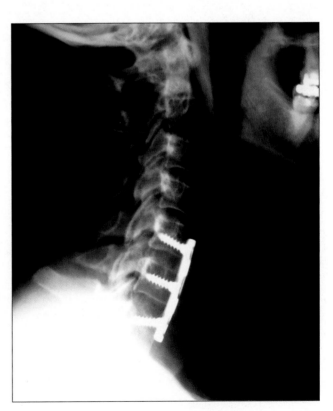

FIGURE 10

Evidence

Bohlman HH, Emery SE, Goodfellow DB, Jones PK. Robinson anterior cervical discectomy and arthrodesis for cervical radiculopathy: long-term follow-up of one hundred and twenty-two patients. J Bone Joint Surg [Am]. 1993;75:1298-307.

The authors' results in this study suggest that the Robinson anterior cervical discectomy and arthrodesis with an autogenous iliac-crest bone graft for cervical radiculopathy can relieve pain and resolve neurologic deficits in a high percentage (93%) of patients.

Emery SE, Bohlman HH, Bolesta MJ, Jones PK. Anterior cervical decompression and arthrodesis for the treatment of cervical spondylotic myelopathy: two to seventeen-year follow-up. J Bone Joint Surg [Am]. 1998;80:941-51.

In this case review of 108 patients with cervical spondylotic myelopathy, the authors conclude that anterior decompression and arthrodesis with autogenous bone-grafting is a safe procedure associated with a high rate of neurologic recovery, functional improvement, and pain relief.

Hilibrand AS, Fye MA, Emery SE, Palumbo MA, Bohlman HH. The impact of smoking upon the outcome anterior cervical arthrodesis by interbody and strut grafting. J Bone Joint Surg [Am]. 2001;83:668-73.

In this retrospective study of 190 patients, the authors found that a much higher fusion rate was achieved after corpectomy and strut grafting (93%) than after multilevel discectomy and interbody grafting (63%). Therefore, strut grafting should be considered after multilevel anterior cervical decompression to increase the likelihood of successful fusion.

Hilibrand AS, Fye MA, Emery SE, Palumbo MA, Bohlman HH. Increased rate of arthrodesis with strut grafting after multilevel anterior cervical decompression. Spine. 2002;27:146-51.

In this study of 190 patients, the authors concluded that smoking had a significant negative impact on healing and clinical recovery after multilevel anterior cervical decompression and fusion with autogenous interbody graft but not with autogenous iliac-crest or fibular strut grafts. Therefore, strut grafting should be performed in patients who are unable or unwilling to stop smoking prior to surgical treatment.

Hilibrand AS, Schwartz DM, Sethuraman V, Vaccaro AR, Albert TJ. Comparison of transcranial electric motor and somatosensory evoked potential monitoring during cervical spine surgery. J Bone Joint Surg [Am]. 2004;86:1248-53.

The authors in this study of 427 patients report that transcranial electric motor evoked potential monitoring appears to be superior to conventional somatosensory evoked potential monitoring for identifying evolving motor tract injury during cervical spine surgery.

Ozgen S, Naderi S, Ozek MM, Pamir MN. A retrospective review of cervical corpectomy: indications, complications and outcome. Acta Neurochir (Wien). 2004;146:1099-105; discussion 1105.

In this retrospective, single-center study of 72 patients undergoing cervical corpectomy, the authors found that an overall favorable outcome was achieved in 88% of cases. They conclude that cervical corpectomy is an effective method for treating traumatic lesions, degenerative disease, tumors and infectious processes involving the anterior and middle portions of the cervical spine.

Anterior Resection of Ossification of the Posterior Longitudinal Ligament

Kern Singh, Alpesh A. Patel, and Alexander R. Vaccaro

Controversies

- Patients younger than 65 years of age, with physical signs of myelopathy with a paucity of neurologic deficits
- Rapidly progressive myelopathy and severe medical comorbidities (coronary artery disease, chronic obstructive pulmonary disease, diabetes mellitus, peripheral vascular disease)

Indications

- Ossification of the posterior longitudinal ligament (OPLL) causing moderate to severe myelopathy
- OPLL localized to vertebrae C2-T1
- Segmental OPLL with localized anterior thecal sac compression

Examination/Imaging

- A lateral radiograph will determine sagittal alignment (lordotic, neutral, kyphotic).
- Hyperintense foci reflecting cord edema, myelomalacia, or gliosis (on T_2-weighted magnetic resonance imaging [MRI]) may portent a poor prognosis (Figs. 1 and 2).
- Computed tomographic myelography is the best diagnostic tool to accurately assess cord dimensions and the amount of osseous compression from the OPLL (Fig. 3).

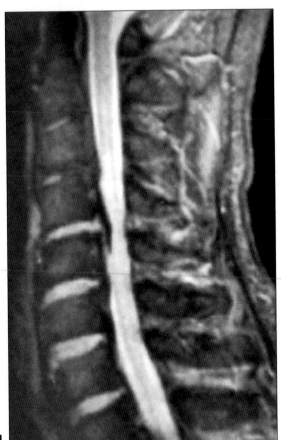

FIGURE 1

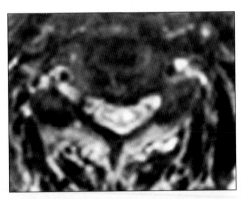

FIGURE 2

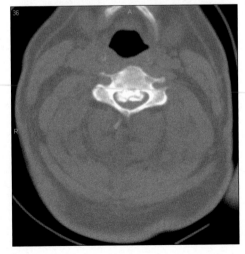

FIGURE 3

Treatment Options

- In the setting of neutral or lordotic cervical alignment, laminectomy and posterior instrumented fusion or laminoplasty may be an alternative procedure.

PEARLS

- *Awake fiberoptic intubation and positioning if the patient's symptoms are worsened during preoperative cervical extension*

- *If MEP monitoring is available, intubation and positioning can be done with the patient under aenesthesia.*

- *Continuous intraoperative somatosensory evoked potential (SSEP) monitoring of median/ ulnar and posterior tibial potentials*

PITFALLS

- *Changes in SSEP or MEP monitoring may signal excessive flexion or extension of the neck, traction, or rotation/compression of the shoulder, elbow, or wrist.*

- *To avoid SSEP "drop out," inhalation anesthetics are maintained at concentrations below 0.4% or a balanced narcotic technique is used.*

Equipment

- Fiberoptic camera
- SSEP and MEP neuromonitoring sensors

Controversies

- In the absence of attainable electrophysiologic monitoring, a neutral cervical posture should be attained.

Surgical Anatomy

- Vertebral artery
  - Identify location on MRI. Arteries may have an anomalous path within the vertebral bodies (2.7%).
  - Endovascular repair of the vertebral artery is preferred if possible.
  - Stent placement is feasible if the injury is less than 6 hours old.
  - Direct repair or indirect pressure/occlusion may result in greater morbidity to the patient.
- Spinal cord and nerve root
  - There is a 2–10% incidence of quadraparesis/ quadriplegia and a 5–17% incidence of root injury (typically C5).
  - Root injuries are less frequently attributed to direct manipulation than to rapid cord migration (untethering effect).

Positioning

- Place the patient in the supine position on a radiolucent operating room table with the head/neck in neutral position.
- After intubation, the head/neck can be extended safely if motor evoked potential (MEP) monitoring is available.

Instrumentation

- Microscope or loupe magnification with excellent lighting

Controversies

- Losing track of the midline orientation is common. Consider an anteroposterior (AP) plain radiograph if orientation is in question.

Portals/Exposures

- A horizontal incision is used in the majority of cases and begins from the midline to the anterior aspect of the sternocleidomastoid. Multilevel cases can be performed through an oblique incision.
- The skin and subcutaneous tissue are undermined slightly and the platysma is divided with electrocautery in a horizontal fashion.
- The underlying sternocleidomastoid is identified laterally while the strap muscles are found medially.
- The deep cervical fascia is divided between the sternocleidomastoid and the strap muscles with blunt dissection carried down to the pretracheal fascia.
- While blunt dissection occurs, care is taken to constantly palpate and retract the carotid sheath laterally.
- Once the vertebral midline is identified, the prevertebral fascia is incised and the medial edges of the longus colli muscles are elevated. The longus colli muscles are carefully mobilized laterally using a small Cobb elevator and electrocautery.
- Self-retaining retractors are placed under the longus colli muscle.
- A localizing radiograph is obtained to confirm the operative level.

Procedure

STEP 1: PREPARATION OF DISK SPACES AND/OR CERVICAL CORPECTOMY

- Identify uncinates to define midline and lateral borders of vertebral body.
- Resect anterior osteophytes
- Perform sharp anulotomy followed by radical disketomy with curettes over the necessary number of segments.
- Identify the posterior longitudinal ligament (PLL) following posterior annulus resection
- Perform corpectomy using rongeurs and a side-cutting burr.
  - The uncinates define the lateral extent of decompression.
  - The PLL, as identified in diskectomy, defines the depth of corpectomy.
  - Use bone wax to control bleeding.

Instrumentation/ Implantation

- 3-mm Leksell rongeur
- 3-mm high-speed burr

Controversies

- Avoid placement of bone wax on potential graft host bone junctions.

PITFALLS

- *Avoid the use of Kerrison punches or rongeurs with a prominent footplate.*

- *Asymmetric or incomplete decompression due to loss of midline orientation*

- *Dural tear and cerebrospinal fluid (CSF) leak during release of adhesion between OPLL and dura or due to removal of ossified dura*

Instrumentation/ Implantion

- Diamond-tipped burr
- Loupe or microscope magnification
- Micronerve hook, currettes

Controversies

- Removal of ossified dura will lead in most cases to a CSF leak. An option would be to thin the ossified dura and perform a release of the OPLL along the lateral gutters bilaterally to allow the dura to gently float anteriorly.

STEP 2: TAKEDOWN OF OPLL

- Use a diamond-tipped burr to thin the OPLL.
- Identify and open nonossified portions of the PLL using microsurgical curettes, a sharp blade, or a nerve hook.
- Dissect a plane between the OPLL and the dura.
- Elevate the thinned OPLL off the dura using a nerve hook or microsurgical curettes (Fig. 4). Release dural adhesions with a nerve hook or microsurgical curettes (Fig. 5).

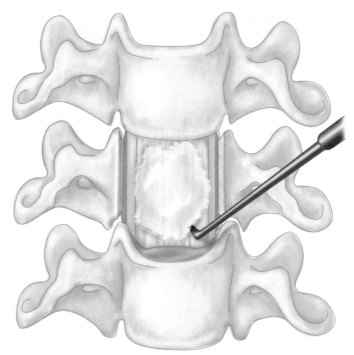

FIGURE 4

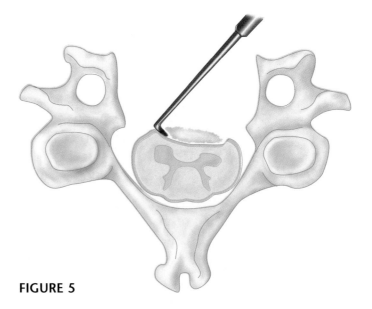

FIGURE 5

PEARLS

- *Avoid overdistraction with graft.*

- *Consider posterior instrumented fusion to augment multilevel reconstructions.*

PITFALLS

- *Graft subsidence*

- *Graft dislodgement*

- *Plate dislodgement*

Instrumentation/ Implantation

- Anterior cervical plates

Controversies

- Dynamic versus static cervical plates for multilevel decompression

STEP 3: GRAFT PLACEMENT, ANTERIOR PLATING

- Careful end plate and graft preparation is necessary to create parallel surfaces for optimum fusion.
- Anterior cervical plating is then performed with screws directed into the vertebral body directed away from the graft-endplate interface.
- Check lateral radiograph to confirm graft and plate position as well as sagittal alignment.

Postoperative Care and Expected Outcomes

- Dural tear and CSF leak
  - Primary repair: 6.0 Gore-Tex suture
  - Augmented repair
    - Fascial autograft (sternocleidomastoid) or allograft (bovine fascia)
    - Fat autograft
    - Duragen
    - Fibrin glue
  - Drain
    - A drain is tunneled subcutaneously to the level of the clavicle, well distal to the incision to prevent fistula formation with the primary wound through a drain tract in close proximity to the dural leak.
    - A lumbar drain or lumboperitoneal shunt is often placed to decrease pressure on the dural repair. Drainage should average around 15 ml/hr.
    - Postoperatively, the patient's head is elevated approximately 45°.
    - The drain is continued until minimal output is noted.
  - Antibiotics: ceftriaxone (improved CSF penetration)
  - Positioning: supine with head of bed elevated 45°
- Prior to extubation, a patient thought to have potential airway swelling must fulfill the following criteria:
  - Direct fiberoptic evaluation of the trachea and vocal cords to assess for significant swelling.
  - Indirect assessment of swelling by deflating the endotracheal cuff and listening for air leak.
- Depending on the extent of anterior cervical decompression, a hard cervical collar or a halo vest may be used postoperatively for immobilization.

- Postoperative swelling can be severe. Hematoma collection can additionally affect the airway. The patient should be placed in an upright sitting position and closely monitored for airway dysfunction.
- Resolution of myelopathic symptoms may or may not occur. Prevention of further myelopathic degeneration is the goal.

Evidence

Curylo LJ, Mason HC, Bohlman HH, Yoo JU. Tortuous course of the vertebral artery and anterior cervical decompression: a cadaveric and clinical case study. Spine. 2000;25:2860-4.

Cadaveric study examining course of vertebral arteries as well as location of transverse foramen relative to anatomic landmarks. Of 222 specimens, 2.7% demonstrated an intraosseous arterial course. Three clinical cases are reviewed; one case involved intraoperative laceration of the aberrant artery during corpectomy.

Belanger TA, Roh JS, Hanks SE, Kang JD, Emery SE, Bohlman HH. Ossification of the posterior longitudinal ligament: results of anterior cervical decompression and arthrodesis in sixty-one North American patients. J Bone Joint Surg [Am]. 2005;87:610-5.

Sixty one patients with an average of 4 years' postoperative follow-up are reported; 56 of 61 patients showed neurologic improvement. Complications included dural tear in eight patients, with five of eight developing CSF fistula; eight patients with new neurologic deficit; three graft extrusions; and one pseudarthrosis. Fifty-eight of 61 showed bony fusion at the most recent follow-up.

Jain SK, Salunke PS, Vyas KH, Behari SS, Banerji D, Jain VK. Multisegmental cervical ossification of the posterior longitudinal ligament: anterior vs posterior approach. Neurol India. 2005;53:283-5.

Review of 27 patients with multilevel OPLL (greater than four levels) managed with either anterior decompression or posterior decompression (laminaplasty or laminectomy and fusion). No differences in outcomes were noted. Anterior decompression demonstrated a much higher number of complications, including neurologic worsening, dural tear and CSF leak, graft extrusion, and respiratory distress.

Yamaura I, Kurosa Y, Matuoka T, Shindo S. Anterior floating method for cervical myelopathy caused by ossification of the posterior longitudinal ligament. Clin Orthop Rel Res. 1999;259:27-34.

Surgical technique is reviewed for decompression of the spinal cord by release of the OPLL. The authors reported a 71% average recovery rate based on Japanese Orthopaedic Association criteria.

Anterior Cervical Disk Arthroplasty

Rick C. Sasso and Paul A. Anderson

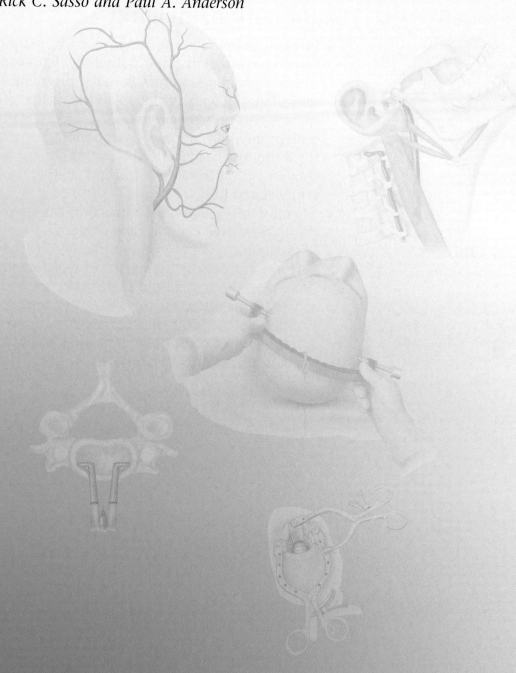

PITFALLS

- *Kyphosis and sagittal plane deformity*

- *Spondylolisthesis and instability*

- *Severe degeneration with limited range of motion*

- *Large osteophytes and facet joint arthritis*

Controversies

- Myelopathy
- Multilevel pathology
- Axial neck pain
- Adjacent to fusion

Treatment Options

- Anterior cervical diskectomy and fusion
- Allograft versus anterior iliac crest autograft
- Anterior cervical locking plate versus no plate

Indications

- Single-level cervical herniated nucleus pulposus (HNP) causing radiculopathy or myelopathy
- Single-level uncovertebral osteophyte causing radiculopathy or myelopathy

Examination/Imaging

- Physical examination must correlate to magnetic resonance imaging (MRI) pathology. For example, physical examination may reveal a profound left C7 radiculopathy with severe weakness of the left triceps muscle and severe pain in a C7 radicular pattern in a patient in whom aggressive nonoperative treatment for 3 months has failed. MRI in this patient may show a large central-to–left-sided HNP at C6-7 (Fig. 1A and 1B).
- Selective nerve root sleeve injection can help identify the target nerve causing radiculopathy.
- Preoperative computed tomography (CT) scan is performed to assess the extent of osteophytes and determine the template disk size (Fig. 2A and 2B).
  - The templates assess the size of the implant preoperatively. The appropriate size is determined from the vertebral body with the smallest anteroposterior (AP) diameter.

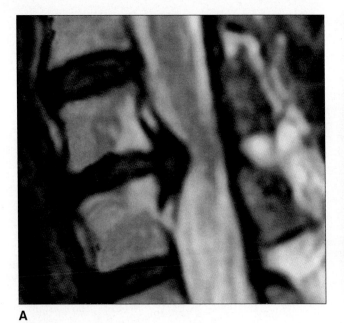
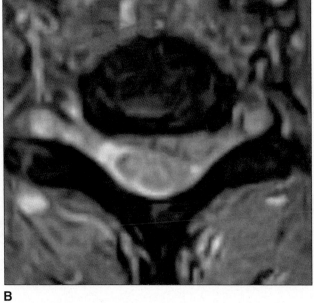

A **B**

FIGURE 1A-B

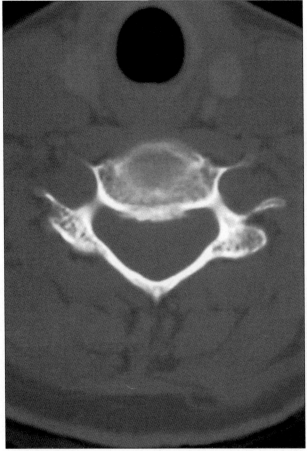
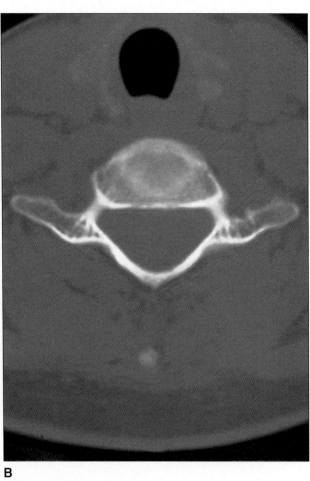

A **B**

FIGURE 2A-B

- A magnification template is placed onto the image (Fig. 3A), and a CT scan magnification scale is used to determine appropriate ratio (Fig. 3B; 50%). The 50% template is then used to determine the appropriate implant size (Fig. 3C).

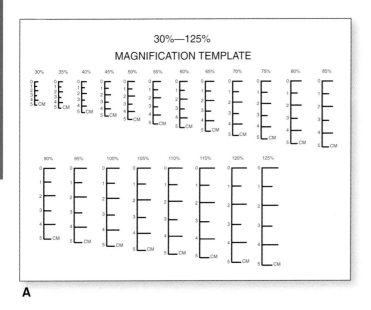

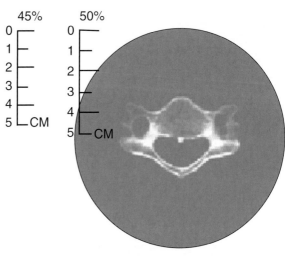

A

B

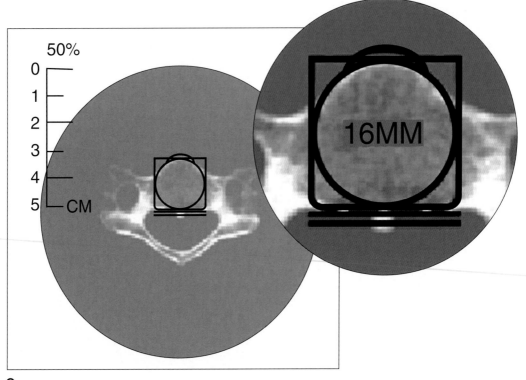

C

FIGURE 3A-C

Surgical Anatomy

- Remove the C6/7 disk.
- Decompress the left (and right) C7 neuroforamina as well as the spinal cord.
- Reconstruct the C6/7 disk with an artificial disk (Bryan Cervical Disk arthroplasty) (Fig. 4A and 4B).

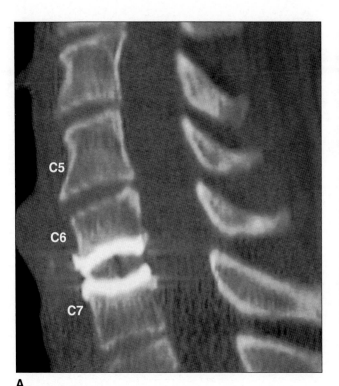

A

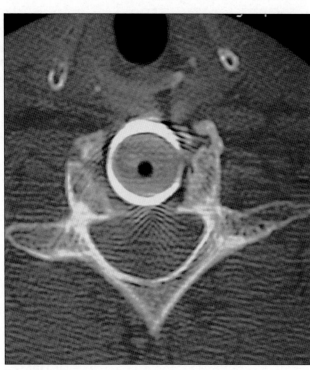

B

FIGURE 4A-B

Equipment

- Fluoroscope
  - Initial AP: verify that target disk segment is not rotated.
  - Lateral: assure the position of the incision and ability to visualize the posterior aspect of the disk space.
- Fluoroscope will be kept in lateral position during procedure to verify milling depth and size of implant.

Controversies

- The head may be placed in a doughnut headrest.
- A head halter chin strap may be used to help stabilize the head throughout the procedure.
- The back of the head should not be posterior to the shoulders. The neck should be in physiologic position with the head level or slightly anterior to the shoulders (as if standing with the back against a wall).

Positioning

- The patient is placed in supine (Fig. 5).
- The patient's neck is placed in neutral (not extension) during milling for arthroplasty.
- A radiolucent operating table is needed for both AP and lateral fluoroscopy.

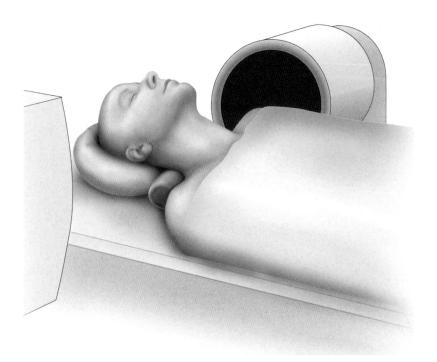

FIGURE 5

Instrumentation

• Standard hand-held retractors

Controversies

• Whether to use a left- versus a right-sided approach continues to be a controversial topic. Although cadaveric studies demonstrate less strain on the recurrent laryngeal nerve with a left-sided approach, multiple large clinical studies have not shown any difference in complications. Right-handed surgeons may find a right-sided approach easier. Certainly, approaching from the side opposite the HNP allows a more full and complete view and access to the pathologic foramen.

Portals/Exposures

■ A standard anterior approach to the cervical spine is made through a transverse incision in an existing skin crease (Fig. 6).

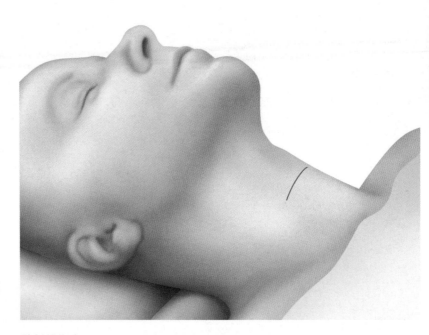

FIGURE 6

Instrumentation/ Implantation

- Transverse centering tool

Controversies

- It is imperative to decompress the contralateral nerve root if a motion-sparing device is implanted. This is not as important if a fusion is done because the lack of motion salvages an incomplete decompression.

Procedure

STEP 1

- Remove the C6/7 disk using a transverse centering tool (Fig. 7) and determine the midline. The transverse centering tool keys off of the uncovertebral joints to assist in determining the exact midline.

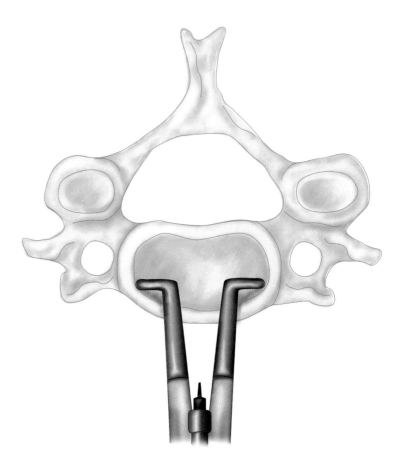

FIGURE 7

Instrumentation/Implantion

• Alignment guide
• Milling guides

Controversies

• A lateral radiograph can be taken to assure that the alignment guide is flush with the lower end plate before inserting anchor posts.

STEP 2

■ Determine appropriate height with an alignment guide positioned in the disk space with the cephalad and caudal milling guides, and attach both milling guides (Fig. 8).

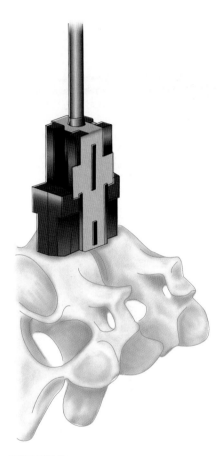

FIGURE 8

PEARLS

• *Use a depth gauge through the milling guide to reaffirm that the implant is of appropriate size (Fig. 9).*

• *Place a rasp and conduct a milling trial to assure proper end plate preparation and distraction.*

PITFALLS

• *Posterior uncovertebral osteophytes should have been removed during the decompression. The rasp and trial will determine if adequate decompression was performed.*

Instrumentation/ Implantation

• Verify trial position with lateral radiograph. This will assure the milling diameter has been chosen properly.

Controversies

• Should the PLL be removed routinely? The proper function of the disk does not depend upon whether the PLL is intact or removed. In order to assure adequate nerve root decompression (the main reason you are doing this operation), it is necessary to remove the PLL at least laterally over the takeoff of the nerve root.

STEP 3

■ Drill pilot holes through the milling guide, and place the 4.0-mm anchor posts with the anchor post screwdriver.
■ Remove the alignment guide.
■ Apply distraction device to the anchor posts.

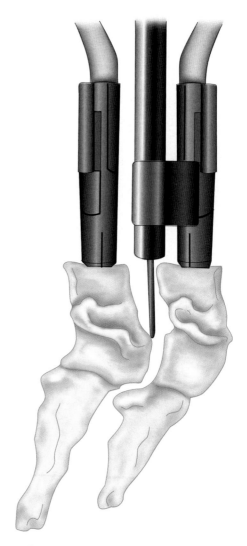

FIGURE 9

Controversies

- Should aggressive range-of-motion exercises begin immediately postoperatively?

STEP 4

- In small increments, mill the upper and lower end plates until the tool is at the final position.

STEP 5

- Fill Bryan Cervical Disk with saline and place into milled disk space.

Postoperative Care and Expected Outcomes

- No cervical collar is needed.
- Start normal motion immediately.
- Prescribe a nonsteroidal anti-inflammatory drug (NSAID) of choice for 2 weeks postoperatively.

Evidence

Anderson PA, Sasso RC, Rouleau JP, Carlson CS, Goffin J. The Bryan Cervical Disc: wear properties and early clinical results. Spine J. 2004;4(6 Suppl):303S-9S.

Goffin J, Van Calenbergh F, van Loon J, Casey A, Kehr P, Liebig K, Lind B, Logroscino C, Sgrambiglia R, Pointillart V. Intermediate follow-up after treatment of degenerative disc disease with the Bryan Cervical Disc Prosthesis: single-level and bi-level. Spine. 2003;28:2673-8.

Anderson PA, Rouleau JP, Bryan VE, Carlson CS. Wear analysis of the Bryan Cervical Disc prosthesis. Spine 2003;28:S186-94.

Puschak TJ, Sasso RC. Use of artificial disk replacement in degenerative conditions of the cervical spine. Curr Opin Orthop. 2004;15:175-9.

CERVICAL SPINE
Posterior Approaches

Occipital-Cervical Fusion

Howard B. Levene and Jack I. Jallo

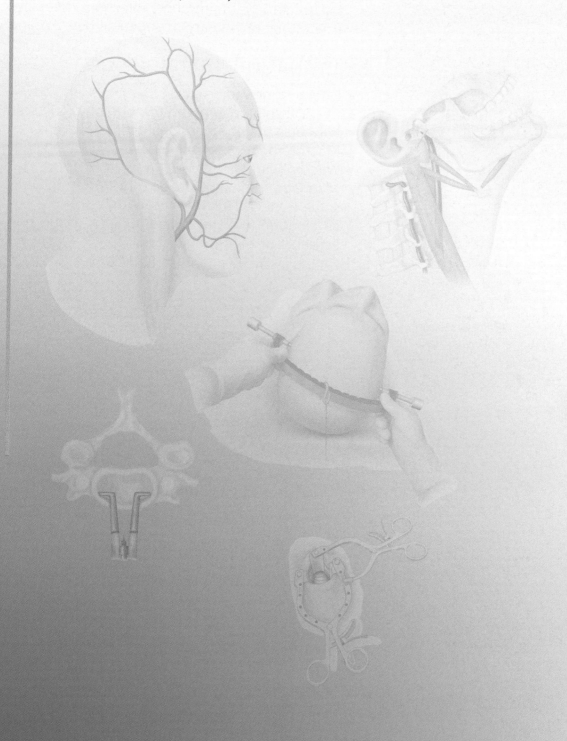

Controversies

- Need for halo preoperatively
- Need for halo postoperatively

Treatment Options

- External fixation (halo) only
- Combined approach (anterior resection of dens, posterior fusion)
- Various occipital-cervical fusion devices (bone and wire, loop and wire, screw and rods, in-out option for occipital screw)

Indications

- Acute occipital-cervical instability: trauma (Fig. 1A and 1B)
- Chronic occipital-cervical instability: degenerative, inflammatory/autoimmune, infectious, neoplastic (metastatic or primary), congenital (Fig. 2A and 2B)

Examination/Imaging

- Lateral spine radiograph
- Cervical spine computed tomography (CT) scan with two- and three-dimensional reconstructions
- Measurement of reference lines (Chamberlain line, Wackenheim line, etc.)
- Magnetic resonance imaging (MRI) of the cervical spine (especially with myelopathy) (Fig. 3)
- Myelogram (CT and radiographic) if MRI is not available or is contraindicated

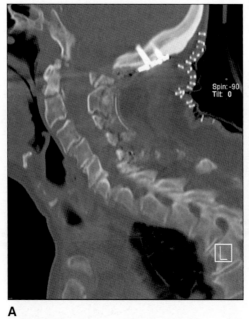
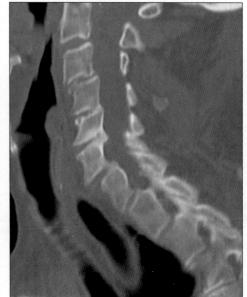

FIGURE 1A-B **A** **B**

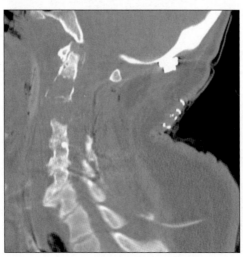
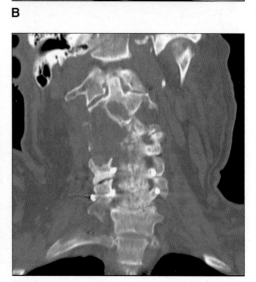

FIGURE 2A-B **A** **B**

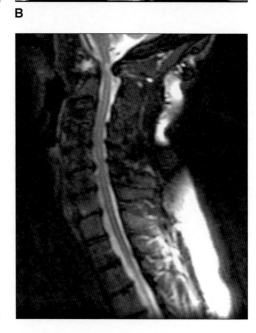

FIGURE 3

Surgical Anatomy

- Occiput/inion (Fig. 4)
- Vertebral arteries (Fig. 5)
- Condyle joints and C1 and C2 bony anatomy (C2 screw placement)
- Lateral masses (C3-6 lateral mass screw placement) (Fig. 6A and 6B)

Ideal Screw Locations

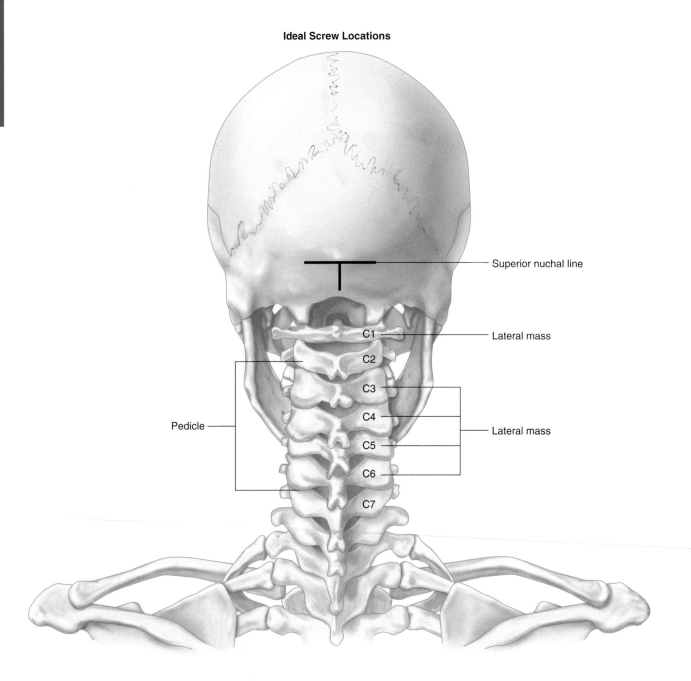

FIGURE 4

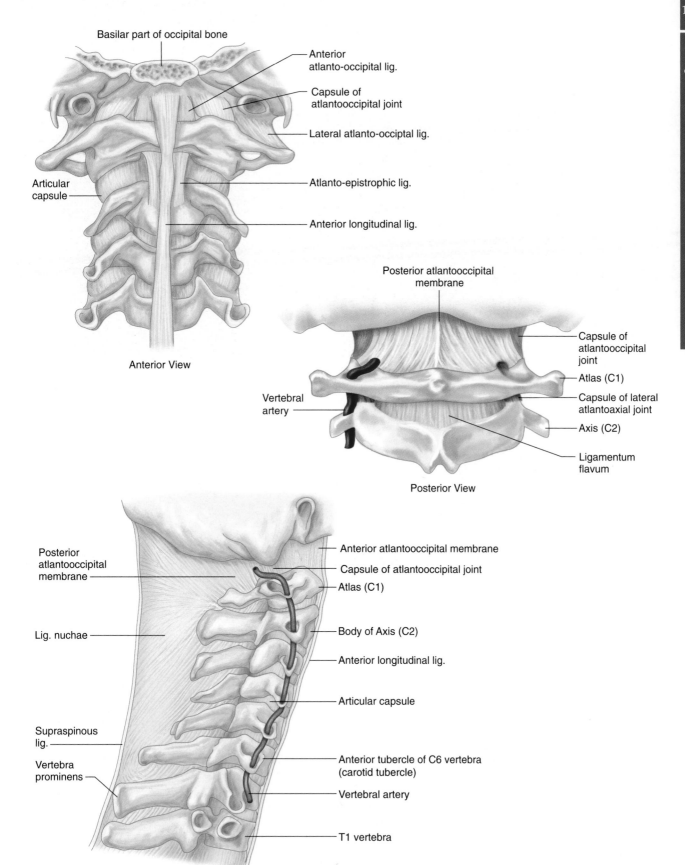

Basilar part of occipital bone

Anterior atlanto-occipital lig.

Capsule of atlantooccipital joint

Lateral atlanto-occiptal lig.

Articular capsule

Atlanto-epistrophic lig.

Anterior longitudinal lig.

Anterior View

Posterior atlantooccipital membrane

Capsule of atlantooccipital joint

Atlas (C1)

Vertebral artery

Capsule of lateral atlantoaxial joint

Axis (C2)

Ligamentum flavum

Posterior View

Posterior atlantooccipital membrane

Lig. nuchae

Supraspinous lig.

Vertebra prominens

Anterior atlantooccipital membrane

Capsule of atlantooccipital joint

Atlas (C1)

Body of Axis (C2)

Anterior longitudinal lig.

Articular capsule

Anterior tubercle of C6 vertebra (carotid tubercle)

Vertebral artery

T1 vertebra

Right Lateral View

FIGURE 5

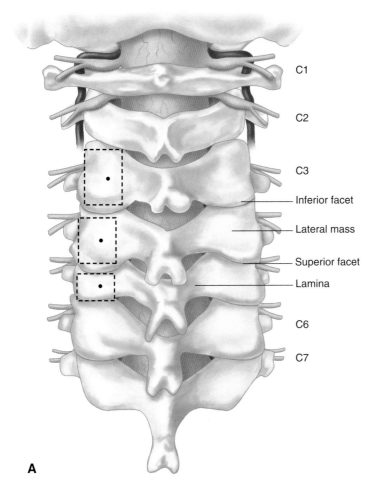

C1

C2

C3

Inferior facet

Lateral mass

Superior facet

Lamina

C6

C7

A

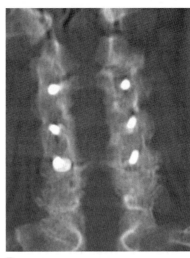

B

FIGURE 6A-B

Positioning

- Place patient in prone in 3-point pin fixation.
- Alternatively, the patient can be placed in prone in a halo ring affixed to the table (Fig. 7).
- Another option is continuous traction.

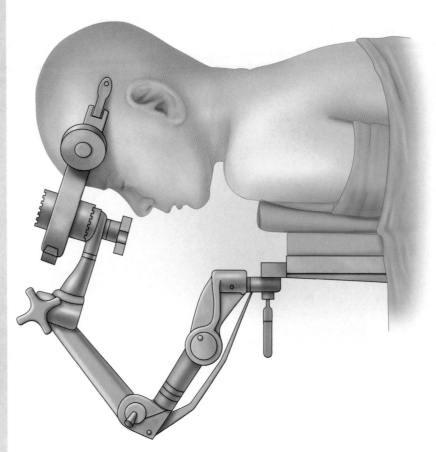

FIGURE 7

Equipment

- Fluoroscopy for pedicle/lateral mass screws

Controversies

- Use of cervical traction is advocated by Menenzes (Menezes and Sonntag, 1996).

Instrumentation

- Wire-based systems
- Screw/rod-based systems

Portals/Exposures

- Inion to C5 (Fig. 8). Lateral masses to C3 at minimum must be exposed.

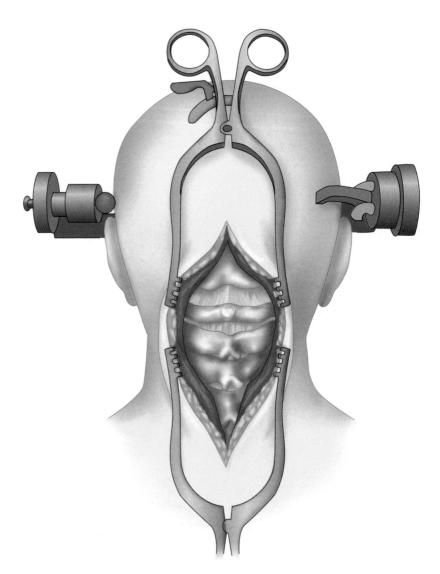

FIGURE 8

Controversies

- Menezes advocates using traction and avoiding pin fixation (Menezes and Sonntag, 1996).

Controversies

- The choice of screw fixation is variable. Options include fusion to C1, to C2, or distally.

Procedure

STEP 1

- Position the patient on gel rolls, in pins, in a prone, neutral position (see Fig. 7).
- Shave and mark from the inion down the midline to C5.
- Prepare in the usual sterile fashion.

STEP 2: EXPOSURE OF INION TO C5

- Dissect using sharp, blunt, and electrocautery down the midline through the following layers (see Fig. 8):
  - Superficial fascia. Identify the midline raphe.
  - Identify the spinous process and the prevertebral fascia.
  - Dissect bilaterally down the spinous processes. Preserve the ligamentum nuchae as much as possible.
  - Take care to identify the spinous process of C2 and the ring of C1. Dissection here must be very cautious so as to avoid entering the occipital, C1, or C2 spaces or the C1/2 interspace.
  - Expose laterally to identify lateral masses.
  - Expose anteriorly to identify the inion.
- Bony exposure of occiput to C2 lateral masses must be achieved at minimum. Expose lower lateral masses as needed.

STEP 3: INSTRUMENTATION

- Place the Kiel plate midline (Fig. 9).
- Place an isthmus or pedicle screw at C2. (Expose the lateral masses of distal vertebra as needed.)

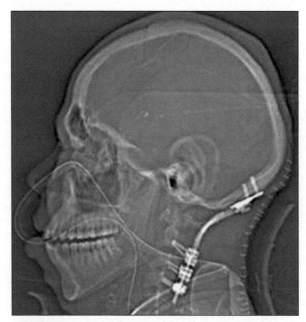

FIGURE 9

Controversies

- Use of autologous bone versus allograft bone. Autologous bone has high fusion rates and higher comorbidities.

- Contour the rods to the approximate neutral position of the occipitocervical junction. The rod bend will to approximately a 130° angle, but this will vary per patient.
- Connect the rods to the Kiel plate and screw.
- Pack the construct with autologous/allograft material to encourage fusion.

STEP 4
- Close layers sequentially.
- Drain as needed.

Postoperative Care and Expected Outcomes

- Place the patient in a hard collar for 2–4 weeks with CT/radiographic follow-up until fused.
- After 12 weeks, flexion/extension views should be obtained to determine if fusion is noted radiographically.
- Approximately 80% fusion rates are expected.
- Complications include infection, neurovascular compromise from instrumentation, subdural or subarachnoid hematoma due to instrumentation placement, cerebrospinal fluid flow abnormalities due to instrumentation placement, pullout of screws/plate/instrumentation, and fracture/migration of instrumentation.

Controversies

- Not all surgeons advocate use of a hard cervical collar postoperatively.

Evidence

Abumi K, Takada T, Shono Y, Kaneda K, Fujiya M. Posterior occipitocervical reconstruction using cervical pedicle screws and plate-rod systems. Spine. 1999;24:1425-34.

Deutsch H, Haid RW Jr, et al. Occipitocervical fixation: long-term results. Spine. 2005;30:530-5.

Dvorak MF, Sekeramayi F, et al. Anterior occiput to axis screw fixation. Part II: a biomechanical comparison with posterior fixation techniques. Spine. 2003;28:239-45.

Lee SC, Chen JF, et al. Complications of fixation to the occiput—anatomical and design implications. Br J Neurosurg. 2004;18:590-7.

Menezes AH, Sonntag VKH. Principles of Spinal Surgery. New York: McGraw-Hill, 1996.

Oda I, Abumi K, et al. Biomechanical evaluation of five different occipito-atlanto-axial fixation techniques. Spine 1999;24:2377-82.

Schmidek HH, Sweet WH. Schmidek & Sweet's Operative Neurosurgical Techniques: Indications, Methods, and Results. Philadelphia: WB Saunders, 2000.

Vaccaro AR, Betz RR, et al. Principles and Practice of Spine Surgery. St. Louis: CV Mosby, 2003.

Vender JR, Rekito AJ, et al. The evolution of posterior cervical and occipitocervical fusion and instrumentation. Neurosurg Focus 2004;16:e9.

Winn HR, Youmans JR. Youmans Neurological Surgery. Philadelphia: WB Saunders, 2004.

Posterior C1–C2 Fusion Techniques: Harms Technique and Magerl Technique

Joseph M. Zavatsky, John A. Handal, Minn Saing, Alexander R. Vaccaro, and Joon Y. Lee

Harms Technique: Posterior C1-2 Polyaxial Screw and Rod Fixation (Harms and Melcher, 2001)

Indications

- Atlantoaxial instability due to
  - Fractures of the odontoid (types II and III)
  - Rotatory subluxation: C1/C2
  - Unstable os odontoideum
  - Postodontoidectomy without basilar invagination
  - Malignancy
- Nonunions
  - Odontoid (types II and III)
  - Failed posterior C1–C2 fusion
- C1-2 osteoarthritis

Examination/Imaging

- Neurologic and musculoskeletal examination.
- Preoperative imaging should include plain radiographs (Fig. 1A), computed tomography (CT) (Fig. 1B), and magnetic resonance imaging (MRI) (Fig. 1C) and magnetic resonance angiography (MRA) of the cervical spine.
  - Radiographs should include anteroposterior (AP), lateral, open-mouth, and supervised dynamic lateral flexion and extension views. Combined lateral mass displacement in excess of 7 mm or an atlantodens interval greater than 3 mm suggests transverse ligament disruption.
  - A CT scan with axial, sagittal, and coronal thin-cut (1-mm) reconstruction images through the upper cervical spine is an important part of preoperative planning.
    - It provides accurate detail of the bony anatomy and any associated injuries.
    - It delineates the position of the foramen transversarium through which the vertebral artery runs.
    - It allows you to measure the length of the screws that will be utilized in the C1 lateral mass and C2 pedicle.
  - Approximately 20% of patients requiring atlantoaxial fusion using the transarticular or

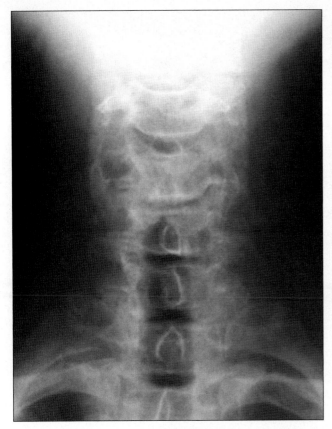
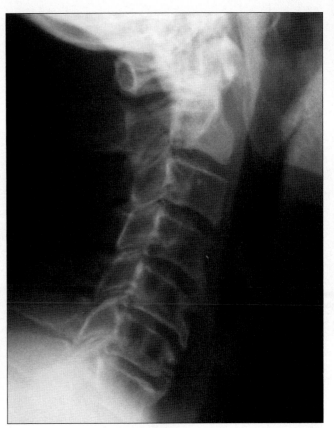
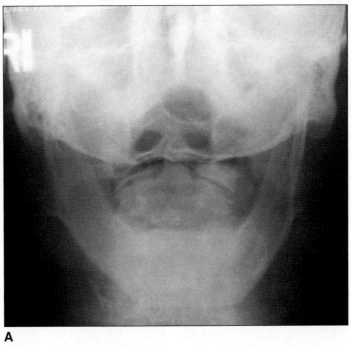

A

FIGURE 1A

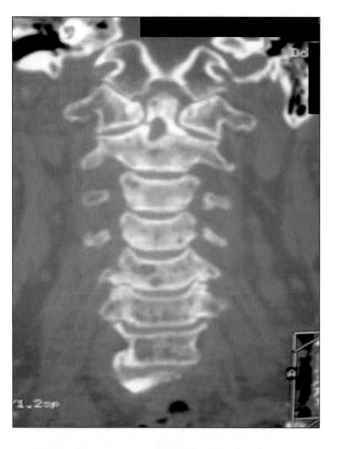
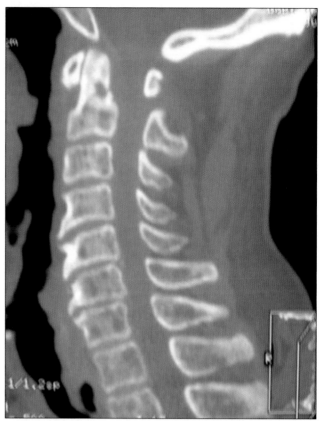
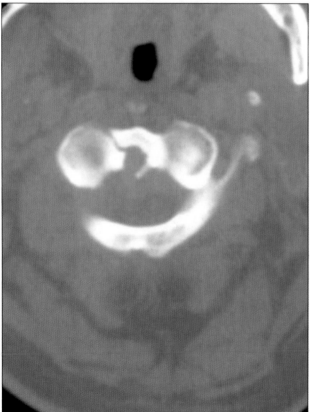
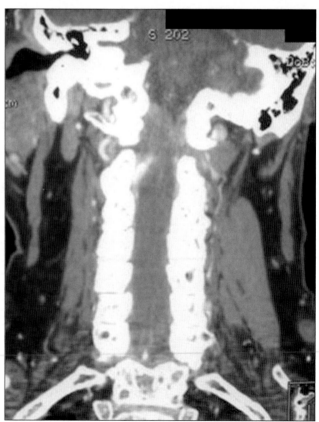

B

FIGURE 1B *Continued*

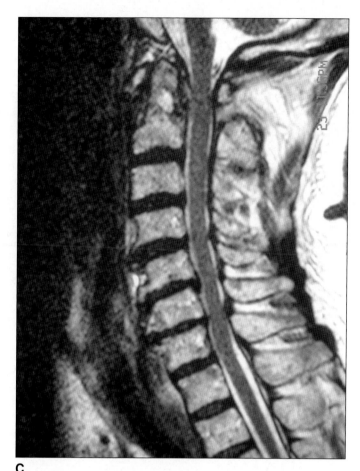

C

FIGURE 1C *Continued*

Treatment Options

- C1-2 transarticular facet screws (Magerl technique)
- Gallie "bone block" graft placed posteriorly between the arches of C1 and C2, secured with sublaminar wires
- Brooks "wedge" bone graft secured to the posterior lamina with sublaminar wires
- Halifax interlaminar clamp

Harms technique show anatomic variations in the path of the vertebral artery and osseous anatomy that would preclude screw placement (Jun, 1998; Madawi et al., 1997). In addition to evaluating vertebral artery dominance, CT or MRA can delineate the spatial relationship of the vertebral artery relative to the C1 lateral mass and C2 pedicle.

- MRI allows enhanced visualization of any soft tissue injuries including injury to the transverse atlantal ligament, as well as visualization of the spinal cord.
  - ◆ Odontoid fractures with transverse atlantal ligament injury can be addressed with a posterior fusion. Anterior odontoid screw fixation alone will not restore atlantoaxial stability secondary to transverse ligamentous disruption.
  - ◆ In rheumatoid patients, it is also useful to identify a pannus posterior to the odontoid that could compress the cord with any posterior translation of the dens.

Surgical Anatomy

- The posterior arch of C1 and the C1-2 facet joint are key anatomic landmarks for the placement of C1 lateral mass screws. The dorsal root ganglion of C2 lies just posterior to the starting point of the C1 lateral mass screw and must be gently retracted caudally for adequate exposure (Fig. 2A). The starting point for the C1 screw is at the midpoint of the inferior portion of the C1 lateral mass at its junction with the posterior arch. A more superior and medial trajectory of the screws, when compared to transarticular screws, decreases the risk of vertebral artery injury (Fig. 2B and 2C).

- The ponticulus posticus or congenital arcuate foramen is a common bony anomaly of the atlas

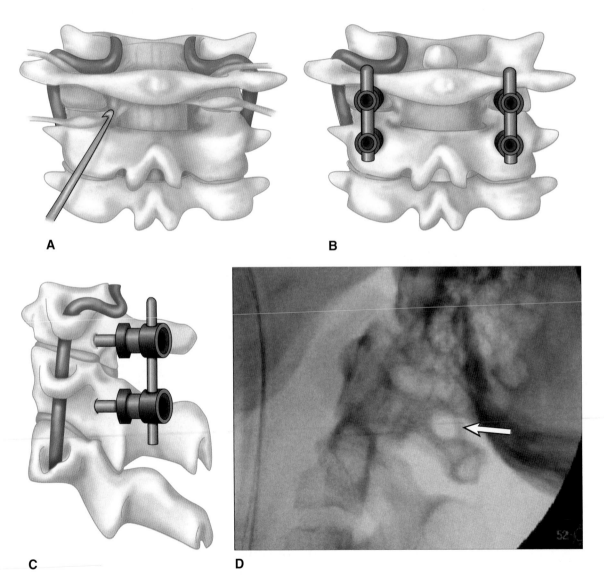

A

B

C

D

FIGURE 2A-D

(Young et al., 2005) (Fig. 2D). It is a bony arch on the cephalad aspect of the C1 lamina that contains the vertebral artery. If present, it can easily be confused with the lamina of C1, and so must be identified during the posterior dissection and placement of C1 lateral mass screws to prevent vertebral artery injury.

Positioning

- After an awake fiberoptic nasotracheal intubation is performed, a nasogastric tube is inserted for intraoperative gastric drainage.
- If the patient is immobilized in a halo-vest orthosis, a rigid Philadelphia collar is placed on the patient prior to halo-vest removal. In coordination with anesthesia, the surgeon stands at the head of the hospital bed and stabilizes the patient's neck. The patient is cautiously repositioned in the prone position on the operating table with the torso on bolsters or a four-poster frame. The halo-ring adapter can be attached to the Mayfield adapter. If the halo-ring adapter is removed, the patient is placed in Mayfield tongs prior to prone positioning. After repositioning the patient prone, the Mayfield tongs are fixed to the operating table using a Mayfield headholder with the neck in a neutral position (Fig. 3).

PEARLS

- *An open-mouth view is obtained by placing an appropriate-size roll of sterile gauze in the patient's mouth to facilitate a clear open-mouth view.*

- *In very osteopenic bone, inverse (negative) radiologic images can be utilized for better bony visualization.*

- *On the lateral C-arm image, the posterior occiput should be flexed off the posterior arch of C1 to facilitate screw placement at C1.*

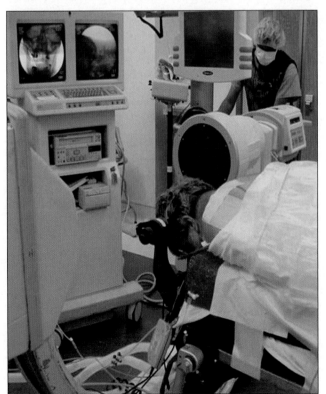

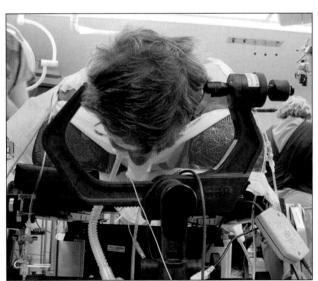

FIGURE 3

Equipment

- A C-arm fluoroscope should be positioned at the head of the operating table, with the bed being turned 180° using an extended endotracheal tube and the feet of the patient being toward the anesthesiologist.
- Mayfield headholder
- Bolsters or a four-poster frame

- All bony prominences are well padded, and the patient's arms are secured by the side using a folded sheet that is tucked beneath them.
- Using a fluoroscopic C-arm, proper alignment of the atlantoaxial bony structures is confirmed with the radiograph centered at the C1-2 articulation.
  - The lateral fluoroscopic image must not be oblique at C1-2, or misdirection of the drilling path may result in erroneous screw placement.
  - The appropriate C1 and C2 radiographic landmarks are visualized. The lateral wall of the C1 lateral mass and medial wall of the C2 pedicle are important landmarks defined on the open-mouth view.
  - The C-arm gantry is canted in the cephalad or caudad direction until all bony landmarks are clearly identified.
- If necessary, adjustments can be made while the patient is in the Mayfield headholder to obtain cervical reduction. Reduction should be confirmed by fluoroscopy. If possible, extreme positions of neck flexion or extension should be avoided.
- Somatosensory evoked potential and transcranial motor evoked potential monitoring are neurophysiologic spinal cord monitoring methods that can be utilized intraoperatively. Baseline readings can be obtained before and after placing the patient in the prone position.

Portals/Exposures

- An electric razor, followed by a straight razor, are used to remove all hair from the patient's occipital, suboccipital, and neck regions. The posterior iliac crest is also shaved in a similar fashion for bone graft harvesting.
- The skin surfaces of the neck and posterior iliac crest are wiped cleaned with isopropyl alcohol, prepped with Betadine, and draped in a sterile fashion.
- Using the inion of the occiput cranially, and the protuberance of the vertebral prominens caudally, the midline is identified and marked from the occiput to C3-4 with a sterile marker.
- The subcutaneous skin of the planned skin incision can be infiltrated with 0.5% lidocaine containing epinephrine diluted 1:100,000.
- A 10-blade scalpel is used to sharply incise the skin in the midline from the occiput to C3-4.

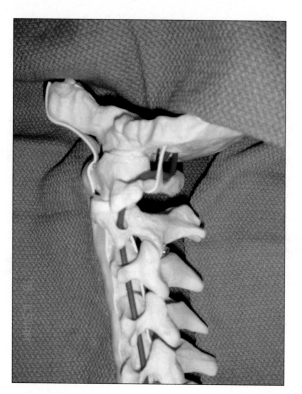

FIGURE 4

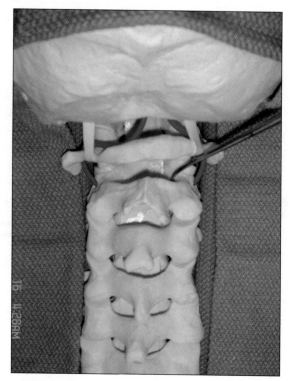

FIGURE 5

- Bovie electrocautery is used for the subcutaneous dissection down to and through the underlying ligamentum nuchae. Midline dissection of the nuchal ligament provides a relatively avascular dissection and decreases the risk of injury to the greater and third occipital nerves. Self-retaining retractors are inserted for adequate visualization.
- At the cephalad end of the incision, a 1.5-cm fascial cuff of trapezius, along the nuchal ridge, can be elevated to facilitate lateral exposure of C1-2, but this is not usually necessary.
- The midline tubercle of the arch of C1 and the larger bifid spinous process of C2 are used as palpable landmarks during dissection. Starting at the midline, the periosteum of C1 and the tip of the spinous processes of C2 are incised sharply.
- Careful subperiosteal dissection is continued from C2 to C1, starting in the midline and proceeding laterally. Periosteal elevators can facilitate the subperiosteal dissection of the paraspinous muscles as they are swept laterally.
- The lateral masses of C2 are exposed with care not to disturb the C2-3 facet capsules.
- The C1-2 joint can be exposed with dissection over the superior surface of the C2 isthmus and pedicle.

Significant venous bleeding can be encountered with dissection around the cavernous venous plexus surrounding the C2 nerve. This can effectively be controlled with bipolar electrocautery, thrombin-soaked Gelfoam, and cotton pledgets.

■ To decrease the risk of injuring the vertebral artery on the superior surface of the C1 lamina, do not dissect further than 15 mm laterally from the midline in the adult patient. If present, the ponticulus posticus or congenital arcuate foramen must be identified during the posterior dissection because it can easily be confused with the lamina of C1 (Young et al., 2005).

■ The dissection is complete with exposure of the suboccipital rim of the foramen magnum.

Instrumentation/ Implantation

- Penfield elevator
- Blunt pedicle probe
- High-speed burr
- Pneumatic drill and 2-mm drill bit

Procedure

Step 1

■ The authors' preferred treatment is to drill, measure, and tap all the screw holes prior to the insertion of any screws. Because of the increased risk of venous bleeding with dissection around the C1-2 joint for C1 lateral mass screw placement, the C2 isthmus or pedicle screw holes are completed first.

■ Beginning at C2, a number 4 Penfield elevator is used to define the medial border of the C2 isthmus or pedicle. The starting point for the C2 pedicle screw is in the superior and medial quadrant of the C2 lateral mass (Fig. 5). The entry point for placement of the C2 isthmus or pedicle screw is marked with the 2-mm high-speed burr.

■ The starting hole and drill bit trajectory can be confirmed under C-arm fluoroscopic guidance with open-mouth and lateral views.

■ A C2 pedicle pilot hole is drilled using a 2-mm drill bit in a 20-30° convergent and cephalad trajectory, using the superior and medial aspect of the C2 pedicle as a guide. The integrity of the walls of the pilot drill hole is confirmed with a blunt pedicle probe.

■ A depth gauge can be used to confirm the measurement obtained from the preoperative CT scan of the appropriate-length screw, and this can be checked on a lateral fluoroscopic image.

■ The drill hole is tapped.

■ Step 1 is repeated for the contralateral C2 isthmus or pedicle.

PEARLS

- *Critical landmarks for the accurate placement of C1 lateral mass screws*

  - *The C1-2 joint*

  - *The midpoint and medial and lateral wall of the C1 lateral mass*

- *The ponticulus posticus or congenital arcuate foramen can be confused with the C1 lamina and must be identified to prevent vertebral artery injury during the posterior dissection and placement of C1 lateral mass screws (Young et al., 2005).*

STEP 2

- The dorsal root ganglion of C2 must be carefully retracted caudally to expose the starting point for the C1 lateral mass screw. The starting point for the C1 lateral mass screw is at the midpoint of the C1 lateral mass at its junction with the posterior arch of C1 (Figs. 6 and 7).
- C-arm imaging can be used to verify the midpoint and trajectory of the C1 lateral mass screw.
- A 2-mm high-speed burr is used to mark the starting point for the drill and to prevent the drill from walking off the convex surface of the posterior lateral mass of C1.
- The drill bit is directed in a straight to slightly convergent trajectory in the AP plane, and parallel to the posterior arch of C1 in the sagittal plane. Drill position is confirmed on AP and lateral C-arm fluoroscopic images.
- A depth gauge can be used to confirm the measurement obtained from the preoperative CT scan of the appropriate-length screw, and this can be checked on a lateral fluoroscopic image.
- The drill hole is tapped.
- Step 2 is repeated for the contralateral C1 lateral mass.

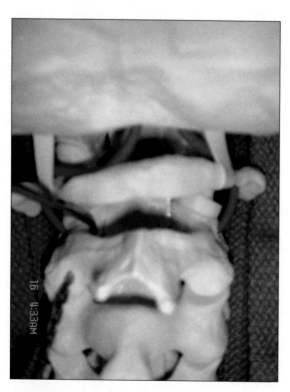

FIGURE 6

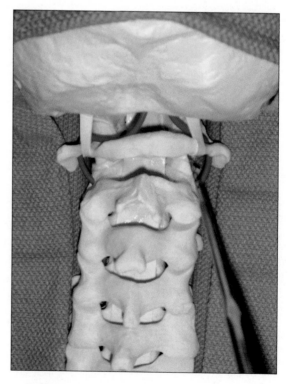

FIGURE 7

Instrumentation/ Implantation

- Variable-length 3.5-mm polyaxial screws

STEP 3

- Bicortical 3.5-mm polyaxial screws of the appropriately measured length are inserted into the C2 isthmus or pedicles.
- Fluoroscopic imaging is used to confirm proper screw placement.
- Bicortical 3.5-mm polyaxial screws of the appropriately measured length are placed into the lateral masses of C1 (Fig. 8). An 8-mm unthreaded portion of the C1 polyaxial screw sits proud above the bony surface of the lateral mass, allowing the polyaxial portion of the screw to sit above the posterior arch of C1. The proud segment of the screw is unthreaded and theoretically minimizes the risk of irritation of the greater occipital nerve.
- Screw position is confirmed on fluoroscopic imaging.

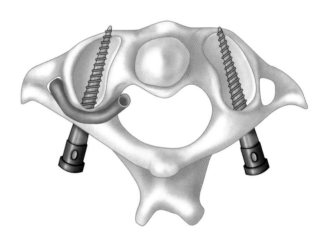

FIGURE 8

STEP 4

- If reduction of C1 is necessary, the patient's head can be repositioned before fixation of the rods to the screws. When performed, the reduction is visualized under fluoroscopy.
- The interconnecting rods are measured and secured with locking nuts (Fig. 9).
- Distraction or compression of the construct can be accomplished at this time.
- The locking nuts are tightened with a torque wrench.
- If bone graft is needed for definitive fusion, a moist sponge is placed in the wound to prevent tissue desiccation.

PEARLS—Cont'd

- *The integrity of the posterior arch of C1 is not necessary for stable fixation.*

- *Patients with rheumatoid arthritis often have instability adjacent to the atlantoaxial region requiring a more extensive fusion. This technique can be incorporated as part of fusions to the occiput and/or the subaxial spine.*

- *An alternative method of C1-2 reduction is to place the C1 screw deeper in the AP plane than the C2 screw and leave the C2 screw more proud. Locking the rod perpendicular to the polyaxial head of C2 allows the surgeon to translate C1 posteriorly as the rod is subsequently secured to the C1 screw. If C1 needs to be displaced anteriorly, the technique of screw prominence can be reversed.*

Instrumentation/ Implantation

- Variable-length interconnecting rods
- Locking nuts for polyaxial screws
- Torque wrench

Instrumentation/ Implantion

- Cobb elevators
- Osteotomes
- Gouges

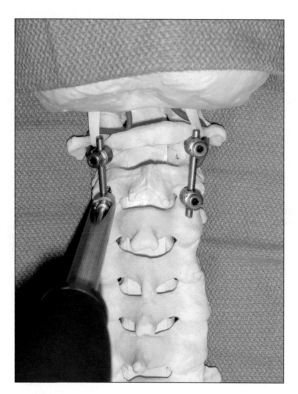

FIGURE 9

STEP 5

- For definitive fusion, posterior iliac crest bone graft is harvested. The posterior superior iliac crest is palpated and a 5-cm line centered over the crest is marked with a sterile marking pen. A 10-blade scalpel is used to incise the skin. Self-retaining retractors are inserted.
- Bovie electrocautery is used to dissect the subcutaneous tissue down to the junction of the lumbodorsal and gluteus maximus fascia.
- The posterior superior iliac crest is palpated and the fascia is initially reflected using Bovie electrocautery. A subperiosteal dissection is performed using a Cobb elevator at the superior and lateral margins of the crest. Osteotomes are used to harvest a tricortical structural graft that can be laid over the decorticated posterior elements of C1 and C2.
- Small gouges can also be used to harvest cancellous bone graft through the cortical defect.
- The graft is placed in a sterile cup, mixed with the patient's blood, and covered.
- Hemostasis is obtained. The wound is irrigated and the graft site is packed with Marcaine-soaked Gelfoam.
- The retractors are removed and the incision is closed in layers.

STEP 6

- The cervical operative field is irrigated with antibiotic solution, and the irrigation fluid is suctioned from the field.
- If definitive fusion is being performed, the posterior surfaces of C1 and C2 are decorticated with the high-speed burr. Alternatively, decortication of the posterior aspects of C1 and C2 can be performed prior to insertion of the screws and rods.
- The cancellous bone graft surface is placed over the decorticated surfaces of C1 and C2.
- The C1-2 joint surfaces can also be decorticated and packed with bone graft for an intra-articular fusion.

STEP 7

- The wound is closed securely in a layered fashion, obliterating any dead space.
- Steri-Strips are placed perpendicular to the incision and covered by sterile 4 × 4 gauze and a clear Tegaderm dressing.
- Final AP and lateral cervical radiographs are obtained to assess placement of the hardware and alignment of the atlantoaxial region.
- A rigid cervical collar (i.e., Philadelphia or Miami J) is secured in place.
- The patient is removed from the Mayfield headholder. The surgeon or surgical assistant stands at the head of the operating table and is responsible for stabilizing the neck when the patient is repositioned onto the hospital bed in the supine position.

Postoperative Care and Expected Outcomes

- The patient should be taken to the recovery room or the surgical intensive care unit for postoperative recovery.
- Supine and upright lateral cervical radiographs should be obtained in the cervical collar to assess stability on postoperative day 1 (Fig. 10). If atlantoaxial stability had been obtained, the patient can be mobilized.
- A postoperative CT scan can be obtained if there is any question concerning screw placement.
- The patient can be discharged from the hospital when medically stable.
- Rigid cervical collar immobilization is used postoperatively.

PITFALLS

- *Screw malposition can result in*

- *Inadequate purchase resulting in a potentially unstable construct. Rigid external immobilization in a halo-vest orthosis for 10–12 weeks should provide enough atlantoaxial stability to achieve fusion if instability is present.*

- *Dural tear and CSF leak. The authors advocate the primary repair of all dural tears, as well as placement of Gelfoam over the repair.*

PITFALLS—Cont'd

- *Violation of the foramen transversarium can result in vertebral artery rupture, dissection, pseudoaneurysm, or occlusion. Even without direct violation of the arterial wall, the screw threads can contact the artery with normal pulsatile flow and result in injury. If this is discovered intraoperatively or postoperatively, the screw should be removed to decrease the risk of vertebral artery injury.*

- *Intraoperative vertebral artery injury is the most serious complication which can cause serious clinical sequela, including brainstem stroke. If this occurs, the screw should be removed immediately and the site should be packed with pieces of Gelfoam large enough not to be a source of emboli. Bone wax can also be used to help tamponade the bleeding. A direct microvascular repair by a vascular surgeon, after the surrounding bone is skeletonized, is also an option. Irrespective of the method used to tamponade the bleeding, a postoperative angiogram should be obtained to evaluate the integrity of the vertebral artery.*

- Routine outpatient static lateral and supervised dynamic lateral flexion and extension radiographs can be obtained at approximately 6-10 weeks to ascertain stability. If stability is obtained, the cervical collar can be weaned from use. Radiographs subsequently are obtained at 3-month intervals to assess stability and fusion.

- Additionally, a CT scan can be obtained 6–9 months postoperatively to assess fusion and fracture healing.

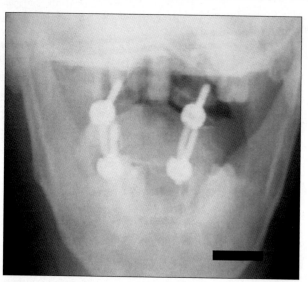

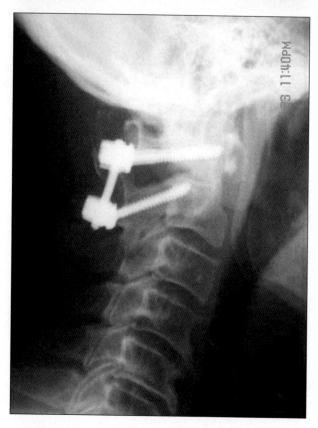

FIGURE 10

Magerl Technique: C1-2 Transarticular Facet Screws (Magerl and Seemann, 1986)

Indications

- Atlantoaxial instability due to
  - Fractures of the odontoid (types II and III)
  - Adjacent fractures of C1 and C2
  - Rotatory subluxation: C1/C2
  - Rheumatoid arthritis
  - Os odontoideum
  - Postodontoidectomy without basilar invagination
  - Congenital malformation (i.e., Klippel-Feil syndrome)
  - Malignancy
- Nonunions
  - Odontoid nonunion (types II and III)
  - Failed posterior C1-C2 fusion
- C1-2 osteoarthritis

Examination/Imaging

- Neurologic and musculoskeletal examination.
- Preoperative imaging should include plain radiographs, computed tomography (CT), and magnetic resonance imaging (MRI) and magnetic resonance angiography (MRA) of the cervical spine (see Fig. 1A, 1B, and 1C).
  - Radiographs should include anteroposterior (AP), lateral, open-mouth, and supervised dynamic lateral flexion and extension views if not contraindicated.
    - Neutral AP and lateral radiographs can evaluate the alignment of C1 and C2.
    - Supervised dynamic lateral flexion and extension views helps determine the reducibility of atlantoaxial subluxation when present.
  - A CT scan with axial, sagittal, and coronal thin-cut (1-mm) reconstruction images through the upper cervical spine is an important part of preoperative planning.
    - It can provide anatomic detail of the lateral mass of C1 and the C2 isthmus and articular processes for optimal placement of transarticular facet screws.

Treatment Options

- Posterior C1-2 polyaxial screw and rod fixation (Harms technique)
- Gallie "bone block" graft placed posteriorly between the arches of C1 and C2, secured with sublaminar wire
- Brooks "wedge" bone graft secured to the posterior lamina with sublaminar wire
- Halifax interlaminar clamp

♦ It delineates the position of the foramen transversarium, through which the vertebral artery runs.
♦ It allows for the evaluation of adequate bone stock of the atlas for sufficient distal fixation of the screws.

- Approximately 20% of patients requiring atlantoaxial fusion show anatomic variations in the path of the vertebral artery and osseous anatomy that would preclude screw transarticular screw placement (Jun, 1998; Madawi et al., 1997). In addition to evaluating vertebral artery dominance, MRA can delineate the course of the vertebral artery through the foramen transversarium and its spatial relationship to the surrounding bony architecture. This can help determine if a screw can be placed safely with minimal risk to the vertebral artery.
- MRI permits visualization of any soft tissue injuries, including injury to the transverse atlantal ligament, as well as visualization of the spinal cord.
  ♦ Odontoid fractures with transverse atlantal ligament injury can be addressed with a posterior approach. Even with union, anterior odontoid screw fixation alone will not restore atlantoaxial stability secondary to ligamentous disruption.
  ♦ When present in rheumatoid patients, a pannus posterior to the odontoid could have a mass effect that could compress the cord with any posterior translation of the dens.
- Noninvasive MRA can be utilized to evaluate vertebral artery injury, patency, and/or dominance.

Surgical Anatomy

- The cephalad orientation of the C1-C2 transarticular screw and the final position of the neck necessary for adequate atlantoaxial alignment may require percutaneous placement of the transarticular facet screws.
- The ponticulus posticus or congenital arcuate foramen is a common bony anomaly of the atlas (Young et al., 2005). It is a bony arch on the cephalad aspect of the C1 lamina that contains the vertebral artery. If present, it can easily be confused with the lamina of C1, and so must be identified during the posterior dissection to prevent vertebral artery injury.

Equipment

- A C-arm fluoroscope positioned at the patient's head, which is located opposite the radiologist
- Mayfield headholder
- Four-poster frame

Positioning

- After awake fiberoptic nasotracheal intubation is performed, a nasogastric tube is inserted for intraoperative gastric drainage.
- If the patient is immobilized in a halo-vest orthosis, a rigid Philadelphia collar is placed on the patient prior to halo-vest removal. In coordination with anesthesia, the surgeon stands at the head of the hospital bed and stabilizes the patient's neck. The patient is cautiously repositioned in the prone position on the operating table with the torso on bolsters or a four-poster frame. The halo-ring adapter can be attached to the Mayfield adapter. If the halo-ring adapter is removed, the patient is placed in Mayfield tongs prior to prone positioning. After repositioning the patient prone, the Mayfield tongs are fixed to the operating table using a Mayfield headholder with the neck in a neutral position.
- All bony prominences are well padded, and the patient's arms are secured by the side using a folded sheet that is tucked beneath them.
- Using a fluoroscopic C-arm, proper alignment of the atlantoaxial bony structures is confirmed with the radiograph centered at the C1-2 articulation. The lateral fluoroscopic image must not be oblique at C1-2, or incorrect drill path trajectory may result.
- If necessary, adjustments can be made while the patient is in the Mayfield headholder to obtain reduction, which should be confirmed by fluoroscopy. If possible, extreme positions of the neck should be avoided.
- Somatosensory evoked potential and transcranial motor evoked potential monitoring are neurophysiologic spinal cord monitoring methods that can be utilized intraoperatively. Baseline readings can be obtained before and after placing the patient in the prone position.

Portals/Exposures

- An electric razor, followed by a straight razor, are used to remove all hair from the patient's occipital, suboccipital, and neck regions. If transarticular screw fixation with bone graft and sublaminar wiring is being performed, the posterior iliac crest is also shaved in a similar fashion for bone graft harvesting.

- The skin surfaces of the neck and posterior iliac crest are wiped cleaned with isopropyl alcohol, prepped with Betadine, and draped in a sterile fashion.
- Using the inion of the occiput cranially, and the protuberance of the vertebral prominens caudally, the midline is identified and marked from the occiput to C3-4 with a sterile marker.
- The subcutaneous skin of the planned skin incision can be infiltrated with 0.5% lidocaine containing epinephrine diluted 1:100,000.
- A 10-blade scalpel is used to sharply incise the skin in the midline from the occiput to C3-4.
- Bovie electrocautery is used for the subcutaneous dissection down to and through the underlying ligamentum nuchae. Midline dissection of the nuchal ligament provides a relatively avascular dissection and decreases the risk of injury to the greater and third occipital nerves. Self-retaining retractors are inserted for adequate visualization.
- The midline tubercle of the arch of C1 and the larger spinous process of C2 are used as palpable landmarks during dissection. Starting at the midline, the periosteum of C1 and the tip of the spinous processes of C2 are incised sharply.
- Careful subperiosteal dissection is continued from C3 to C1, starting in the midline and proceeding laterally. Periosteal elevators can facilitate the subperiosteal dissection of the paraspinous muscles as they are swept laterally. The lateral masses of C3 and C2 are exposed with care not to disturb the C2-3 facet capsules.
- The C1-2 joint can be exposed with dissection over the superior surface of the C2 pedicle. The capsule of the C1-2 facet is reflected from caudal to cephalad using caution not to injure the C2 nerve and surrounding vessels. Significant venous bleeding can be encountered with dissection around the cavernous venous plexus surrounding the C2 nerve. This can effectively be controlled with bipolar electrocautery, thrombin-soaked Gelfoam, and cotton pledgets.
- To decrease the risk of injuring the vertebral artery on the superior surface of the C1 lamina, do not dissect further than 15 mm from the midline laterally in the adult patient.

Instrumentation/ Implantation

- Cobb elevators
- Osteotomes
- Oscillating saw
- Gouges
- Curettes

Procedure

STEP 1

- If posterior bone graft and sublaminar wiring are going to be utilized with transarticular screw fixation, bone graft harvesting and passage of the C1 sublaminar wire should be completed prior to the insertion of the transarticular screws.
- After the dissection, the C1-2 posterior arch interspace and graft size are approximated. A moist sponge is placed in the wound to prevent tissue desiccation while harvesting the bone graft.
- The posterior superior iliac crest is palpated and a 5-cm line centered over the posterior superior iliac crest is marked with a sterile marking pen. A 10-blade scalpel is used to incise the skin. Self-retaining retractors are inserted.
- Bovie electrocautery is used to dissect the subcutaneous tissue down to the junction of the lumbodorsal and gluteus maximus fascia.
- The posterior superior iliac crest is palpated and the fascia is initially reflected using Bovie electrocautery. A subperiosteal dissection is performed using a Cobb elevator at the superior and lateral margins of the crest. Osteotomes and an oscillating saw are used to obtain a tricortical strut graft of the appropriate size.
- A 1.5 × 4-cm tricortical strut graft is obtained. Small gouges are then used to harvest additional cancellous bone graft.
- The wound is irrigated and the graft site is packed with Marcaine-soaked Gelfoam. The retractors are removed and the incision is closed in layers.
- Any soft tissue on the graft is removed with a small Cobb elevator or curette. The graft is placed in a sterile cup, mixed with the patient's blood, and covered.

Instrumentation/ Implantion

- Straight and curved microcurrettes
- Woodson dissector
- Kerrison rongeurs

STEP 2

- To prepare for the passage of the sublaminar wire, the ligamentum flavum and soft tissues on the underlying surfaces of the posterior arches of C1 and C2 are elevated off the superior and inferior surfaces of the lamina using straight and curved microcurrettes.
- A Woodson dissector can be used to carefully free any adherent portions of dura.
- A 2-mm Kerrison rongeur is used to remove the ligamentum. Venous plexus bleeding deep to the ligamentum can be controlled with bipolar electrocautery, thrombin-soaked Gelfoam, and pledget packing.

Instrumentation/ Implantation

- Penfield elevators

Instrumentation/ Implantation

- 16- or 18-gauge double-looped wire
- A wire-passer or 00 silk suture

STEP 3

- A number 4 Penfield elevator is used to define the medial border of the C2 isthmus. Care must be taken not to violate the dura with the elevator. The Penfield elevator can be used to protect the C2 nerve root and venous plexus with gentle rostral retraction. The removal of any ligamentum flavum adjacent to the C2 lamina will improve visualization of the C2 isthmus and atlantoaxial joint, and help with orientation for transarticular screw placement.
- Step 3 is repeated for the contralateral C2 isthmus.

STEP 4

- Using the Gallie technique, a C1 sublaminar wire is passed prior to the placement of the transarticular screws. A smooth arch is bent into the end of 16- or 18-gauge double-looped wire and conformed to approximate both the length and thickness of the C1 lamina.
- The wire is carefully passed beneath the C1 lamina. This maneuver can be facilitated by the use of 00 silk suture or a wire-passer. Using both hands, the wire is pulled beneath the C1 lamina. One hand pulls and advances the sublaminar wire, while the other hand provides constant gentle tension on the other end of the wire. This keeps the wire flush against the underside of the lamina, decreasing the risk of impinging the wire upon the cord.

STEP 5

- Atlantoaxial alignment is necessary for accurate placement of C1-2 transarticular screws (Fig. 11). This is confirmed using lateral C-arm fluoroscopy.

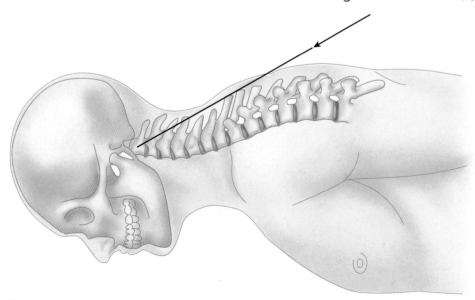

FIGURE 11

- If necessary, anterior atlantoaxial subluxation can be manually realigned intraoperatively with gentle traction on the C1 sublaminar wire and pressure on the axis.
- Posterior atlantoaxial subluxation can be realigned with flexion repositioning of the patient's head in the Mayfield tongs. Alternatively, posterior atlantoaxial subluxation can be reduced with the placement of the bone block graft between C1 and C2. After placement, the graft can be manually manipulated against the posterior arch of C1 to obtain reduction. Reduction can be maintained after the C1 sublaminar wire is secured around the spinous process of C2 and the bone block graft.
- The cephalad angle required to place the C1-2 transarticular screw can make placement difficult. To facilitate screw placement, the C2 spinous process can be grasped with a towel clip and gently elevated dorsally. This presents the C2 pedicle at a better angle for accurate placement of the transarticular screws.
- The position of the neck can also influence the trajectory necessary to obtain optimal placement of the transarticular screws. Percutaneous placement of the C1-2 facet screws may be necessary if intraoperative atlantoaxial alignment precludes the drilling or placement of the screws through the wound created by the posterior cervical dissection.

Instrumentation/ Implantation

- Pointer tunneler
- Soft tissue protection sheath

Step 6

- If the trajectory requires a percutaneous approach, a stab incision is made with a 15-blade scalpel through the skin in the paraspinal region of T2-3.
- A pointer tunneler is placed into the soft tissue protection sheath and inserted through the stab incision made at T2-3. The soft tissue protection sheath has a large handle that can be used to manipulate and guide the instrument's trajectory through the soft tissues.
- The tip of the tissue sheath is placed against the inferior articular process of C2 and the pointer tunneler is removed from the tissue sheath.

STEP 7

- The drill guide is inserted into the soft tissue sheath.
- If the percutaneous technique is not required, the drill guide can be inserted directly into the soft tissue sheath and placed against the C2 inferior articular process starting point.
- The starting point for screw entry is in the C2 fossa, 2 to 3 mm lateral to the junction of the lamina and lateral mass, and approximately 2 to 3 mm superior to the inferior edge of the C2 inferior articular process (Figs. 12 and 13).
- C-arm fluoroscopy is used to identify all bony atlantoaxial structures and guide the trajectory of the drill guide. The drill is aimed on lateral fluoroscopy toward the superior half of the anterior C1 lamina and is guided intraoperatively by the medial border of the C2 isthmus.

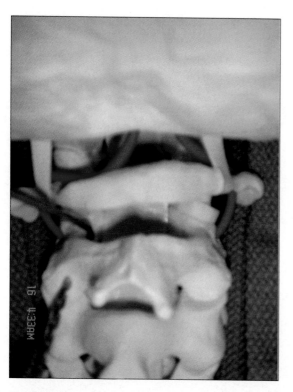

FIGURE 12

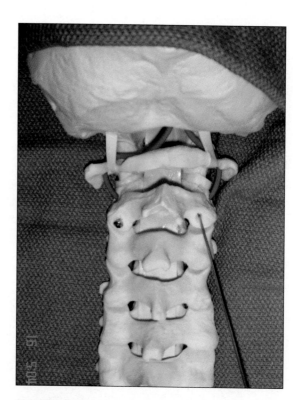

FIGURE 13

PEARLS

- *To decrease the risk of vertebral artery injury, the drill must not be directed laterally, and must follow the medial wall of the C2 isthmus.*

- *Intraoperative bony landmarks, the preoperative thin-cut (1-mm) axial CT scan, and AP and lateral fluoroscopic imaging can all aid in accurate drill bit and C1-2 transarticular screw placement.*

- *Screw fixation with a solid 3.5-mm stainless steel screw is the authors' preferred method for transarticular screw placement (Fig. 15).*

Instrumentation/ Implantation

- Drill bit
- Drill bit guide
- Penfield elevators

- The drill is advanced through the pars interarticularis of C2, along the central axis of the C2 isthmus in a 0-10° convergent trajectory in the AP plane.
- A number 4 Penfield elevator can be used to protect the C2 nerve root and venous plexus with gentle rostral retraction. This allows visualization of the drill as it passes across the posterior edge of the atlantoaxial facet joint into the lateral mass of C1. The tip of the drill should engage the anterosuperior margin of the C1 lateral mass (Fig. 14).
- C-arm fluoroscopy is used to confirm correct drill bit placement.

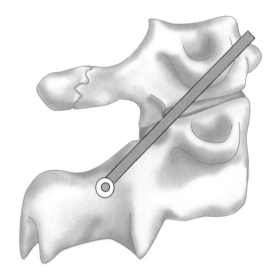

FIGURE 14

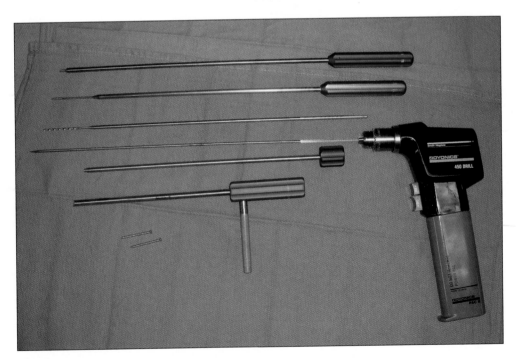

FIGURE 15

Instrumentation/ Implantion

- Drill bit
- Ruler
- Tap
- Fully threaded 3.5-mm cortical screws

Instrumentation/ Implantation

- High-speed burr

Instrumentation/ Implantation

- Leksell rongeur
- Kerrison rongeur

Instrumentation/ Implantion

- Heavy needle driver
- Wire cutters

STEP 8

- The near cortex is tapped through the tissue sheath.
- A fully threaded 3.5-mm cortical screw of appropriate length (usually 40–45 mm) is inserted using the screwdriver under fluoroscopic visualization. The anterior cortex of the C1 lateral mass may be purchased with the screw.
- Screw placement is confirmed with C-arm fluoroscopic imaging.
- Steps 5–8 are repeated for the contralateral C1-2 transarticular screw.

STEP 9

- The posterior cortical margin of the arch of C1 and the lamina and spinous process of C2 are decorticated with the burr.

STEP 10

- Using a Leksell rongeur, the tricortical strut graft is converted into a bicortical graft by removing the rounded cortical edge.
- The graft is temporarily placed between the posterior arches of C1 and C2 for final sizing and to approximate the midline of the graft. The Leksell rongeur is used to make any final modifications for optimal sizing of the graft.
- A Leksell rongeur is used to notch the midline on the inferior aspect of the graft to accommodate the spinous process of C2 for a secure graft fit.

STEP 11

- The graft is placed back in between the atlas and axis with the notch of the graft sitting on the spinous process of the axis for a secure fit.
- The C1 sublaminar loop of wire is passed below and secured in a notch made on the undersurface of the C2 spinous process (Fig. 16).

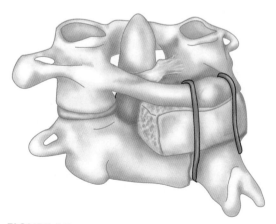

FIGURE 16

- The free ends of wire are wrapped around the bone graft and secured. A heavy needle driver is used to twist the free ends of wire together and tighten them snugly around the graft.
- Any excess wire is cut with wire cutters and removed. The cut ends of wire are carefully laid flush against the strut graft.

Instrumentation/ Implantation

- High-speed burr

Step 12

- The posterior cortical surfaces of the C1 posterior arch and C2 lamina are decorticated with the high-speed burr.
- The bone dust and shavings from the burr are left in the operative field, and cancellous bone graft morsels are placed over the posterior decorticated surfaces of C1 and C2.

Step 13

- The wound is closed securely in a layered fashion, obliterating any dead space.
- Steri-Strips are placed perpendicular to the incision and covered by sterile 4 × 4 gauze and a clear Tegaderm dressing.
- Final AP and lateral cervical radiographs are obtained to assess placement of the hardware and alignment of the atlantoaxial region.
- A rigid cervical collar (i.e., Philadelphia or Miami J) is secured in place.
- The patient is removed from the Mayfield headholder. The surgeon or surgical assistant stands at the head of the operating table and is responsible for stabilizing the neck when the patient is repositioned onto the hospital bed in the supine position.

Postoperative Care and Expected Outcomes

- The patient should be taken to the recovery room or the surgical intensive care unit for postoperative recovery.
- Supine and upright lateral cervical radiographs should be obtained in the cervical collar to assess stability on postoperative day 1 (Fig. 17). If atlantoaxial stability had been obtained, the patient can be mobilized.
- A postoperative CT scan can be obtained if there is any question concerning screw placement.
- The patient can be discharged from the hospital when medically stable.

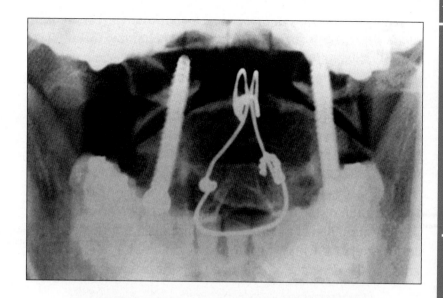

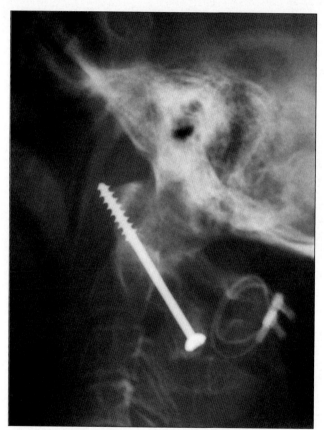

FIGURE 17

- Rigid cervical collar immobilization is used for approximately 6–10 weeks postoperatively.
- Routine outpatient static lateral radiographs can be obtained 6 weeks postoperatively to ascertain stability. Radiographs can be obtained at 12-week intervals to assess stability and fusion. Supervised

PITFALLS

- *Screw malposition can result in*

  - *Inadequate purchase resulting in a potentially unstable construct. Rigid external immobilization in a halo-vest orthosis for 10-12 weeks should provide enough atlantoaxial stability to achieve fusion if instability is present.*

  - *Dural tear and CSF leak. The authors advocate the primary repair of all dural tears, as well as placement of Gelfoam over the repair.*

  - *Violation of the foramen transversarium may result in vertebral artery rupture, dissection, pseudoaneurysm, or occlusion. Even without direct violation of the arterial wall, the screw threads can contact the artery with normal pulsatile flow and result in injury. If this is discovered intraoperatively or postoperatively, the screw should be surgically removed to decrease the risk of vertebral artery injury.*

  - *Intraoperative vertebral artery injury is the most serious complication, which can cause serious clinical sequela, including brainstem stroke. If this occurs, the screw should be removed immediately and the site should be packed with pieces of Gelfoam large enough not to be a source of emboli. Bone wax can also be used to help tamponade the bleeding. A direct microvascular repair by a vascular surgeon, after the surrounding bone is skeletonized, is also an option. Irrespective of the method used to tamponade the bleeding, a postoperative angiogram should be obtained to evaluate the integrity of the vertebral artery.*

dynamic lateral flexion and extension radiographs can be obtained at the end of the initial 10-week healing period to further assess atlantoaxial stability. If stability is obtained, the cervical collar can be weaned from use.

- Additionally, a CT scan can be obtained 6-9 months postoperatively to assess fusion and fracture healing.

Evidence

Harms J, Melcher R. Posterior C1-C2 fusion with polyaxial screw and rod fixation. Spine. 2001;26:2467-71.

Henriques T, Cunningham B, Olerud C, et al. Biomechanical comparison of five different atlantoaxial posterior fixation techniques. Spine. 2000;25:2877-83.

Jun BY. Anatomic study for ideal and safe posterior C1-C2 transarticular screw fixation. Spine. 1998;23:1703-7.

Madawi A, Solanki G, Casey AT, et al. Variation of the groove in the axis vertebra for the vertebral artery: implications for instrumentation. J Bone Joint Surg Br. 1997;79:820-3.

Magerl F, Seemann P-S. Stable posterior fusion of the atlas and axis by transarticular screw fixation. In Kehr P, Weidner A (eds). Cervical Spine I. New York: Springer-Verlag, 1986:322-7.

Naderi S, Crawford NR, Song GS, et al. Biomechanical comparison of C1-C2 posterior fixations: cable, graft, and screw combinations. Spine. 1998;23:1946-55; discussion 1955-6.

Tan M, Wang H, Wang Y, et al. Morphometric evaluation of screw fixation in atlas via posterior arch and lateral mass. Spine. 2003;28:888-95.

Young JP, Young PH, Ackermann MJ, et al. The ponticulus posticus: implications for screw insertion into the first cervical lateral mass. J Bone Joint Surg Am. 2005;87:2495-8.

Cervical Spine: Lateral Mass Screw Fixation

Kern Singh and Alexander R. Vaccaro

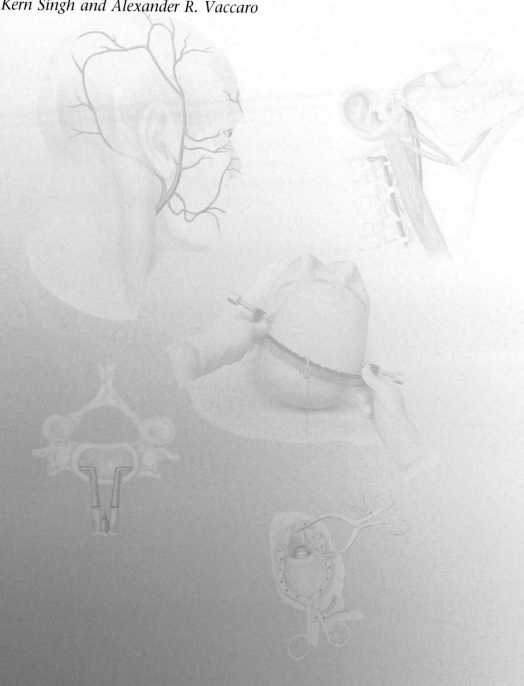

Controversies

- In severe osteopenia/osteoporosis, lateral mass fixation may be inadequate. It may be supplemented with posterior wiring if posterior elements are present and/or with pedicle screw fixation if the anatomy allows.

Treatment Options

- Posterior wiring
- Posterior hook fixation
- Posterior cervical pedicle screw fixation

Indications

- Acute and chronic instability
  - Posterior element fractures
  - Posterior ligamentous injuries
  - Post-laminectomy instability
- Destruction of bony anatomy secondary to neoplasm
- Stabilization after multisegment anterior decompression and fusion (long anterior fusions for tumor, infection, ankylosing spondylitis)
- Pseudarthrosis following anterior cervical fusion

Examination/Imaging

- Fine-cut (2-mm) computed tomography with two-dimensional reconstruction allows for assessment of the lateral mass quality in the lower cervical spine.
- T_2-weighted sagittal magnetic resonance imaging (Fig. 1).

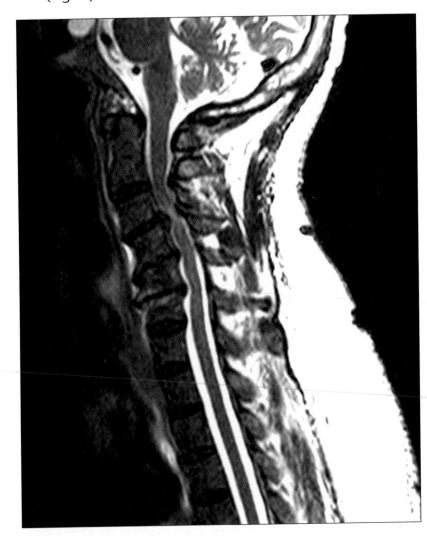

FIGURE 1

Surgical Anatomy (Fig. 2)

- Nerve root injury can occur if the screw trajectory is incorrect, if the screw penetration is too deep (bicortical screw purchase), or if there is significant past pointing of the drill.
- Vertebral artery injury is an exceedingly rare complication that may occur if the trajectory is medial and the screw penetration is too deep.
  - If brisk, pulsatile arterial bleeding is encountered from the drill hole, hemostasis should be obtained using bone wax, thrombogenic agents, and, potentially, placement of a screw in the hole. Postoperative angiography should be obtained to determine the status of the injured vertebral artery.

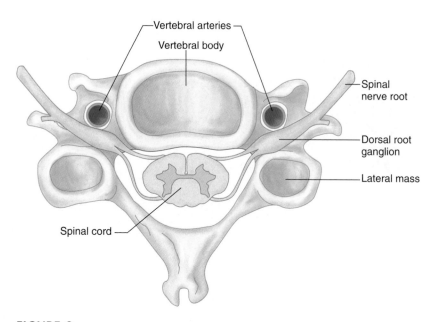

FIGURE 2

Equipment

- Mayfield tongs
- Lateral plain radiography to visualize cervical alignment

Controversies

- Placing instrumentation without appreciating cervical alignment may lead to loss of horizontal gaze, or the need for compensatory mechanisms to maintain horizontal gaze, in the postoperative period.

Positioning

- Mayfield tongs are applied, rigidly fixing the head to the table in the prone position (Figs. 3 and 4).
- The neck is slightly extended. If this may compromise spinal canal capacity to a detrimental degree, lordosis may be obtained following a decompression by having an unscrubbed assistant readjust the head holder to improve cervical lordosis.
- The arms and elbows are placed adjacent to the torso and are well padded to prevent pressure ulcers.
- The shoulders are pulled down by adhesive tape.
- The knees are flexed to prevent distal migration of the patient.

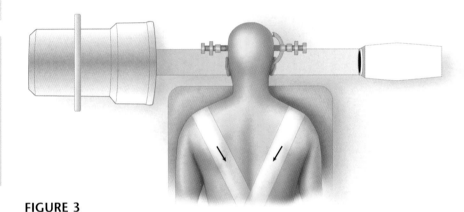

FIGURE 3

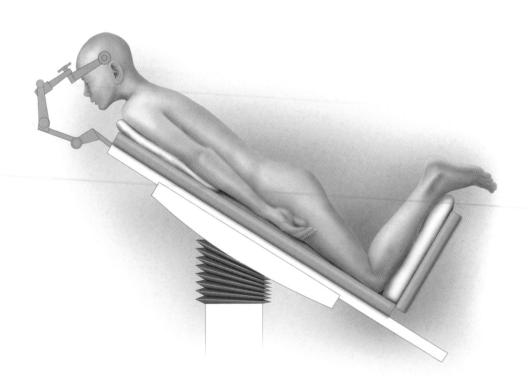

FIGURE 4

Instrumentation

• Bovie electrocautery
• Cobb elevator

Controversies

• The use of minimal incision portals may decrease postoperative neck discomfort and accelerate rehabilitation.

Portals/Exposures

■ A midline vertical skin incision can be made (as necessary) extending from the occipital protuberance past the spinous process of the seventh cervical vertebra (prominent vertebra).

■ The nuchal ligament is divided in the midline and incised as far as the tips of the spinous processes.

■ The deep muscle layer is stripped off the spinous processes close to the bone with the aid of electrocautery (Fig. 5).

■ Subperiosteral dissection is carried to the lateral boundary of the articular masses.

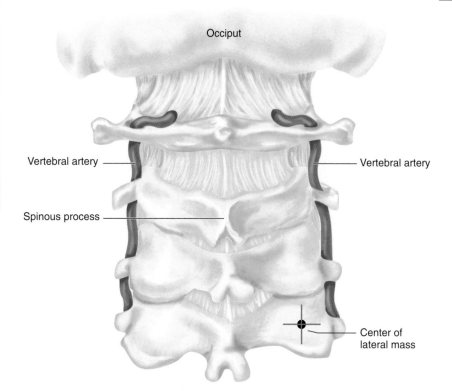

FIGURE 5

Instrumentation/ Implantation

• 2-mm round-tip burr, drill, or Kirschner wire

Controversies

• Roy-Camille technique may be used for screw entry point (Fig. 6B). The starting point for the screw insertion is located at the midpoint of the lateral mass. The screw is directed 10° lateral with no cranial-caudal inclination. This technique may lead to cephalad articular joint violation.

Procedure

STEP 1: DETERMINING THE ENTRY POINT

■ The entry point for screw insertion is located 1 mm medial to the midpoint of the lateral mass. The direction of the screw is 15° cephalad and 30° lateral for C3-6 (Fig. 6A).

STEP 2: DRILLING THE SCREW HOLE

■ Holes are drilled with a 2.4-mm drill bit using the drill guide.
■ The drill depth can be increased in 2-mm increments.
■ A depth gauge is used to confirm the appropriate screw length.

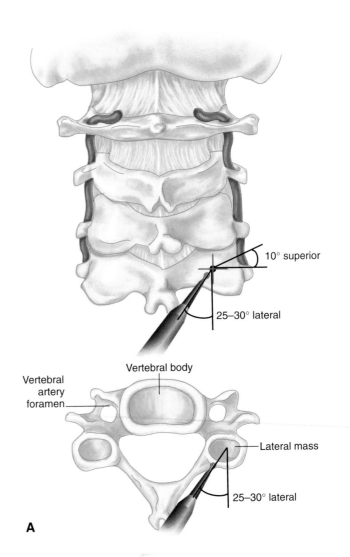

A

FIGURE 6A

PEARLS

- *To ensure optimal screw anchorage in the lateral masses, bicortical screw placement is recommended.*

- *To avoid nerve root iritation when performing bicortical screw placement, screw length should be selected 2 mm shorter than measured.*

PITFALLS

- *Past pointing of the drill may result in nerve root irritation.*

- *Improper drill trajectory may result in injury to the spinal cord or vertebral artery.*

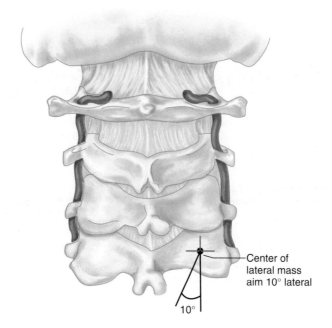

Center of lateral mass aim 10° lateral

10°

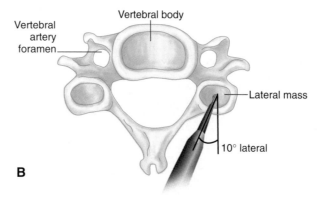

Vertebral body

Vertebral artery foramen

Lateral mass

10° lateral

B

FIGURE 6B   *Continued*

Instrumentation/ Implantation

- Tap
- Polyaxial screws

STEP 3: TAPPING AND SCREW INSERTION

- The tap size may equal the outer screw diameter or be slightly undersized. A self-tapping screw may avoid the need for an additional tapping step.
- An appropriate-sized screw is then placed in the same trajectory as the tap (Fig. 7).

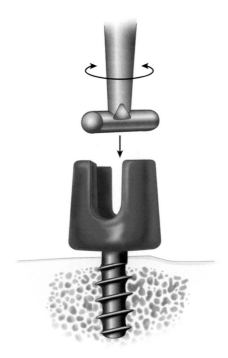

FIGURE 7

STEP 4: ROD INSERTION

- The determined length of rod is cut using the rod cutter (Fig. 8A) and bent utilizing the rod bender (Fig. 8B).
- Contouring of the rod is performed in gentle and multiple steps until the desired shape is achieved.

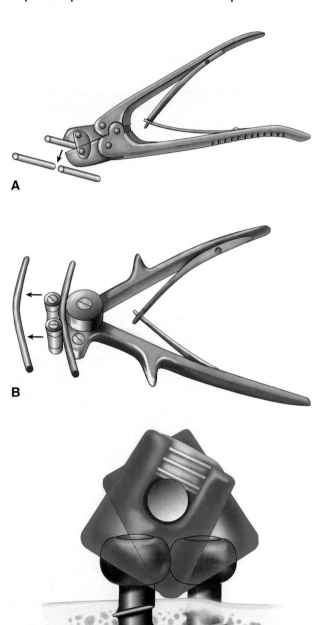

A

B

C

5mm

FIGURE 8A-C

Postoperative Care and Expected Outcomes

- Depending on the length and extent of the entire surgical procedure, the pathology, and bone quality, the required postoperative care may differ significantly (Fig. 9).
- Patients are routinely monitored in the hospital overnight.
- A soft collar orthosis may be used in the setting of short segment reconstructions in degenerative disease. A hard collar is routinely applied in the postoperative period for approximately 6 weeks in degenerative pathologies, depending on the degree of preoperative instability. Rigid external fixation with a halo-vest orthosis is rarely indicated except in severe osteoporosis, questionable compliance, neoplasms, and certain traumatic lesions.
- Deep or superficial wound infections should be addressed at an early stage. Extensive infections may require hardware removal and rigid external immobilization.

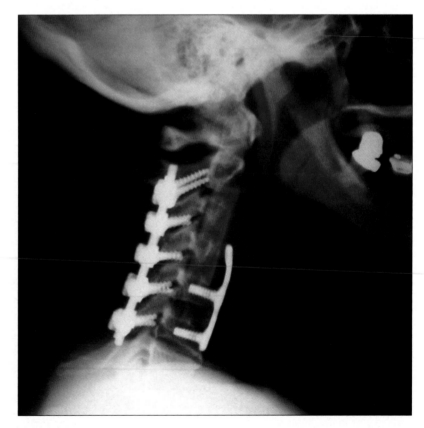

FIGURE 9

- Postoperative neurologic deterioration resulting from hardware malpositioning requires hardware revision or removal.
- Failure of bony fusion may result in instrumentation failure, necessitating hardware revision.

Evidence

Merrola AA, Castro BA, Alongi PR. Anatomic consideration for standard and modified techniques of cervical lateral mass screw placement. Spine J. 2002;2:430-5.

The study indicates that there are significant differences in potential neurovascular injury, which are dependent on the technique used for screw entry, the level instrumented, and the angle of screw trajectory in the parasagittal plane.

Xu R, Haman Sp, Ebraheim NA, Yeasting RA. The anatomic relation of lateral mass screws to the spinal nerves: a comparison of the Magerl, Anderson, and An techniques. Spine. 1999;24:2057-61.

The results of this study indicate that the potential risk of nerve root violation is higher with the Magerl and Anderson techniques than with the An technique.

Cervical Pedicle Screw Fixation

Moe R. Lim, Joon Y. Lee, and Kuniyoshi Abumi

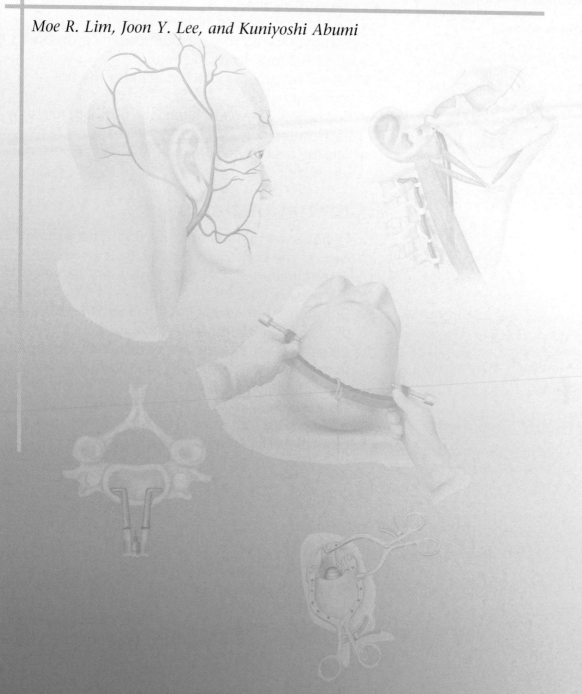

Controversies

- Controversial as a first-choice method of cervical fixation due to the risks of neurovascular complications with inaccurate screw placement

Treatment Options

- Lateral mass screw fixation in the subaxial cervical spine (C3-C6) when sufficient native bone stock permits
- Isthmus screw fixation for C2 when sufficient width of the isthmus permits

Indications

- Cervical instability (traumatic, iatrogenic, neoplastic, or inflammatory) with disruption or destruction of the posterior elements which precludes the use of standard fixation
- First-choice method of fixation for C7
- Congenitally narrow C2 isthmus which precludes use of C2 isthmus screw fixation
- Severe osteopenia which precludes the use of standard fixation
- Correction of cervical kyphosis (post-laminectomy or post-traumatic)
- Salvage fixation for previous anterior or posterior surgeries

Examination/Imaging

- Oblique view radiographs demonstrate an axial view of the contralateral pedicle, allowing the determination of the inner and outer diameters of the pedicle (Fig. 1).
- Computed tomography (CT) allows the assessment of pedicle morphometry, allowing the surgeon to determine appropriate screw diameter, length, and transverse plane trajectory. The normal axial view appearance of a subaxial cervical pedicle is shown in Figure 2A and contrasted with a congenitally narrow pedicle (Fig. 2B) which is insufficient to support a cervical pedicle screw.

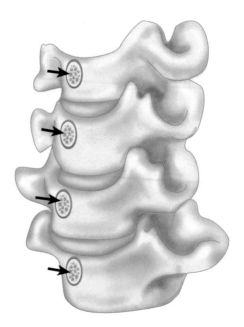

FIGURE 1

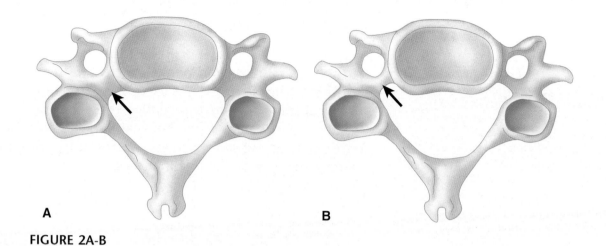

A   **B**

FIGURE 2A-B

- Preoperative CT angiography or magnetic resonance angiography (MRA) is necessary to determine the presence of a unilaterally dominant or anomalous vertebral artery. Figure 3A demonstrates asymmetry of the vertebral foramen on standard CT, suggestive of a right-sided dominant vertebral artery. The MRA (Fig. 3B) confirms the presence of a right-side dominant vertebral artery. If there is absence of a left sided vertebral artery or if it is non-functional than cervical pedicle screw fixation is contraindicated on the right side.

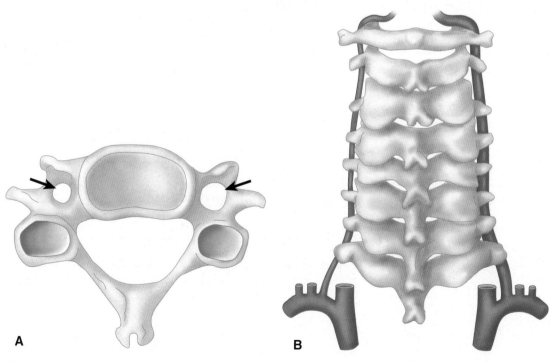

A   **B**

FIGURE 3A-B

Equipment

• Mayfield headholder

Surgical Anatomy

■ Knowledge of the relationship of the vertebral artery to the lateral mass and pedicle is crucial.
■ Figure 4 shows a posterior view of a dissected cervical spine specimen revealing the anatomic relationships between the cervical pedicles and the structures at risk during screw insertion: the vertebral artery, nerve roots, and spinal cord.

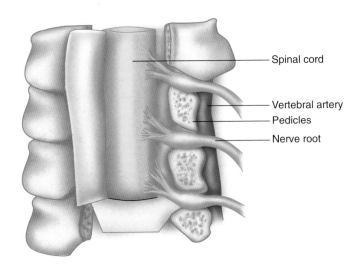

Spinal cord

Vertebral artery
Pedicles
Nerve root

FIGURE 4

Positioning

■ The patient is placed prone on a standard operating room table with two vertical laminectomy gel rolls and a Mayfield head holder (Fig. 5). The neck is positioned in the "sniffing" position with flexion of the upper cervical spine and extension of the subaxial segments.
■ The shoulders are taped down, the knees are flexed, and the feet are supported by pillows.
■ The table is brought into a slight reverse-Trendelenburg position.

Portals/Exposures

■ A standard posterior cervical exposure is performed to the most lateral aspect of the articular masses (Fig. 6).

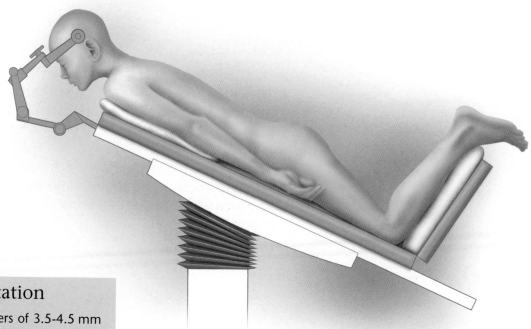

Instrumentation

- Screw diameters of 3.5-4.5 mm diameter are recommended, depending on pedicle size seen on preoperative imaging. Although 3.5 mm screws are adequate in most cases, larger 4.0 or 4.5 mm screws are recommended for the vertebrae with large pedicles to achieve maximal fixation.
- Screw lengths of 18-24 mm are recommended, depending on the anatomy of the specific pedicles seen on preoperative cross-sectional imaging studies.

PEARLS

- *A notch can be identified at the lateral margin of the C2 articular mass. For C2, the pedicle is approximately located just below the notch.*

- *The amount of medial angulation necessary in the transverse plane trajectory can be confirmed by using a Penfield 4 to palpate the medial aspect of the pedicle within the spinal canal.*

PITFALLS

- *A lateral or straight-ahead transverse plane trajectory places the vertebral artery at risk.*

FIGURE 5

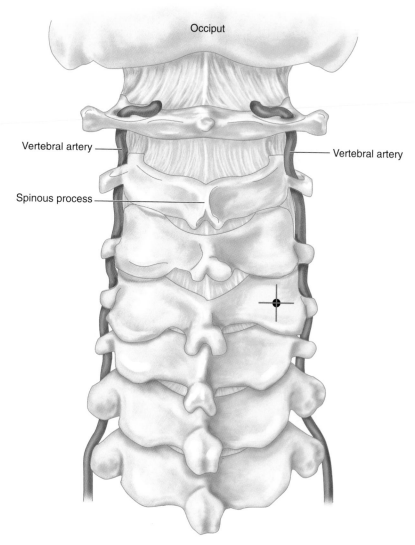

Occiput

Vertebral artery

Vertebral artery

Spinous process

FIGURE 6

Instrumentation/Implantation

- Constrained type screw-rod or -plate connections are necessary for short segment stabilization and for correction of deformities.

Procedure

STEP 1: C2 PEDICLE SCREW PLACEMENT

- The screw insertion point is on the cranial margin of the C2 lamina. The relationship of the vertebral artery to the screw trajectory must be considered (Fig. 7).
- The sagittal plane trajectory is determined by fluoroscopy or navigational guidance.
- The transverse plane trajectory is 15-25 degrees medial.

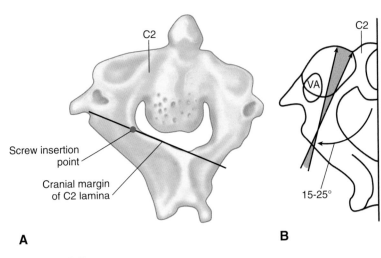

A

B

FIGURE 7A-B

Instrumentation/Implantion

• Constrained type screw-rod or -plate connections are necessary for short segment stabilization and for correction of deformities.

STEP 2: C3-7 PEDICLE SCREW PLACEMENT

■ For C3-7, the insertion point is slightly lateral to the center of the lateral mass and close to the inferior margin of the inferior articular facet of the cephalad segment (Fig. 8).

■ The sagittal plane trajectory is determined by fluoroscopy or navigational guidance

■ The transverse plane trajectory is 25-45 degrees medial.

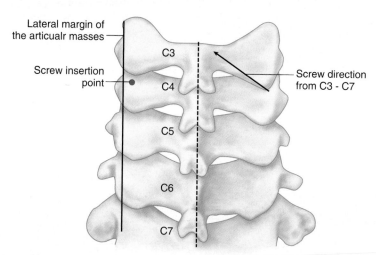

A

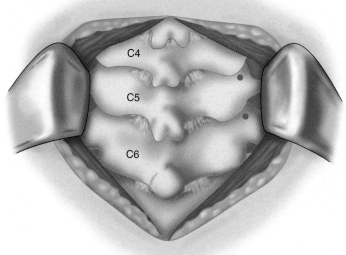

B

FIGURE 8A-B

PEARLS

- *The transverse plane trajectory is approximately perpendicular to the ipsilateral lamina.*

- *The sagittal plane trajectory can be determined by noting the angle formed by the C7 spinous process and the C7 upper endplates on a lateral radiograph. With clear view of the C7 spinous processes in the exposed spine, this sagittal plane angle can be recreated to approximate the sagittal plane trajectory of the pedicle.*

STEP 3: FREEHAND C7 PEDICLE SCREW PLACEMENT

- C7 pedicle screws can be placed safely without fluoroscopic/navigational guidance due to the absence of the vertebral artery at this level.
- A lateral radiograph is used to determine the angle between the upper endplate of C7 and the spinous process of C7 to approximate the sagittal plane trajectory (Fig. 9A).
- A C6-7 laminoforaminotomy is performed.
- The C7 pedicle is directly palpated to determine starting point and trajectory. The use of C2 isthmus screws and subaxial lateral mass screws circumvents the need for fluoroscopic guidance (Fig. 9B).

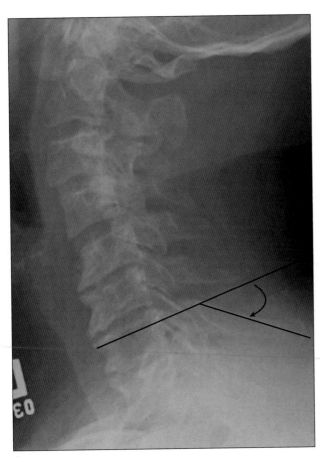
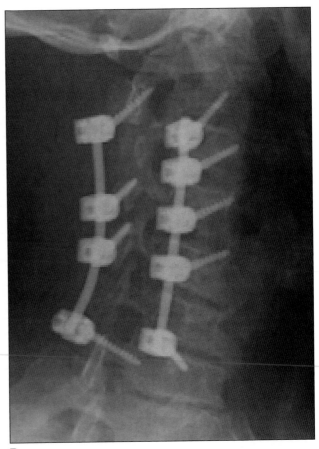

A **B**

FIGURE 9A-B

Step 4: Screw Insertion Technique

- The cortex at the point of insertion is penetrated with a high-speed burr.
- A small pedicle probe is used to cannulate the pedicle followed by tapping the tract.
- The screws are inserted with lateral fluoroscopic guidance to confirm direction and insertion depth (Fig. 10).

Postoperative Care and Expected Outcomes

- Routine post-operative care is recommended.
- If bone stock and screw purchase are sufficient, no external immobilization is necessary. Other wise, we recommend a hard cervical collar for 6 weeks.
- At 6 weeks, physical therapy is initiated to regain strength of the paravertebral musculature.

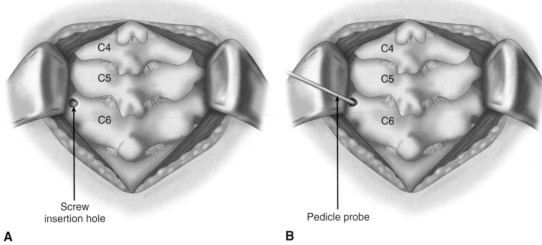

A — Screw insertion hole

B — Pedicle probe

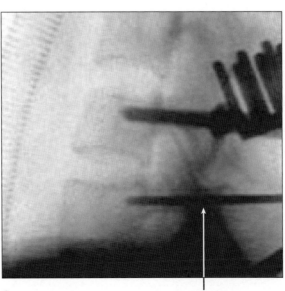

C — Pedicle probe

FIGURE 10A-C

Evidence

Abumi K, Shono Y, Ito M, Taneichi H, Kotani Y, Kaneda K. Complications of pedicle screw fixation in reconstructive surgery of the cervical spine. Spine. 2000;25:962-9.

In this retrospective study of 180 patients and 712 screws, the authors found on CT that 6.7% of the screws breached the pedicles. Only 4% of these breaches caused radiculopathy. The vertebral artery was injured in 1 patient. Bleeding was stopped with bone wax, and no neurologic compromise resulted.

Johnston T, Lautenschlager E, Marcu D, Karaikovic E. Cervical pedicle screws vs. lateral mass screws: a flexion-extension fatigue analysis. Poster #45. Presented at the Meeting of the Cervical Spine Research Society, San Diego, December 2005.

In this cadaveric study, the authors found a lower rate of loosening and higher strength after fatigue testing in subaxial cervical screws compared to lateral mass screws.

Neo M, Sakamoto T, Fujibayashi S, Nakamura T. The clinical risk of vertebral artery injury from cervical pedicle screws inserted in degenerative vertebrae. Spine. 2005;30:2800-5.

In this retrospective study of 18 patients and 86 screws, the authors found a 29% rate of cortical breach. In five of the nine patients in whom the screws critically violated the transverse foramen, CT angiography showed continuity of the vertebral artery in all cases.

Rhee JM, Kraiwattanapong C, Hutton WC. A comparison of pedicle and lateral mass screw contruct stiffnesses at the cervicothoracic junction: a biomechanical study. Spine. 2005;30:e636-40.

In this cadaveric study, the authors found that C7 pedicle screw fixation provides the greatest normalized stiffness for fixation of the cerviothoracic junction. To achieve a similar degree of stiffness using lateral mass screws, an additional level of fixation into C6 was necessary.

Posterior Cervical Osteotomy Techniques

Neel Anand and Brian Perri

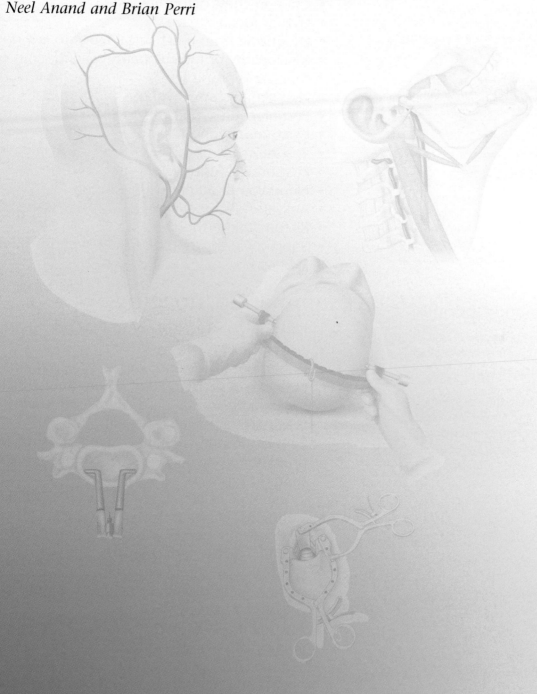

Treatment Options

- Pedicle Subtraction Osteotomy (PSO)—single, posterior-only approach and focal deformity correction
- Combined anterior-posterior deformity correction—facet osteotomies combined with one or more anterior cervical diskectomies and fusions

Indications

- Mid- or upper cervical kyphosis; may have normal C7 plumb line over sacrum
- Cervical-thoracic kyphotic deformity
  - Degenerative sagittal plane deformity pain
  - Chin-on-chest deformity
  - Loss of forward gaze
  - Dysphagia from mechanical block to jaw opening
  - Myelopathy or radiculopathy secondary to cervical-thoracic kyphosis
  - Post-laminectomy kyphosis
  - Postinfection kyphosis
  - Posttumor kyphosis
  - Posttrauma kyphosis
  - Postsurgical fusion kyphosis
  - Nonunion of anterior spine fusion
  - Ankylosing spondylitis
  - Rheumatoid arthritis
  - Supra-adjacent thoracic fusion kyphosis (junctional kyphosis)

Examination/Imaging

- Full-length scoliosis anteroposterior (AP) and lateral radiographs
  - Chin-brow to vertebral angle is measured to calculate desired angle of deformity correction to obtain a horizontal gaze. Undercorrection is better tolerated than overcorrection.
  - To measure the C7 plumb line, if anterior to sacral promatory, you may need to address lumbar or thoracic kyphosis.
- Cervical AP and lateral neutral, flexion, and extention radiographs
  - To localize region of kyphosis (cervical thoracic junction versus midcervical).
  - Dynamic views help determine intervertebral motion (i.e., movement between spinous processes).
  - AP radiograph is used to assess for coronal imbalance.
- Magneric resonance imaging (MRI) is used to to delineate cord compression and course of vertebral artery (verify entry into transverse foramen of C6 versus anomalous C7 entry point; rule out commonly encountered aberrant course if instrumenting C2 pedicle)

- Computed tomography (CT)
  - To provide detailed anatomic relationships and measurements of cervical and thoracic vertebral anatomy (pedicles, location of vertebral arteries, registration for intraoperative navigation if used)
  - To identify ossification of the posterior longitudinal ligament

Surgical Anatomy

- PSO bone resection includes bilateral lamina, facets, and pedicles with wedge resection of anterior verterbral body (Fig. 1).

Equipment

- Intraoperative somatosensory evoked potentials and continuous electromyography are used to monitor cord and nerve root function, with special attention given at the time of deformity correction.
- Cell-saver is used to salvage blood loss from the osteotomy.
- Minimize use of bone wax during vertebral osteotomy as this may interfere with bone fusion.
- Use thrombin-soaked Gelfoam and cotton pledgets to control bleeding.

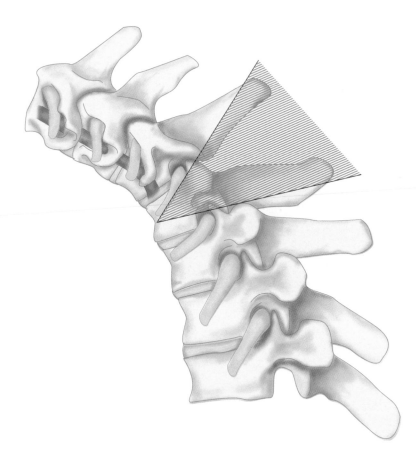

FIGURE 1

- Bony apposition of the posterior elements occurs once the osteotomy is closed. Two nerve roots will exit one foraminal opening (C7 and C8 if the PSO is at C7; C8 and T1 if the PSO is at T1) (Fig. 2).

Positioning

- The patient is positioned in prone with a Mayfield headholder.

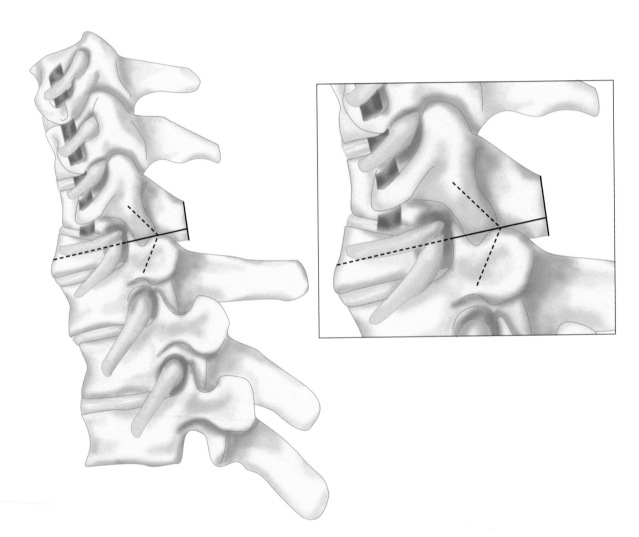

FIGURE 2

Portals/Exposures

■ PSO at C7 or T1—major correction at single level
■ Multiple Smith-Petersen osteotomies—any spine level(s)

Procedure

STEP 1

■ A midline incision is made for the approach from C2 (or C3 if there is good bone quality, dysplastic C2 pedicles, or an anomalous vertebral artery) to T2 (or T3 if the PSO is performed at T1).
■ For a C7 PSO, place polyaxial facet screws from C3 to C6 and polyaxial pedicle screws at C2, T1, and T2
■ For a T1 PSO, place polyaxial facet screws from C3 to C7 and polyaxial pedicle screws at C2, T2, and T3.
■ The PSO level is not instrumented.

STEP 2

■ Bilateral laminectomy and facetectomy is completed at the PSO level, exposing the dura and bilateral nerve roots.
■ Bilateral laminectomy is completed two levels above and two levels below the PSO level. This provides room for the spinal cord shortening after the deformity correction without experiencing compression from posterior bony elements.
■ Bilateral pedicles at the PSO level are sounded and drilled down to the vertebral body. In Figure 3,

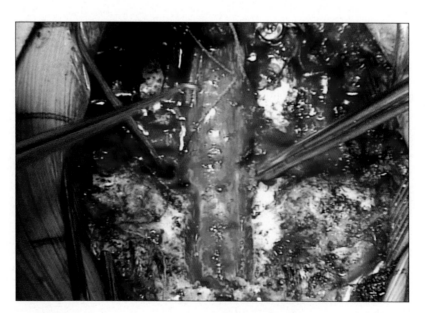

FIGURE 3

bilateral laminectomies have been completed at the PSO level, and two levels above and below. Bilateral C7 and T1 facet joints have been resected for this T1 PSO. The pedicles are drilled bilaterally and the cortical margins are then removed.

- Cortical margins are resected with a combination of thin-lipped rongeur, pituitary rongeur, and curettes.
- A V-shaped wedge of cancellous bone is resected from the vertebral body with a pituitary rongeur and straight and curved curettes. Resection of cancellous bone should be carried out to the anterior cortex. Straight and curved curettes are carried down through the pedicles and into the vertebral body (Fig. 4). The cancellous osteotomy is carefully performed, staying within the margins of the vertebral body. Fluoroscopy is used to verify that the depth of the osteotomy is carried to the cortical margins of the vertebrae.
- A temporary malleable rod is attached to the pedicle screws to prevent anterior translation or sudden movement of the spinal cord before the posterior vertebral cortex is resected.

PEARLS

- *Remove the posterior vertebral cortical bone to complete the osteotomy. Resection of this bone bridge, just ventral to the dural sac, is the last step of the vertebral body osteotomy. This segment of bone maintains an open posterior vertebral window for completion of the vertebral wedge osteotomy. Once the posterior cortex is broken, the posterior vertebral body closes down and access to the vertebral body is decreased.*

- *Lateral intraoperative fluoroscopy is used to verify the depth of the vertebral osteotomy. Sequential images can be taken as the instruments employed for osteotomy are advanced anteriorly. A small curette can be placed anteriorly within the apex of the V-shaped osteotomy and imaged to verify depth, for example.*

- *Asymmetric osteotomy may be performed to correct for both sagittal and coronal deformity.*

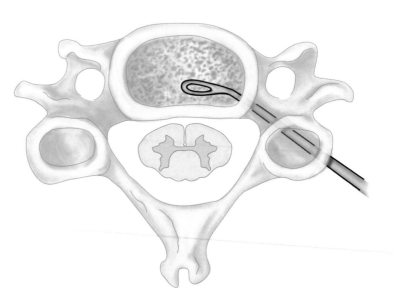

FIGURE 4

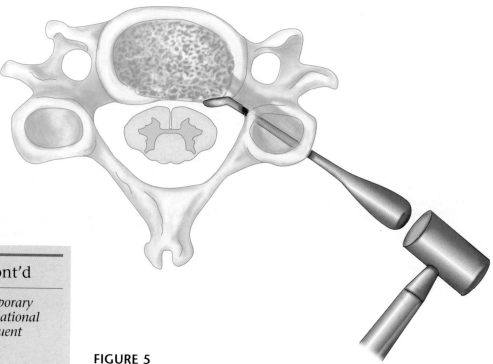

FIGURE 5

Instrumentation/ Implantion

- Midas Rex high-speed drill with an M8, side-cutting drill bit
- Kerrison rongeurs (2 mm, 3 mm)
- Straight and curved curettes
- Pituitary rongeur
- Down-pushing (Epstein) curettes
- Bone wax, Floseal, and thrombin-soaked Gelfoam for hemostatic control

■ Down-pushing Epstein curettes are used to depress the posterior and lateral vertebral cortices into the void of the vertebral body (Fig. 5). This should be performed bilaterally and as the last step in the osteotomy. Following this step, the posterior osteotomy wedge will close down and access to the osteotomy region is limited. A unilateral, temporary, malleable rod should be in place prior to performing this step. This rod will prevent complete collapse of the osteotomy.

Step 3

- The osteotomy is closed by releasing the Mayfield clamps, followed by controlled, manual elevation of the Mayfield headholder, then reclamping of the headholder. Watch the thecal sac and nerve roots to avoid compression injury.
- Obtain a lateral radiograph to check sagittal alignment.
- An appropriately contoured rod is fixed to the pedicle/lateral mass screws on the side opposite the malleable temporary rod.
- The malleable rod is removed and a second contoured rod is attached.
- Further reduction and compression across the osteotomy site is performed with the compression instrumentation (Fig. 6). An infolding of the dura occurs following reduction of the kyphotic deformity.
- Cross-linked attachments can be used to increase stability of fixation.

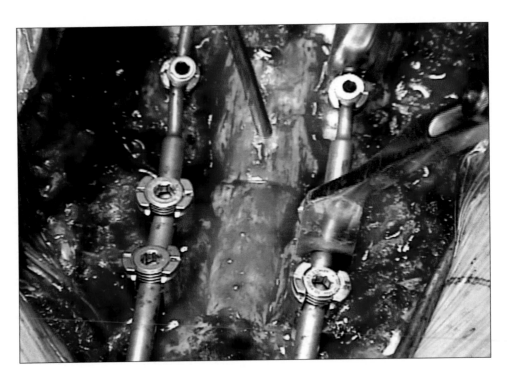

FIGURE 6

Postoperative Care and Expected Outcomes

- A closing-wedge osteotomy creates cervical lordosis.
- Posterior elements are removed at the level of the osteotomy, and laminectomies two levels above and below are performed.
- Bony apposition of anterior, middle, and posterior columns is established.
- Posterior instrumentation stabilizes the spine and maintains compression across the osteotomy site to increase fusion rate and success. A postoperative halo may be used if the patient is osteoporotic.
- Postoperatively, the spinal column is shortened.
- The fulcrum for PSO is the anterior column, so there is less risk for spinal cord injury versus a Smith-Petersen osteotomy, in which the fulcrum is the middle column.

Evidence

Mummaneni PV, Mummaneni VP, Haid RW, Rodts GE, Sasso RC. Cervical osteotomy for the correction of chin-on-chest deformity in ankylosing spondylitis. Neurosurg Focus. 2003;14(1):Article 9.

Webb JK, Sengupta DK. Posterior cervicothoracic osteotomy. In Vaccaro AR, Albert TJ (eds). Spine Surgery: Tricks of the Trade. New York: Thieme, 2003:35-7.

Cervical Laminoplasty

Christopher Brown, Jason E. Lowenstein, and S. Tim Yoon

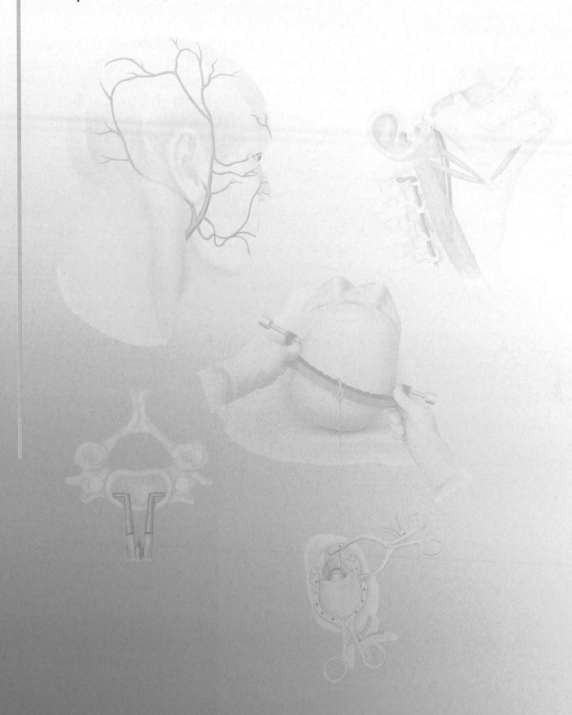

Treatment Options

- **Anterior cervical diskectomy and fusion:** This option is advantageous in the patient with one or two levels of cord compression related to disk degeneration or herniation that causes focal areas of canal narrowing.
- **Anterior corpectomy and fusion:** Patients with cervical spondylosis affecting multiple levels (three or more) or who have retrovertebral compression are candidates for this procedure (especially with overall cervical kyphosis).
- **Laminectomy and fusion:** Patients with multilevel compression and axial neck pain from facet arthrosis are good candidates for this treatment option.
- **Laminoplasty:** This is a motion-preserving procedure (nonfusion) that can be used to treat cord compression at multiple levels. While the procedure usually involves dorsal decompression from C3 to C7, by allowing dorsal cord expansion and drift, it can be used for ventral cord compression lesions such as OPLL.

Differential Diagnosis

- Cervical spondylosis is the predominant cause of cervical myelopathy in patients over the age of 55. With disk degeneration, the height of the disk decreases, leading to bulging of the anulus that narrows the spinal canal. Loss of disk height causes overriding of the uncovertebral joints, leading to osteophyte formation that can further contribute to stenosis of the spinal canal or neural foramen. The overall spinal column shortens, which leads to redundancy and thickening of the ligamentum flavum, which can cause compression of the dorsal aspect of the spinal canal.
- Soft disk herniations can cause both radiculopathy and myelopathy based on the location of herniation, either posterolateral or directly posterior, respectively.
- Infectious diskitis, if left untreated, can lead to an epidural abscess that can cause cord compression leading to myelopathy.
- Loss of normal sagittal alignment can cause compression by stretching the cord over a kyphotic segment.
- Neurogenic disorders (multiple sclerosis, amyotrophic lateral sclerosis, syringomyelia, cerebellar disorders) may mimic symptoms of myelopathy.
- Instability of the cervical spine can cause myelopathic symptoms. Generalized ligamentous laxity as seen in Down syndrome or rheumatoid arthritis can lead to instability and cord compression. Traumatic injuries to the bony or ligamentous stabilizers of the cervical spine can result in progressive deformity and myelopathy.
- Ossification the posterior longitudinal ligament (OPLL) can lead to direct compression of the cord. OPLL is the most common cause of multisegment stenosis in Japan and is found in lower frequency in Western societies. Ossification of the ligament initially occurs at the end plates and then extends throughout the ligament. OPLL can be classified as segmental, continuous, or mixed based on its pattern of ossification (Figs. 1 and 2).

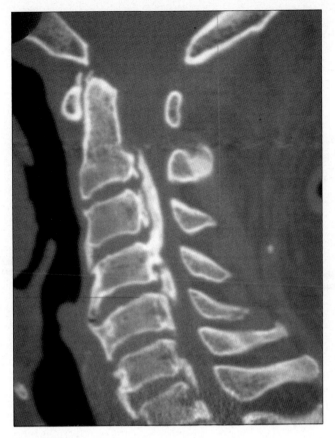

FIGURE 1

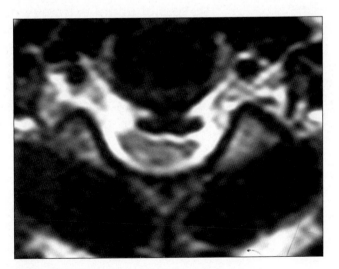

FIGURE 2

Indications

- Cervical spondylitic myelopathy, involving three or more disk levels (Fig. 3)
- Ossification of posterior longitudinal ligament (Fig. 4)
- Congenital/developmental stenosis of the spinal canal
- Spinal cord tumor

Examination/Imaging

PHYSICAL EXAMINATION

- Symptoms of myelopathy
  - The history of the patient's symptoms is often the most important aspect in evaluating a patient with critical spinal cord compression. Pain is often not a significant complaint in myelopathic patients unless there is associated root compression or facet arthrosis. Typical complaints involve disturbance of gait, balance, or manual dexterity. Gait problems are related to balance problems causing clumsiness or frequent falls. Patients may describe an unsteady gait that has necessitated the need for assistive devices such as a cane or walker.
  - Myelopathic patients often complain of hand numbness and sometimes volunteer a history of Lhermitte's sign. Other complaints are related to loss of upper extremity dexterity. Complaints related to changes in their handwriting, grasping small items, buttoning clothing, and manipulating small objects are common.
  - Bowel and bladder problems are usually late complaints and indicate severe, prolonged compression that may not improve with operative treatment.
- Signs of myelopathy
  - The physical examination begins with careful observation of the patient's gait. A broad-based, shuffling gait can be highly suggestive. Patients may be unable to perform a heel-toe walk or have very poor balance while performing toe rises.
  - Hyperactive reflexes, clonus, and a positive Babinski's sign are all signs of upper motor neuron compression. Patients with concomitant polyneuropathy or peripheral nerve or root entrapment (severe diabetes or multilevel stenosis) may not have these reflexes.

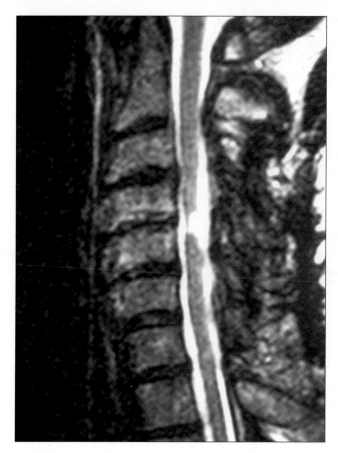

FIGURE 3

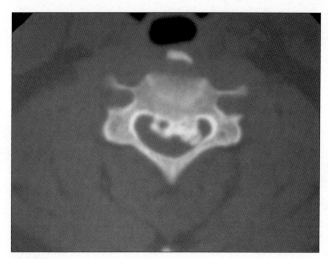

FIGURE 4

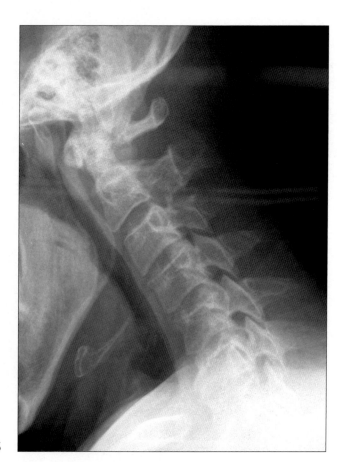

FIGURE 5

- Pathologic reflexes may be present based on the level of compression. The scapulohumeral reflex is present with compression above the C3 level. The inverted radial reflex is present with compression at the C5-6 level. Hoffmann's reflex also indicates spinal cord compression, but can be positive in normal individuals.
- Patients may have intrinsic atrophy of the hand that is most evident in the first dorsal interosseous muscle compartment.

IMAGING

- Anteroposterior and lateral flexion/extension radiographs provide information about the sagittal alignment of the cervical spine, amount of motion, and relative spondylosis.
- Magnetic resonance imaging shows the amount of compression as well as any signal changes within the cord.
- Computed tomography with and without contrast shows the bony anatomy in great detail. It is the study of choice for evaluating OPLL (Fig. 6) and aids in preoperative planning if instrumentation is to be used.

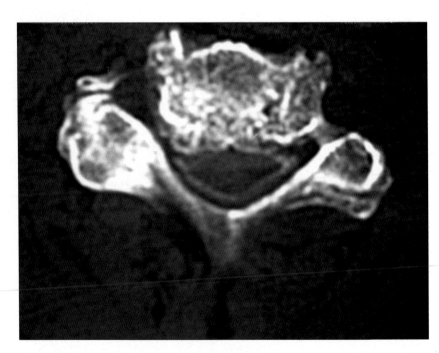

FIGURE 6

Positioning

- Intubation is done with special precautions in the setting of spinal cord compression. The exact technique can be tailored to fit the situation and can involve care in not extending the neck more than what was comfortable for the patient in active range of motion prior to sedation or fiberoptic assistance.
- A Mayfield headholder (Fig. 7) is applied to the skull to reduce risk to soft tissues and provide the most stable fixation of the head to the operative table.
- The patient is placed in the prone position with chest bolsters that allow the abdomen to be free.
- The bed is placed in reverse Trendelenburg position to place the cervical spine in a more horizontal position and to decrease venous bleeding.

Portals/Exposures

- A posterior longitudinal incision from C2 to T1 with a midline approach to the spinous processes is performed.
- A subperiosteal dissection is performed to expose the C3 to C7 lamina extending out to the middle of the lateral masses.
- The extensor muscle attachment to the C2 spinous process is carefully preserved. The inferior surface of the C2 lamina is usually broad and should be exposed to aid in visualization of the C3 lateral mass.

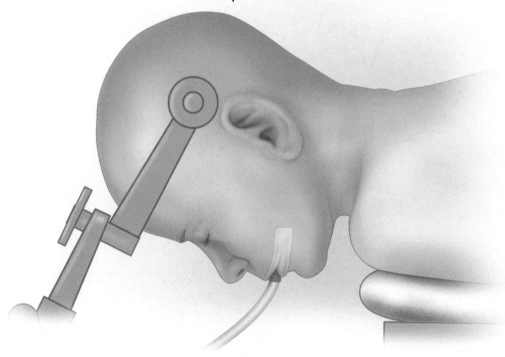

FIGURE 7

Procedure

STEP 1. TROUGH PREPARATION

- The spinous processes are amputated (Fig. 8). This aids in exposure, reduces the displacement of posterior musculature, and can provide bone graft to keep the lamina open.
- The trough location is identified at the junction of the lamina and lateral mass (Fig. 9).
- A low-aggression 4-mm high-speed burr is used to form the trough (Figs. 10 and 11).
- For the opening side, three layers of bone are removed, the outer and inner cortices and inner cancellous region.
- Troughs are made no deeper than the 4-mm diameter of the burr. After descending to that depth, the burr should be directed medially.
- At the caudal end of the lamina, the ligamentum flavum provides a protective barrier. However, this is not the case at the cranial end of the lamina,

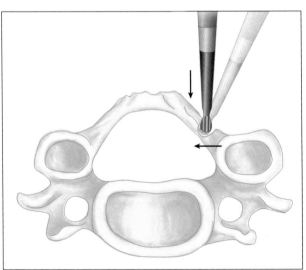

FIGURE 9

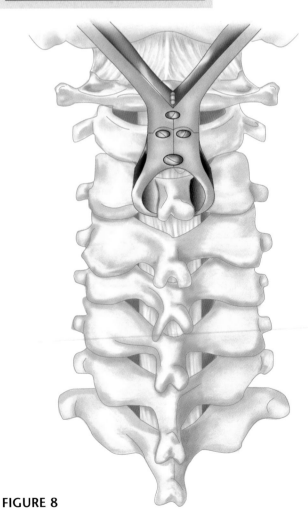

FIGURE 8

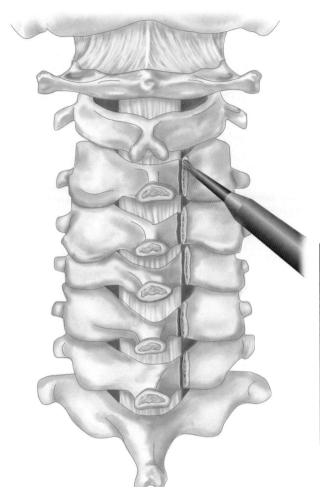

FIGURE 10

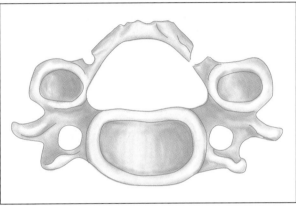

FIGURE 11

where the surgeon may choose to switch to a 3-mm diamond burr to remove the inner cortex and avoid causing brisk epidural bleeding.

- As the bone is thinned, the surgeon should use a delicate instrument such as a microcurette or Penfield elevator to identify any bone bridges still attaching the lamina to the lateral masses. The attachments can then be removed with a microcurette or 1-mm Kerrison punch.
- Care should be used at this time to avoid creating significant epidural bleeding.
- The hinge side is prepared opposite the opening side at the same anatomic junction of the lamina and lateral mass. It entails removal of the outer cortex and cancellous layer, leaving the inner cortex intact. This provides a pliable yet firm hinge that yields to moderate pressure without breaking the inner cortex (Figs. 12 and 13).

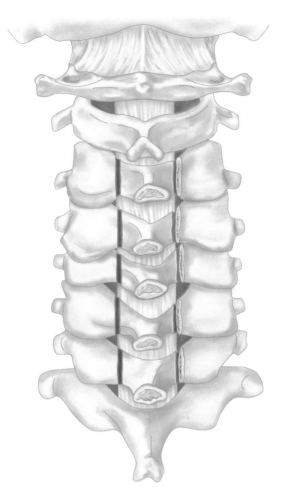

FIGURE 12

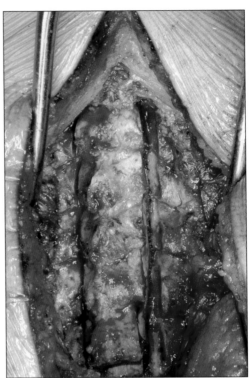

FIGURE 13

STEP 2. OPENING THE LAMINOPLASTY

■ The ligamentum flavum is released at both the C2-3 and C7-T1 interspaces after removal of the spinous process (Fig. 14). Commonly this step is performed prior to trough preparation as this step can weaken the hinge, but it can also be performed in the reverse order. Some surgeons prefer not to release the ligamentum flavum in this location to give further stability to the hinged bone once opened.

■ Proceeding from caudal to cranial, a nerve hook or curved curette is used to elevate the lamina on the opening side (Fig. 15).

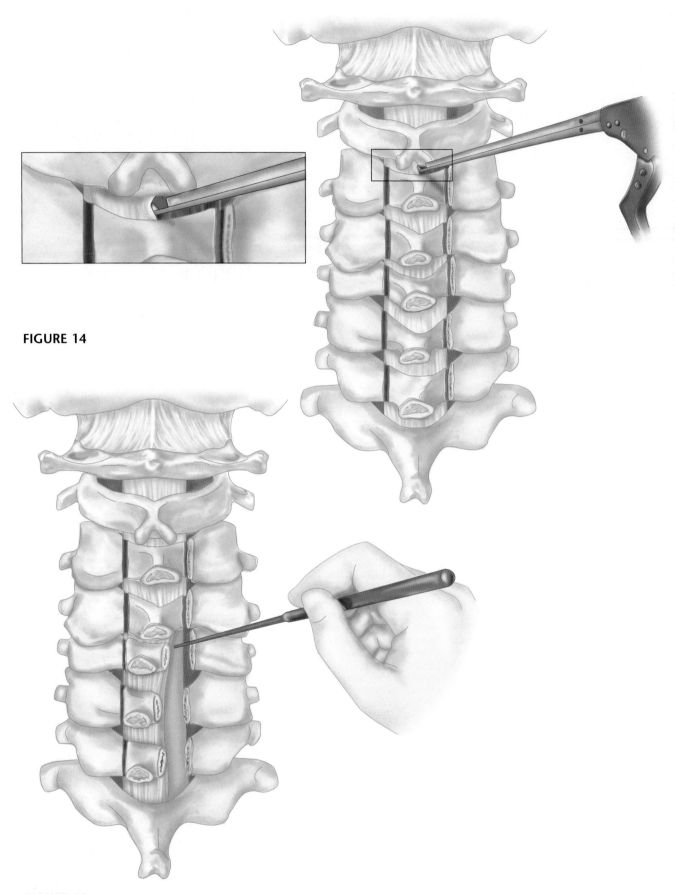

FIGURE 14

FIGURE 15

- Bipolar forceps are used for cauterization of epidural veins. A Kerrison punch can be used to divide ligamentous and facet capsule attachments (Figs. 16 and 17).

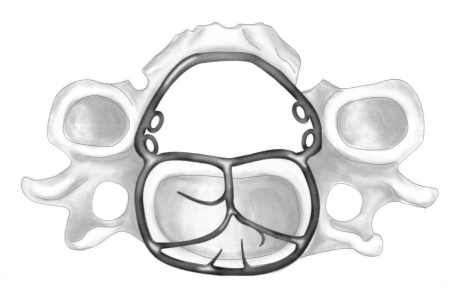

FIGURE 16

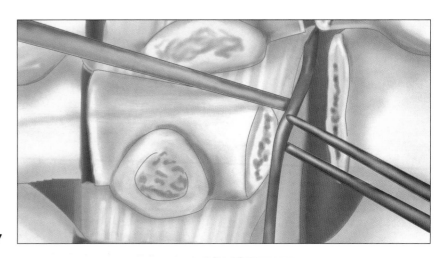

FIGURE 17

STEP 3. POSTERIOR ARCH RECONSTRUCTION

- The laminoplasty door is held open using a variety of techniques.
  - Autogenous spinous processes can be used. C6 and C7 are usually suitable (Fig. 18)
  - Allograft (rib) or machined cortical graft (Figs. 19, 20, and 21) can be more convenient to use than autograft spinous processes

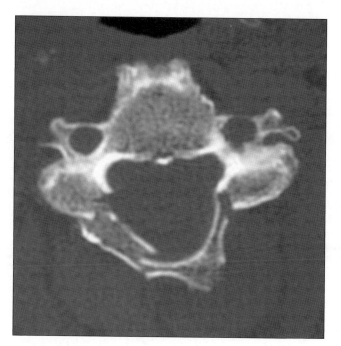

FIGURE 18

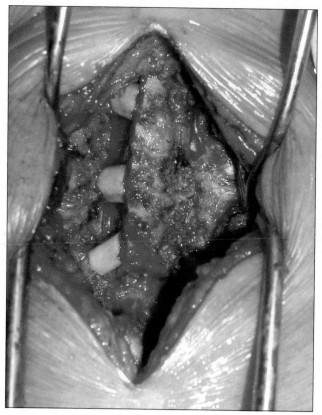

FIGURE 19

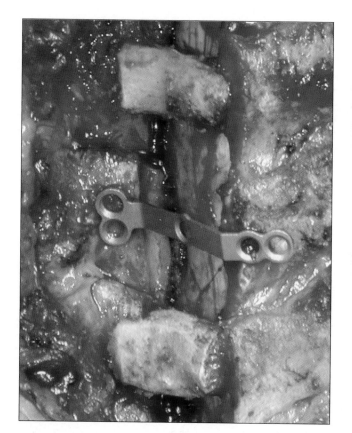

FIGURE 20

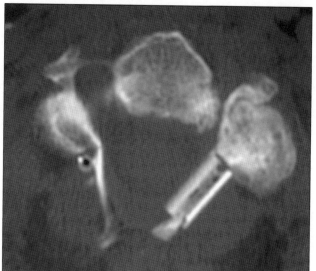

FIGURE 21

- Tethering (suture, arthroscopic anchor)
- Rigid internal fixation (open-door plates) (Figs. 22, 23, 24, 25, and 26)
■ The hinge side undergoes bony healing that permanently holds the posterior arch open.

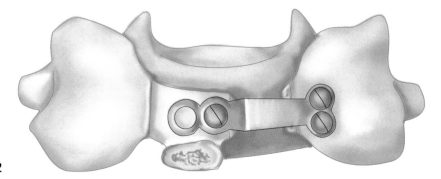

FIGURE 22

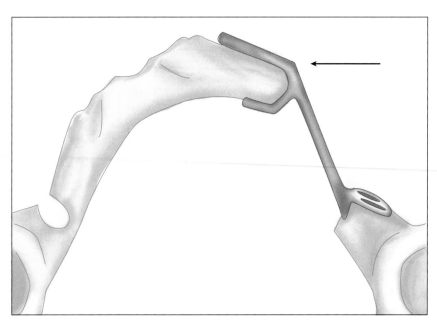

FIGURE 23

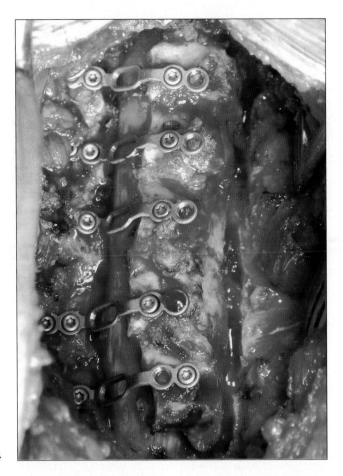

FIGURE 24

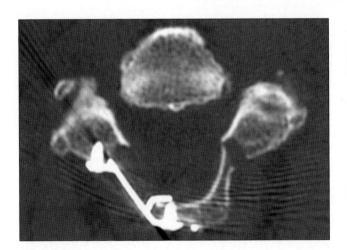

FIGURE 25

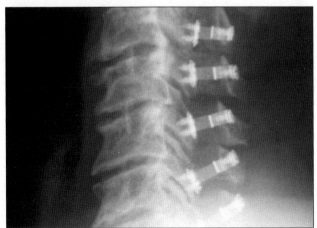

FIGURE 26

STEP 4. FRENCH DOOR LAMINOPLASTY

- French door laminoplasty is an alternative technique to the open-door procedure described previously.
- This entails a midline spinous process and lamina division using a low-aggression burr.
- Bilateral hinges are made at the junction of the lamina and facet (Fig. 27).
- The French doors are then held open.
- Sutured bone graft is employed.
- Rigid internal fixation is achieved with a plate (Figs. 28 and 29).

STEP 5. WOUND CLOSURE

- A deep drain is placed.
- Layered fascial and subcutaneous closure is performed with a subcuticular skin closure.

Postoperative Care and Expected Outcomes

- A soft cervical collar is worn for comfort.
- Immediate active range of motion is encouraged.
- Drain output is monitored, and the drain is usually removed 24-48 hours postoperatively.
- The patient is weaned from the cervical collar over 2-4 weeks.

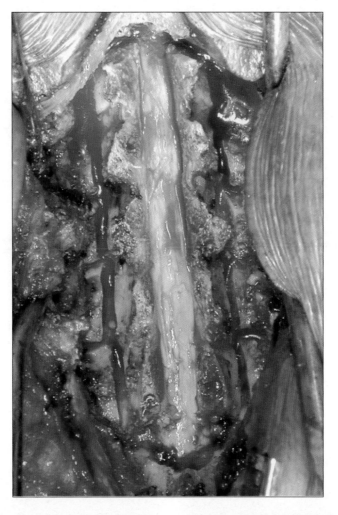

FIGURE 27

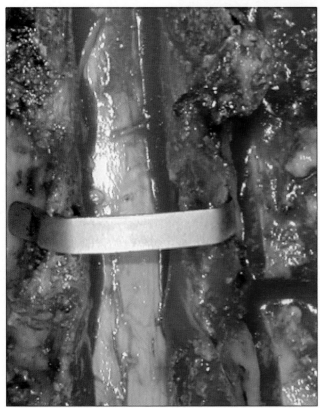

FIGURE 28

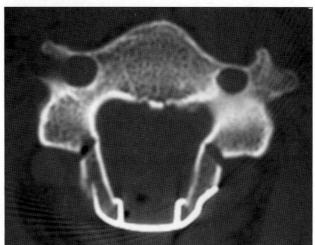

FIGURE 29

Evidence

Edwards CC 2nd, Heller JG, Murakami H. Corpectomy versus laminoplasty for multilevel cervical myelopathy: an independent matched-cohort analysis. Spine. 2002;27:1168-75.

Emery SE, Bohlman HH, Bolesta MJ, Jones PK. Anterior cervical decompression and arthrodesis for the treatment of cervical spondylotic myelopathy: two to seventeen-year follow-up. J Bone Joint Surg Am. 1998;80:941-51.

Geck MJ, Eismont FJ. Surgical options for the treatment of cervical spondylotic myelopathy. Orthop Clin North Am. 2002;33:329-48.

Hosono N, Yonenobu K, Ono K. Neck and shoulder pain after laminoplasty: a noticeable complication. Spine. 1996;21:1969-73.

Yonenobu K, Hosono N, Iwasaki M, Asano M, Ono K. Laminoplasty versus subtotal corpectomy: a comparative study of results in multisegmental cervical spondylotic myelopathy. Spine. 1992;17:1281-4.

THORACIC SPINE

Anterior Thoracic Diskectomy and Corpectomy

Kyle Fox, Max C. Lee, and Daniel H. Kim

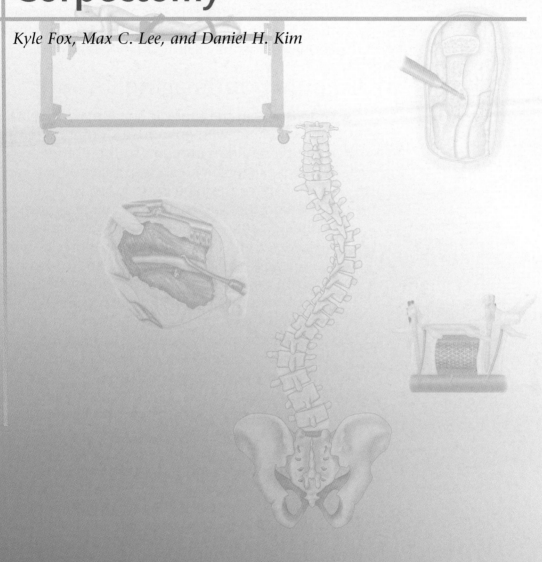

Controversies

- An alternative to an open thoracic discectomy is the thoracoscopic approach because of the potential advantages of less soft tissue disruption and pulmonary dysfunction. However, certain limitations exist with thorocoscopy such as lack of training, lack of equipment, or the unique complications related to the thoracoscopic approach.
- Relative contraindications to thoracoscopic spine surgery may also be present, which include extensive adhesions, emphysema, restricted cardiopulmonary function, prior chest trauma, or prior thoracotomy. These relative contraindications may prevent safe collapse of the ipsilateral lung.

Treatment Options

- Thoracic laminectomy
- Transpedicular approaches
- Costotransversectomy
- Lateral extracavitary approach
- Thoracoscopic approaches
- Thoracotomy

Indications

- Spinal cord compression
- Progressive spinal deformity
- Mechanical instability from tumor, trauma, or infection
- Thoracic corpectomy may be necessary for the treatment of vertebral osteomyelitis, metastatic tumors of the vertebrae, vertebral body fractures, and large, densely calcified herniated disks.

Examination/Imaging

- Lesions within the thoracic spine may present with subtle findings with an insidious onset. Often pain is the presenting symptom, so the history and physical examination can help rule out any cardiac or pulmonary causes requiring further work-up.
  - "Benign thoracic pain" is known as thoracic disk disease causing mid-dorsal or unilateral chest pain. However, disease involving the thoracic spine can also cause chest pain, thoracic and/or lumbar region pain, pain wrapping around the trunk, lower extremity pain, and groin pain.
  - Patients presenting with only pain can often experience a delay in diagnosis until the signs and symptoms of myelopathy develop, such as sensory impairment, including dysesthesia, paresthesias, or complete sensory loss; bladder dysfunction, such as urgency, frequency, and/or incontinence; spasticity; hyperreflexia; and lower extremity paresis.
- Following a thorough history and neurologic examination, neuroradiologic evaluation then ensues.
  - Magnetic resonance imaging (MRI) often adequately demonstrates herniated disks, nerve root compression, cord compression, tumors, and infection.
  - Computerized tomography (CT) scans can confirm MRI findings of a soft versus hard disk, neuroforaminal compromise, central canal compromise, and further evaluation of the bony anatomy should instrumentation be considered.
  - If further evaluation is still needed or MRI is contraindicated, a CT myelogram may be performed.
- Further preoperative work-up may include somatosensory evoked potentials (SSEPs) and electromyographic studies. These tests provide a

baseline for the significance of cord compression and radiculopathy, respectively, which is used as an adjunt to intraoperative monitoring.

■ If respiratory issues are a concern, pulmonary function testing may be necessary. Pulmonary function testing also can provide a baseline if postoperative pulmonary dysfunction occurs.

■ Angiographic evaluation of the artery of Adamkiewicz (great anterior radiculomedullary artery) may be obtained preoperatively. This artery originates as the left intercostal or lumbar artery in 68-73% of the cases and at the level of the 9th–12th intercostals artery in 62-75% of the cases (Yoshioka et al; 2006). Because the artery of Adamkiewicz does not always originate from one of the large intercostal arteries, preoperative evaluation of its precise origination helps avoid the potential for postoperative spinal cord ischemia. In addition to conventional angiography, evaluation can be accomplished via magnetic resonance or CT angiogram.

Positioning

■ The standard open thoracotomy procedure can be accomplished via a right- or left-sided approach and should be primarily dictated by the site of pathology.

• A right-sided approach is preferable for upper and middle thoracic lesions as there is more working space over the spinal surfaces behind the azygos vein as compared with that of the aorta.

• For lower thoracic lesions, a left-sided approach is preferable as the liver may cause the hemidiaphragm to rise and obstruct the operative field.

■ A double-lumen intubation should be performed with a fiberoptic bronchoscope. There should be one-lung ventilation with a tidal volume of 10-20 mg/kg in the dependent lung in the lateral decubitus position. SSEPs may be used and can affect anesthetic choices.

■ After adequate preparation by the anesthesiologist, the patient may then be placed in the lateral decubitus position with the side dependent on the location of the pathology and choice of entry (Fig. 1).

PEARLS

• *Alternatives for positioning include a radiolucent table with a beanbag or bolsters to position patients laterally. The table can be broken below the level of pathology in order to distract open the level of pathology.*

• *Ensure that the patient's spine is perfectly perpendicular to the floor when placing screw instrumentation.*

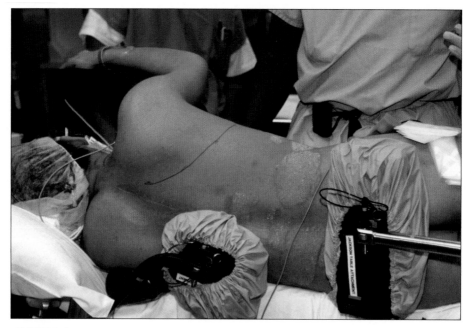

FIGURE 1

- A Jackson spinal table is used with four-point support at the symphysis, sacrum, scapula, and chest. Axillary roll padding is often used for the dependent axilla. The lower legs should be flexed and pressure points padded appropriately. The upper arm is placed in abduction and elevated to avoid obstruction.
- The surgeon often stands posterior to the patient with the first assistant standing on the opposite side of the surgeon. The position of the primary surgeon is the surgeon's choice.
- C-arm fluoroscopy should be utilized to guide this procedure with lateral spine images. The C-arm should be placed accordingly, with the C-arm monitor visible to the surgeon on the opposite side.
- After the C-arm is placed and the relevant spinal anatomy and ipsilateral scapula are outlined on the skin with a marking pen, the entire lateral chest wall is prepared and draped for a full thoracotomy procedure.

Portals/Exposures

- The incision should be fluoroscopically planned. The vertebral level(s) are localized directly onto the superficial skin surface.
- The incision should be approximately 12-15 cm in length on the rib of the vertebra one to two segments above where the most rostral instrumentation is to be placed. However, the incision may need to be extended to provide adequate exposure for multiple levels, with the goal of using the smallest incision that safely allows the surgeon to work.

Procedure

STEP 1

- The incision is made on the skin over the relevant rib as planned. The rib is then resected or a rib spreader is placed between ribs.
- The parietal pleura is sectioned after the correct levels are identified. This dissection is begun at the dorsal medial aspect of the vertebral body and extended cranially and caudally until healthy structures are encountered.
- If a neoplastic process is present, normal anatomic landmarks may be obscured, so one may benefit from performing a diskectomy above and below the tumor area. This will help with orientation and provides a frame of reference. As the disks are avascular, they are rarely infiltrated with tumor and can serve as boundaries for the vertebrectomy.
- Then, the segmental vessels are identified and ligated/clipped at the level of the midvertebral body.
- Tumor devascularization is achieved by working in a gradual centripetal direction.

STEP 2. RIB RESECTION VERSUS RETRACTION

- If entry into the spinal canal is required to perform a decompression, the choice of rib resection versus rib cut and retraction must be made.
- The rib head and the proximal 2-3 cm of rib adjacent to the spinal pathology are removed to expose the involved pedicle. This resection may be accomplished with Cobb periosteal elevators, curved curettes, and Kerrison rongeurs. Also, rib cutters and drills may be used. Rib resection sometimes can be avoided simply by cutting the rib and retracting accordingly.

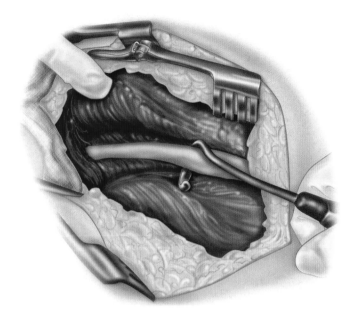

FIGURE 2

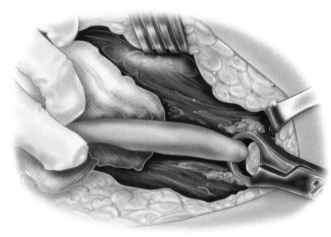

FIGURE 3

- The lower border of the pedicle should first be identified with a blunt nerve hook (Fig. 2).
- The pedicle may be removed with Kerrison rongeurs in a ventral-to-dorsal direction, exposing the lateral thecal sac (Fig. 3).
- If spinal cord decompression is needed, the posterior longitudinal ligament is opened and resected with visualization of the dura mater.

STEP 3

- After the pedicle is removed and the dura is visualized, the standard diskectomy procedure may be performed.
- The anulus fibrosus is incised with a Cobb periosteal elevator.
- The contents of the disk space are then safely curetted and removed with pituitary rongeurs.
- Osteophytes, calcified disk material, and vertebral body end plates are removed using microdissectors, burrs, or disk rongeurs.

STEP 4

- When performing a corpectomy, the disk just rostral and the disk just caudal should be incised to properly delineate the boundaries of the corpectomy.
- A large cavity is created in the middle of the vertebral body via burrs, curettes, osteotomes, and/or rongeurs until the posterior cortex is reached. Then, the posterior cortex plus the posterior longitudinal ligament are removed together via angled curettes and Kerrison rongeurs (Figs. 4 and 5).
- Pathology extending into the spinal canal should be dissected away from the spinal cord into the vertebral body cavity.
- Finally, an angled curette or a drill is used to remove cartilage and decorticate the vertebral body end plates.

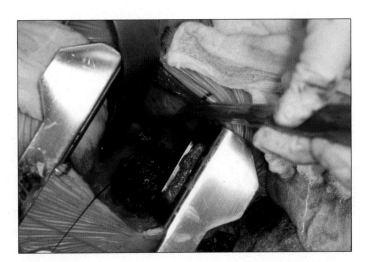

FIGURE 4

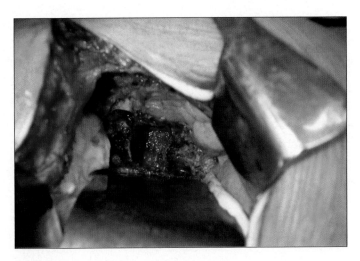

FIGURE 5

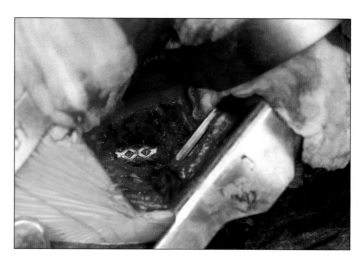

FIGURE 6

STEP 5. GRAFT PLACEMENT

- A graft is then inserted into the corpectomy site. This may be a bone strut, a titanium cage, an expandable cage, or a stackable cage (Fig. 6).
- If a nonautologous bone graft source is used, the cage or graft may be packed with a bone graft extender. Autograft materials such as rib or iliac bone may be used versus allograft materials.

STEP 6: INSTRUMENTATION PLACEMENT

- Various systems are available for instrumentation.
- Stabilization is achieved with four bone screws connected to a load-bearing frame plate (Fig. 7).
- Alternatively, staples with screws and a dual-rod system may be used, or a single staple screw/rod construct should a supplementary posterior stabilization be performed (Fig. 8).

STEP 7: CLOSURE

- The thoracic cavity should thoroughly be irrigated to remove all blood clots and debris. The lung and mediastinal contents should be inspected to rule out hemorrhage or air leaks. All tissue layers should be closed with the appropriate sutures.
- One or two chest tubes may be placed into the thoracic cavity and sutured to the skin with silk sutures. One chest tube is positioned at the thoracic cavity apex so that there is adequate lung reinflation, while the other should be placed posteroinferiorly for adequate drainage of fluid. Each chest tube is left on -20 cm H_2O suction initially, with waterseal drainage the following day, and can usually be removed by the second postoperative day.

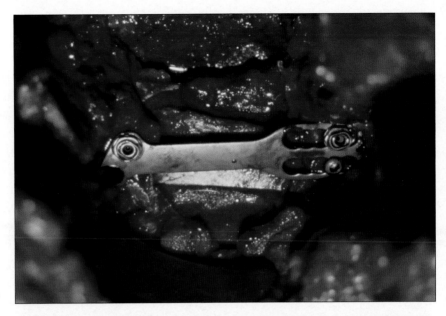

FIGURE 7

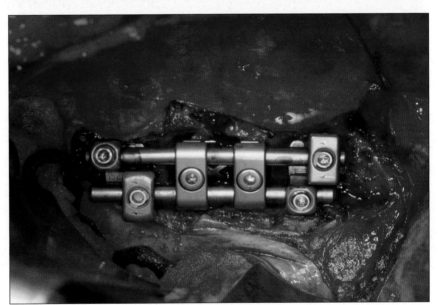

FIGURE 8

Postoperative Care and Expected Outcomes

- As with any surgical intervention, complications exist but often can be avoided with good surgical technique.
  - The anterior approach decreases the chances of spinal cord injury and inadequate decompression versus other approaches because of the exposure it provides and because it eliminates the need for spinal cord manipulation.
  - Because of the close proximity to the spinal cord, decompression can still result in spinal cord injury. Furthermore, despite the adequate

exposure advantage, incomplete diskectomy and/or corpectomy may result in inadequate decompression. Identifying the proper disk and vertebral levels and performing a pedicle-to-pedicle decompression in cases of corpectomy can help avoid these complications.

- If instrumentation is required after the diskectomy and corpectomy, complications related to fusion may occur. If there is lack of fusion or hardware failure, another surgery may be needed to supplement the previous fusion with posterior fusion and fixation. Hardware failure may also cause canal compromise, requiring re-exploration and hardware removal.

▪ Pulmonary complications may occur with an anterior thoracotomy. These complications include pneumonia, pneumothorax, atelectasis, pulmonary embolism, and pleural effusion. Good surgical technique and postoperative evaluation can help prevent these complications but may need to be treated accordingly.

▪ Incisional complications are possible. These typically include diaphragmatic hernia, abdominal sag, wound dehiscence, and infection.

Evidence

Anand N, Regan JJ. Video-assisted thoracoscopic surgery for thoracic disc disease: classification and outcome study of 100 consecutive cases with a 2-year minimum follow-up period. Spine. 2002;27:871-9.

Burke TG, Caputy A. Treatment of thoracic disc herniation: evolution toward the minimally invasive thoracoscopic technique. Neurosurg Focus. 2000;9:e9.

Das K, Rothberg M. Thoracoscopic surgery: historical perspectives. Neurosurg Focus. 2000;9:e10.

McCormick WE, Will SF, Benzel EC. Surgery for thoracic disc disease. Complication avoidance: overview and management. Neurosurg Focus. 2000;9:e13.

Middleton GS, Teach JH. Injury of the spinal cord due to rupture of an intervertebral disc during muscular effort. Glasgow Med. 1911;76:1-6.

Moro T, Kikuchi SI, Konno SI. Necessity of rib head resection for anterior discectomy in the thoracic spine. Spine. 2004;29:1703-5.

Rosenthal D, Dickman CA. Thoracoscopic microsurgical excision of herniated thoracic discs. J Neurosurg. 1998;89:224-35.

Visocchi M, Masferrer R, Sonntag VKH, Dickman CA. Thoracoscopic approaches to the thoracic spine. Acta Neurochir (Wien). 1998;140:737-43.

Wakefield AE, Steinmetz MP, Benzel EC. Biomechanics of thoracic discectomy. Neurosurg Focus. 2001;11:e6.

Yoshioka K, Niinuma H, Ehara S, Nakajima T, Nakamura M, Kawazoe K. MR angiography and CT angiography of the artery of Adamkiewicz: State of the Art. RadioGraphics 2006;26:S63-S73.

Anterior Thoracolumbar Spinal Fusion with Single- or Dual-Rod Instrumentation via Open Approach for Idiopathic Scoliosis

Peter G. Gabos

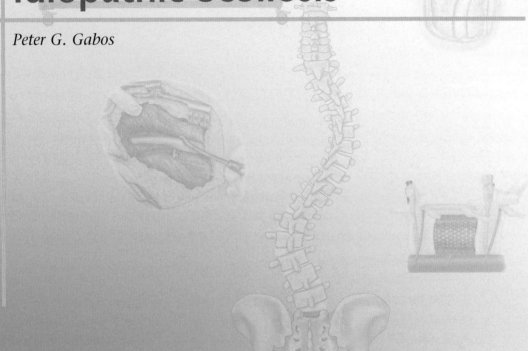

Controversies

- Does sparing a spinal motion segment significantly benefit the patient?
- Are there more risks/complications with anterior surgery?
- Is there better correction of curvature with anterior versus posterior surgery?

Treatment Options

- Posterior spinal fusion with dual-rod instrumentation
- Anterior spinal fusion with single- or dual-rod instrumentation, via open or thoracoscopic technique

Indications

- To halt progression of spinal curvature
- To restore spinal alignment and balance
- To preserve caudal motion segments (typically one to two segments) when compared to posterior spinal fusion
- To prevent the crankshaft phenomenon in skeletally immature patients (Risser 0, open triradiate cartilage)
- To allow for a thoracoscopic approach in selected cases
- Appropriate candidates typically include Lenke type 1 (single structural thoracic) and Lenke type 5 (single structural thoracolumbar/lumbar) curves (Fig. 1A and 1B).

Examination/Imaging

- Clinical assessment of curve location, coronal and sagittal balance, trunk rotation, shoulder asymmetry, pelvic obliquity, integrity of the neuraxis, and any other associated anomalies
- Full-length standing posteroanterior, lateral, and right and left supine bending radiographs to assist in curve classification, assessment of curve flexibility, and selection of fusion levels
- Magnetic resonance imaging in selected cases (e.g., neurologic signs or symptoms, early- or juvenile-onset scoliosis, rapid curve progression, unusual curve pattern)

Positioning

- The surgical approach is always from the convex side of the curvature, in the lateral decubitus position.

Portals/Exposures

THORACIC
- Standard thoracotomy approach gives access to vertebral levels T2 to approximately L1.
- Expanded access can be achieved with the use of a double thoracotomy if absolutely necessary.

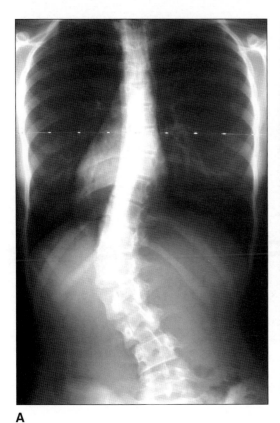 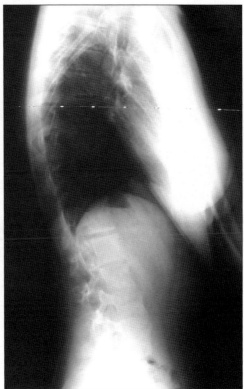

A   **B**

FIGURE 1A-B

Pearls—Cont'd

• *A flat radiolucent table and beanbag positioner are utilized.*

• *When utilized, unobstructed fluoroscopic access is verified prior to prepping and draping.*

• *Neurophysiologic monitoring of spinal cord function, using both somatosensory evoked potential and transcranial motor evoked potential monitoring is recommended to optimize patient safety.*

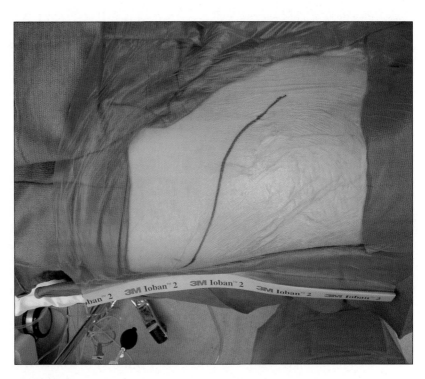

FIGURE 2

PEARLS

- *Thoracic (open technique)*

  - *Single-lung ventilation is not required, but does allow for better visualization during the procedure.*

  - *Standard thoracotomy is utilized, typically choosing the interspace corresponding to the apex of the deformity.*

  - *Constructs spanning more than seven levels may require double thoracotomy.*

  - *To limit incision size and chest wall dissection, disk excision and screw implantation can be done through small percutaneous accessory incisions at the more cephalad or caudad levels.*

- *Thoracolumbar*

  - *Split the costal cartilage at the tip of the 10th rib, maintaining the attachments to the diaphragm (cephalad cartilage tip) and abdominal musculature (caudad cartilage tip).*

  - *Use temporary stay sutures to mark the diaphragm as it is incised, for later reapproximation.*

  - *Reapproximate the split 10th rib costal cartilage to initiate closure.*

- *Lumbar*

  - *Beware of the thinning musculature and superficial location of the peritoneum medially near the rectus sheath.*

  - *Dissection should proceed medial to the psoas muscle.*

THORACOLUMBAR

- A 10th rib thoracoabdominal approach allows the greatest exposure and versatility for fusions crossing the thoracolumbar junction (Fig. 2).

LUMBAR

- An anterior retroperitoneal flank approach gives sufficient access to vertebral levels L1-5.

PEARLS—Cont'd

- *The genitofemoral nerve lies directly on the psoas muscle.*

- *The iliolumbar vein consistently requires ligation when working at the L4-5 level.*

- *Preserve paraspinous sympathetic fibers that do not interfere with the dissection.*

Controversies

- Most surgeons will ligate the segmental vessels overlying each vertebral body. Temporary clamping of individual vessels for several minutes under electrophysiologic monitoring prior to sacrifice should be considered.

Procedure: Thoracolumbar Spine Fusion via an Open Approach Using Single-Rod Instrumentation

STEP 1: ANTERIOR RELEASE AND DISCECTOMY

- Once adequate spinal exposure has been obtained, transection of the anterior longitudinal ligament and complete diskectomy is performed to, or including, the posterior longitudinal ligament.

STEP 2: PLACEMENT OF THE ANTERIOR VERTEBRAL BODY SCREWS

- The entry point of the vertebral body screw is preferentially the junction of the pedicular origin and the vertebral body, crossing the center of the vertebral body and directed perpendicularly across to the far side. At the cephalad and caudad end vertebrae, a staple can be impacted to prevent pullout or plow-through of the screws. At intervening levels, a washer can be placed to help distribute load.

Procedure: Thoracolumbar Spine Fusion via an Open Approach Using Dual-Rod Instrumentation

STEP 1: ANTERIOR RELEASE AND DISKECTOMY

- This is performed in the same manner as described in Step 1 for single-rod instrumentation.

STEP 2: PLACEMENT OF THE ANTERIOR VERTEBRAL BODY SCREWS

- With systems employing a dual-rod construct, there is typically a two-holed tined vertebral staple that is implanted first, which then receives the vertebral body screws (Fig. 4). When positioning these devices, care should be taken not to allow the anterior screw to be too close to the anterior aspect of the vertebral body as vertebral body fracture can occur. The proper staple is selected by identifying the size that maximizes the coverage of the lateral aspect of the vertebral body without violating the adjacent disk space.
- Anteriorly placed devices may also incur more kyphosis, which is undesirable in the lumbar spine. The posterior screw should be placed in a position as posterior is as possible without allowing for canal intrusion.

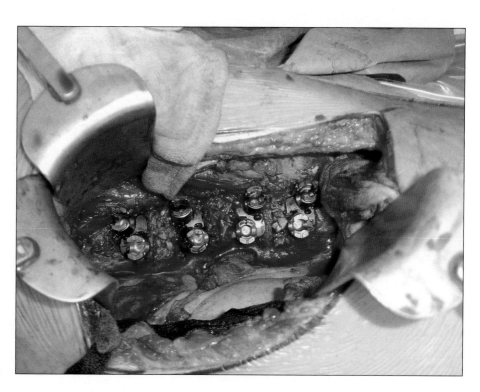

FIGURE 4

Step 3: End Plate Ablation

- This is performed in the same manner as described in Step 3 for single-rod instrumentation.

Step: 4: Placement of Anterior Interbody Supports

- This is performed in the same manner as described in Step 4 for single-rod instrumentation.

Step 5: Rod Placement

- The rods are appropriately contoured to the desired sagittal and coronal plane configuration. The posterior-most rod is reduced to the screws first and captured sequentially. Some degree of rod rotation may be necessary to "fine tune" the correction, which has already largely occurred from the meticulous diskectomy and structural graft placement.
- The anterior screws can be used to further derotate the vertebrae at this point, if necessary. Some final compression of the posterior screws across the disk spaces to firmly compress the grafts prior to final tightening can be performed at this stage. The anterior-most rod is then placed and captured at this point, essentially in situ.
- Some spinal implant systems will employ a cross connector, which can be placed at this point (Fig. 5).

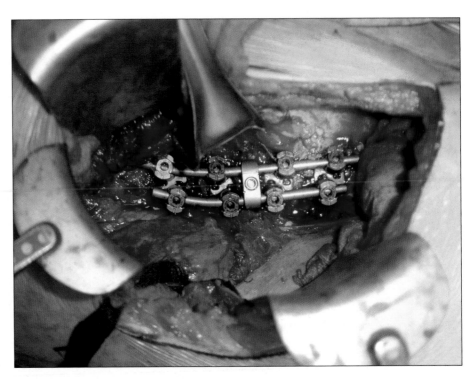

FIGURE 5

STEP 6: PLACEMENT OF CHEST TUBE AND
WOUND CLOSURE

- This is performed in the same manner as described in Step 6 for single-rod instrumentation.

Postoperative Care and Expected Outcomes

- The patient is mobilized beginning on the day following surgery. If single-rod instrumentation is utilized, a spinal orthosis is fashioned and worn for 3-4 months postoperatively. If dual-rod instrumentation is utilized, no brace is employed.
- Activity modifications are necessary for at least the first 6 months postoperatively, with a return to competitive sports at 12 months or when clear evidence of fusion is seen radiographically.
- Radiographs are taken to assess the implant stability, maintenance of correction and maturation of the fusion at 1, 3, 6, and 12 months postoperatively (Figs. 6A, 6B, and 7). Yearly radiographs are obtained thereafter until definitive fusion is seen.

Controversies

- When using a single-rod system with rod diameter greater than 5 mm and multilevel structural interbody support, bracing may not be necessary in the early postoperative phase.

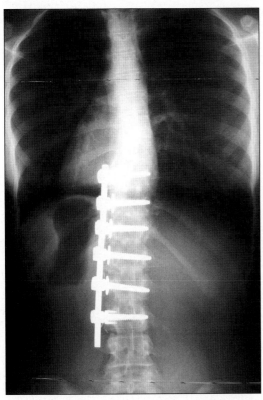

A

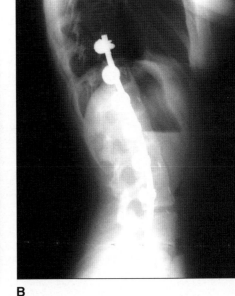

B

FIGURE 6A-B

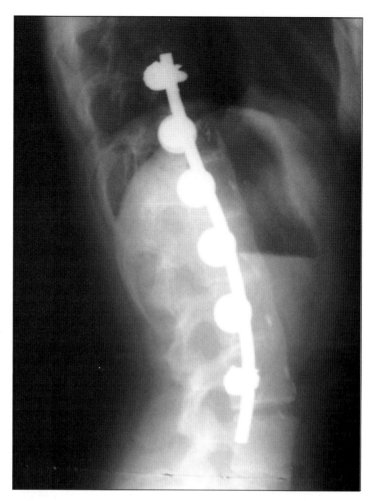

FIGURE 7

Evidence

Fricka KB, Mahar AT, Newton PO. Biomechanical analysis of anterior scoliosis instrumentation: differences between single and dual rod systems with and without structural interbody support. Spine. 2002;27:702-6.

In bovine specimens, dual-rod constructs were stiffer in torsion and flexion-extension loading than single-rod systems. Lateral bending stiffness was similar for both constructs. When structural interbody support (SIS) was added, stiffness in flexion increased significantly in single-rod constructs, approaching that of dual-rod constructs.

Lowe TG, Alongi PR, Smith DA, O'Brien MF, Mitchell SL, Pinteric RJ. Anterior single-rod instrumentation for thoracolumbar adolescent idiopathic scoliosis with and without the use of structural interbody support. Spine. 2003;28:2221-32.

Forty-one patients with adolescent idiopathic scoliosis underwent anterior spinal fusion using a single-rod (6.0 or 6.5 mm) construct. SIS was used in 21 patients, and packed morselized autograft alone was used in 20 patients. There were no rod or screw failures and no obvious pseudarthroses at 3-year follow-up. Results were similar for both groups with respect to curve correction and restoration of sagittal balance, and the Scoliosis Research Society Outcomes Instrument. The use of SIS over morselized autograft did not appear to be of significance when these large-diameter single rods were employed.

Lowe TG, Enguidanos ST, Smith DA, Hashim S, Eule JM, O'Brien MF, Diekmann MJ, Wilson L, Trommeter JM. Single-rod versus dual-rod anterior instrumentation for idiopathic scoliosis: a biomechanical study. Spine. 2005;30:311-17.

In human cadaveric specimens, SIS appeared to contribute the most to construct stiffness in flexion whether single- or dual-rod constructs were employed. In lateral bending, stiffness of single- and dual-rod constructs with and without SIS was equivalent. In torsion, single- and dual-rod instrumentation and SIS contributed to global stiffness. Transverse rod connectors in dual-rod constructs only contributed to stiffness in torsion. In bovine specimens, dual rods were stiffer than single-rod constructs, with SIS playing only a minor role.

Polly DW Jr, Cunningham BW, Kuklo TR, Lenke LG, Oda I, Schroeder TM, Klemme WR. Anterior thoracic scoliosis constructs: effect of rod diameter and intervertebral cages on multi-segmental construct stability. Spine J. 2003;3:213-19.

In bovine specimens, single-rod constructs utilizing a 4-mm and 5-mm rod were tested with a seven-level interbody cage construct and compared to constructs employing only one (apical disk), two (end disks), and three (apical and end disks) levels. Intervertebral cages at every level significantly improved construct stiffness when compared to increasing rod diameter alone. When structural supports were not used, axial compression created the greatest strain.

Potter BK, Kuklo TR, Lenke LG. Radiographic outcomes of anterior spinal fusion versus posterior spinal fusion with thoracic pedicle screws for treatment of Lenke yype I adolescent idiopathic scoliosis curves. Spine. 2005;30:1859-66.

This retrospective review compared curve correction and derotation between 40 curve-matched cohorts of Lenke type 1 curves treated by spinal fusion performed anteriorly with single-rod instrumentation versus posteriorly with thoracic pedicle screw (PSF/TPS) constructs. Anterior surgery allowed for an average of one less vertebral level fused. However, the PSF/TPS group demonstrated greater correction of the main thoracic curve and greater spontaneous correction of the uninstrumented thoracolumbar-lumbar curve, and improved correction of thoracic torsion and rotation.

Rhee JM, Bridwell KH, Won DS, Lenke LG, Chotigavanichaya C, Hanson DS. Sagittal plane analysis of adolescent idiopathic scoliosis: the effect of anterior versus posterior instrumentation. Spine. 2002;27:2350-6.

This retrospective study evaluated the postoperative sagittal profile of 110 consecutive patients with adolescent idiopathic scoliosis. Sixty patients underwent posterior dual-rod instrumented fusion and 50 patients underwent anterior instrumented fusion using a single-rod construct. At a follow-up of 32 months, the proximal junctional (kyphosis) measurement (measured between the proximal-most instrumented vertebra and the segment two levels cephalad) increased most in the posterior group; thoracic kyphosis (T5-12) increased most in the anterior group; and lumbar lordosis was enhanced with either approach. No significant change in the distal junctional measurement (measured between the distal instrumented vertebra and the segment two levels caudal) occurred in either group. The authors conclude that each approach affects the sagittal profile differently, albeit to a small degree. When properly performed, both approaches can give an acceptable sagittal profile.

Smith JA, Deviren V, Berven S, Bradford DS. Does instrumented anterior scoliosis surgery lead to kyphosis, pseudarthrosis or inadequate correction in adults? Spine. 2002;27:529-34.

This retrospective review of 14 consecutive adult patients with scoliosis treated by anterior spinal fusion using a single-rod (6-mm) construct demonstrated no cases of pseudarthrosis, progressive kyphosis, or instrumentation failure. Average correction of the Cobb angle was 66%, and the thoracolumbar sagittal plane alignment was maintained or improved in every patient. The patients scored satisfactorily on the Scoliosis Research Society Outcomes Instrument in the areas of satisfaction, pain, self-image, function, and mental health.

Operative Management of Scheuermann's Kyphosis

Alok D. Sharan and Thomas J. Errico

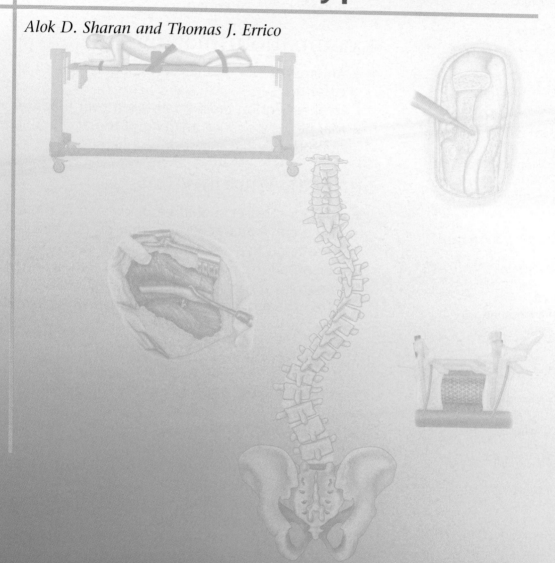

Controversies

- Spondylolisthesis is often associated with Scheuermann's kyphosis.
- An asymptomatic spondylolisthesis does not require treatment.

Treatment Options

- Posterior spinal fusion (hooks, pedicle screws, hybrid constructs)
- Combined anterior/posterior spinal fusion

Indications

- Rigid curves greater than 75 degrees
- Curves that have progressed despite brace treatment
- Painful kyphotic curves that progress despite nonoperative treatment

Examination/Imaging

- Anteroposterior and lateral radiographs on long cassettes
- Hyperextension radiograph taken over a bolster
- Magnetic resonance imaging of thoracic and lumbar spine to rule out a cyst or disk herniation

Surgical Anatomy

- Anterior releases should be performed at the apex of the curve and at all disks that do not become lordotic on hyperextension.
- When performing the anterior diskectomy, it is important to preserve the segmental vessels.
- Often the anterior longitudinal ligament is resected to achieve an adequate release.

Positioning

- For the anterior approach, place the patient in the lateral decubitus position.
  - If a thoracotomy is to be performed, position the patient with the right side up.
  - If a thoracolumbar approach is to be used, position the patient with the left side up.
  - If there is also a scoliosis, position the patient so that the convexity of the curve is up.
- For the posterior approach, place the patient on a four-poster frame.

Procedure

STEP 1: POSTERIOR SPINAL FUSION (PSF)
- At least eight pedicle screws (four levels) should be inserted above and below the apex of the curve.
- A rod should be contoured to normal sagittal alignment.
- The rod is inserted into the proximal screws and cantilevered into the remaining screws (Fig. 2).
- If hooks are used, they should be placed in a claw pattern allowing for compression of the curve.

Equipment

- A padded horseshoe face support is useful to control cervicothoracic extension.

PEARLS

- *The distal end of the instrumentation should end one vertebra caudal to the first lordotic disk space.*

- *The proximal end of the instrumentation should be the proximal vertebra measured in the Cobb angle (Fig. 1).*

- *Performing Smith-Petersen osteotomies can facilitate the reduction of the kyphosis.*

PITFALLS

- *If possible, avoid instrumentation at the apex of the curve as this can become prominent.*

- *An isolated PSF should be used if the kyphosis corrects to less than 50° on the hyperextension radiograph and the patient is skeletally immature; otherwise an anterior spinal fusion should be added.*

Controversies

- Junctional kyphosis can develop if instrumentation is ended proximal or distal to the Cobb levels.
- Isolated PSF can be performed for curves greater than 80° if only pedicle screws are used.
- Pedicle subtraction osteotomies are not typically recommended as they will be performed cephalad to the conus.

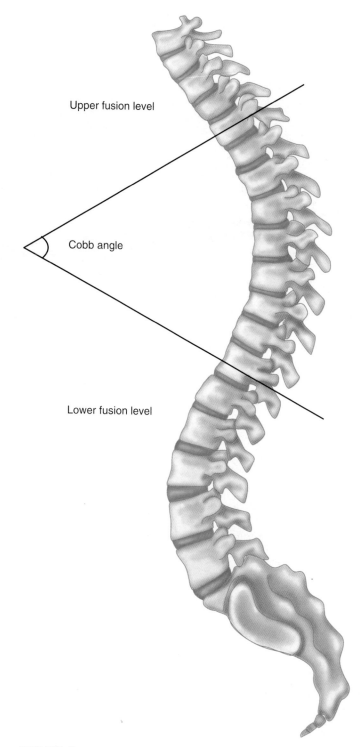

Upper fusion level

Cobb angle

Lower fusion level

FIGURE 1

STEP 2: ANTERIOR SPINAL FUSION

- A strut graft can be placed to provide additional mechanical support.

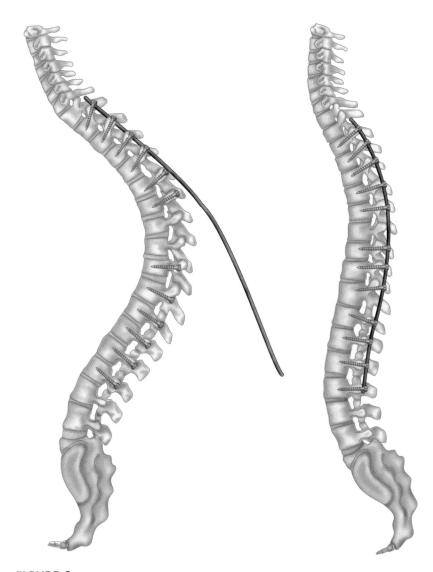

FIGURE 2

Postoperative Care and Expected Outcomes

- Bracing is typically not necessary.
- Patients are maintained in the intensive care unit or a monitored bed overnight.
- Ambulation is encouraged on the first postoperative day.

Evidence

Arlet V, Schlenzka D. Scheuermann's kyphosis: surgical management. Eur Spine J. 2005;14:817–27.

This review article discusses the use of newer segmental instrumentation used to correct kyphosis. The four rod technique as well as various compression techniques are also presented.

Boachie-Adjei O, Sarwahi V. Scheuermann's kyphosis. In Dewald RL (ed): Spinal Deformities: A Comprehensive Text. Thieme Medical Pub, 2003; pp 777–86.

This chapter describes some of the surgical concepts and techniques that are used in correcting kyphosis in Scheuermann's disease.

Murray PM, Weinstein SL, Spratt KF. The natural history and long-term follow-up of Scheuermann kyphosis. J Bone Joint Surg Am. 1993;75:236–48.

This classic article describes the long term followup of 67 patients with Scheuermann's kyphosis followed for an average of 32 years compared to a control group. The patients with Scheuermann's kyphosis had more intense back pain, jobs that require less activity, and less range of motion of extension of their trunk.

Resection of Intradural Intramedullary or Extramedullary Spinal Tumors

James S. Harrop, Ashwini Sharan, John Birkness, and John Ratliff

Treatment Options

- Serial observation
- Radiation therapy (secondary treatment option)

Indications

- Spinal cord compression
  - Weakness
  - Loss of bowel and bladder function
  - Sensory loss
- Symptomatic neuronal/radicular compression
- Progressive growth of lesion on serial imaging
- Persistent pain or radiculopathy
- Spinal deformity

Examination/Imaging

PHYSICAL EXAMINATION

- Cord compression—myelopathy
- Radicular signs or symptoms
- Dermatologic findings in neurocutaneous disorders (e.g., neurofibromatosis)

PLAIN FILMS/COMPUTED TOMOGRAPHY (CT) SCAN

- Typically nondiagnosistic
- Bone erosion or remodeling of osseous elements (scalloping) due to prolonged presence of the lesion
- May use CT to diagnose bony versus soft tissue cord compression

MAGNETIC RESONANCE IMAGING (MRI) WITH GADOLINIUM

- Study of choice
- Differentiates type of intradural lesion
  - Extramedullary—located outside spinal cord
    - Meningioma: dural based, enhances homogenously, calcified
    - Nerve sheath tumor (schwannoma and neurofibroma): dumbbell-shaped lesion that has a separate plane, is extrinsic to the spinal cord, and follows the nerve through the neural foramina (Fig. 1A)
    - Coronal images (Fig. 1B) illustrate path of nerve sheath tumor exiting foramen around pedicle.
  - Intramedullary—located within spinal cord parenchyma (Fig. 2)
    - Expansion of the spinal cord
    - Associated with intraparenchymal cyst or syrinx
    - Primary glial neoplasms (e.g., ependymoma) predominate

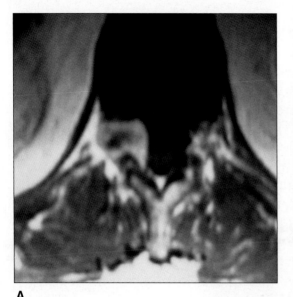

A

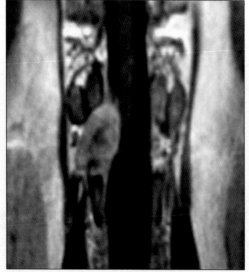

B

FIGURE 1A-B

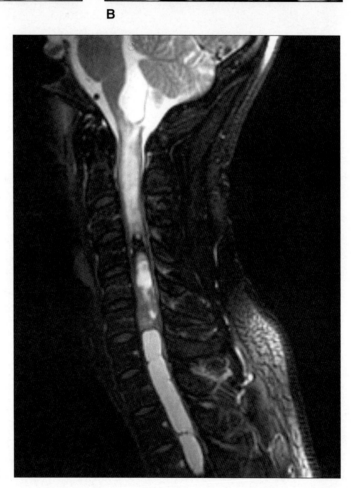

FIGURE 2

Surgical Anatomy

- Spinal column defines boundaries of the spinal canal
  - Anterior—vertebral body
  - Lateral—pedicles
  - Posterior—laminae and spinous process
  - Levels
    - Cervical—7 vertebrae
    - Thoracic—12 vertebrae
    - Lumbar—5 vertebrae
- Spinal meninges or coverings
  - Dura mater
    - Thick fibrous layer
    - Separated from osseous region by a space containing epidural veins and fatty and fibrous tissue.
  - Arachnoid
    - Delicate layer
    - Region where cerebrospinal fluid circulates
  - Pia mater
    - Thin layer
    - Contacts the spinal cord and is adherent to blood vessels entering the spinal cord
- Spinal cord
  - Approximately 45 cm in length
  - Thirty-one pairs of spinal nerves arise from the spinal cord: 8 cervical, 12 thoracic, 5 lumbar, 5 sacral, and 1 coccygeal.
  - Conus medullaris: terminal end of the spinal cord
  - Filum terminalis: fibrous band that continues distally and attaches to the dorsum of the first coccygeal vertebrae
- The spinal cord is a highly organized, somatotopically arranged tissue composed of two functionally and anatomically distinct regions.
  - Gray matter—central portion; consists of neuronal cell bodies and supporting structures
    - Axial plane—central bridge of gray matter connecting each side such that, in an axial section, it resembles the letter H
    - Ventral portion—anterior horn motor cells
  - White matter
    - Encircles gray matter
    - Composed of both myelinated and unmyelinated axonal tracts
- Central canal—in the middle of the H
  - Embryologic remnant from neurulation of the neural plate

- Continuum of the fourth ventricle from the medulla
- Spans the entire length of the spinal cord and terminates as a fusiform terminal ventricle in the conus medullaris
- Lined with cuboidal ependymal cells

Positioning

- General anesthesia with neurophysiologic monitoring
- Prone position with spinal axis in the midline
  - Ensure eyes are not subject to external compression
  - Ensure endotracheal tube is free and not obstructed
  - Pad extremity peripheral nerves over bony protuberances (i.e., ulnar and peroneal)
- Occiput to T_4 lesions (Fig. 3)
  - Application of a Mayfield headholder
  - Neck remains in a neutral position and there is no external compression on the orbit or endotracheal tube
  - Tape shoulder to facilitate imaging

PEARLS

- *Minimizing compression upon the abdomen reduces intra-abdominal pressure and thus epidural venous pressure. This reduces intraoperative blood loss.*

- *Localization of thoracic lesions may be difficult. Either preoperative localizer or radiograph may aid in localizing incision.*

PITFALLS

- *If shoulders are taped, assure that the brachial plexus is not stretched. Intraoperative free-running electromyography or intraoperative upper extremity somatosensory evoked potentials may help limit plexus palsies.*

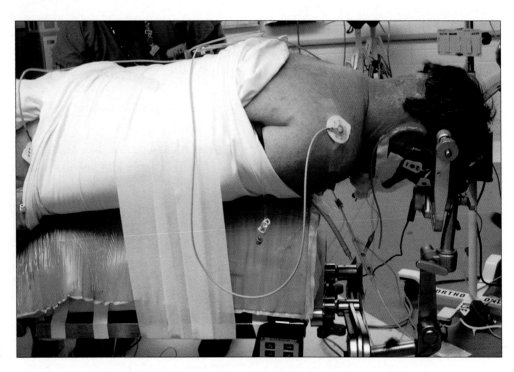

FIGURE 3

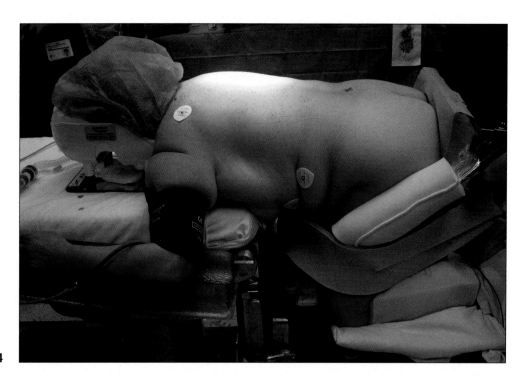

FIGURE 4

- T4 to sacrum lesions (Fig. 4)
  - Andrews frame or laminectomy rolls
  - Abdomen is free of pressure, which provides for a decease in the epidural venous pressure

Portals/Exposures

- Localize midline region and plan extent of laminectomy or bony removal.
- Make a midline incision down to the paraspinal fascia.
- Avascular subperiosteal dissection is continued bilaterally, centered over spinous process and laminae.
  - The retractor system should be low profile and away from the surgical site.
- Use a high-speed drill to resect posterior elements.
  - Drill through the laminae bilaterally at the facet-laminae junction.
  - Resect the rostral and caudal interspinous ligaments.
  - Resect the laminae en bloc and carefully dissect free all dural adhesions (Fig. 5).
- Confirm that the extent of dural exposure is adequate through:
  - Palpation of the lesion
  - Radiographic confirmation
  - Intraoperative ultrasound

Instrumentation

- Retractor with low-profile bar: provides area to attach dural or pial sutures
- Paraspinal muscle hooks: provide exposure and are away from surgical site

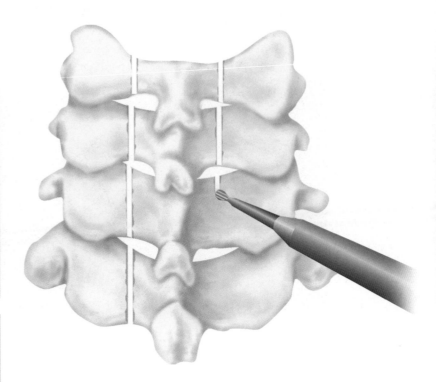

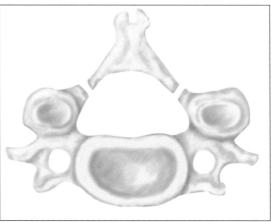

FIGURE 5

- Confirm that hemostasis is excellent particularly at dural margins.

Procedure

STEP 1

- Hemostasis is meticulously maintained, particularly in the epidural region, prior to opening the dura.
- The rostral and caudal extent of the spinal lesion are defined and assured to be within the bony opening.
- Based on preoperative images, a single dural suture is placed through which traction is applied to draw the dura away from the spinal cord.

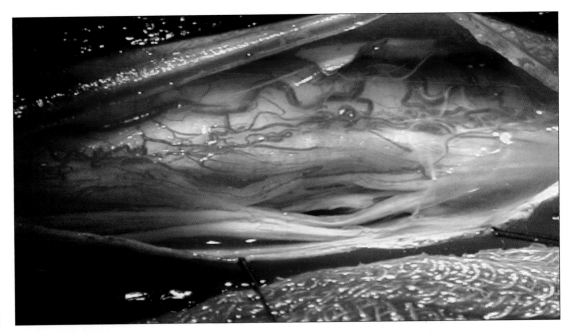

FIGURE 6

Instrumentation/ Implantion

- Operative microscope
- Microdissection instrument set

- A midline or lateral dural incision is made with a sharp instrument.
  - Maintain the arachnoid plane if possible.
  - The arachnoid is opened and spinal fluid allowed to flow freely and decompress the canal.
- Dural tack-up sutures bilaterally maintain the exposure of the spinal lesion and prevent blood products from entering the cerebrospinal fluid (Fig. 6). In addition, the epidural space can be visualized with the use of hemostatic material (Surgicel).

Step 2

- An intraoperative microscope is brought into the surgical field.
  - Provides illumination
  - Higher magnification of field than standard loupes
- Dissection with micro-instrumentation enables the surgeron to
  - Define normal anatomy proximal and distal to the lesion
  - Outline proximal and distal extent of pathologic lesion (Fig. 7A-C)
  - Determine nerve root or parenchymal involvement

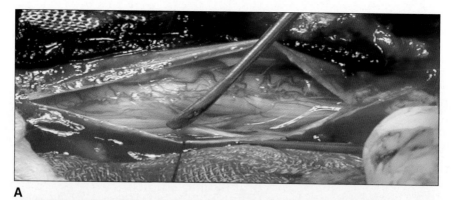

A

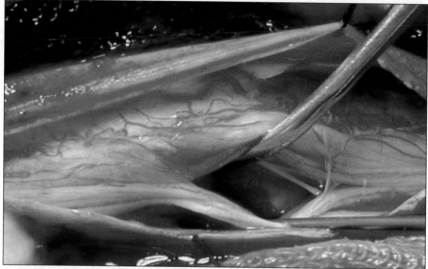

B

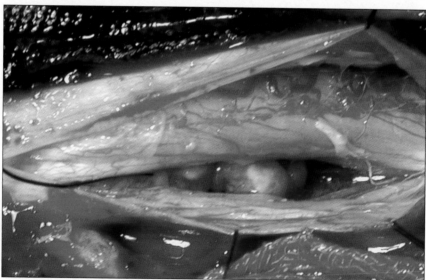

C

FIGURE 7A-C

Instrumentation/ Implantation

- Intraoperative ultrasound
- Microdissection tools

STEP 3

- Extramedullary lesions
  - Mengiomas are dural based and dissected out en bloc and resected.
  - Nerve sheath lesions should be dissected from the spinal cord, and entering and exiting nerve rootlets should be defined (Fig. 8).
  - Neurofibromas and schwannomas may follow the exiting nerve and have a "dumb-bell" appearance on imaging studies.
    - Opening the nerve sheath and debulking may provide for manipulation of the intracanal portion away from spinal cord.
    - Major goal is to remove intracanal portion to prevent or remove cord compression.
  - Neurophysiologic stimulation provides data on nerve conduction and potential sequelae of sacrifice.
- Intramedullary lesions
  - Define lesion with intraoperative ultrasound.
  - Plan cordotomy incision and bipolar coagulation of dorsal vessels along cordotomy section.
  - Make incision parallel to posterior columns along midline raphe.
  - Biopsy lesion and send to pathology.
  - Lengthen cordotomy to extent of lesion to enable removal of rostral and caudal poles.

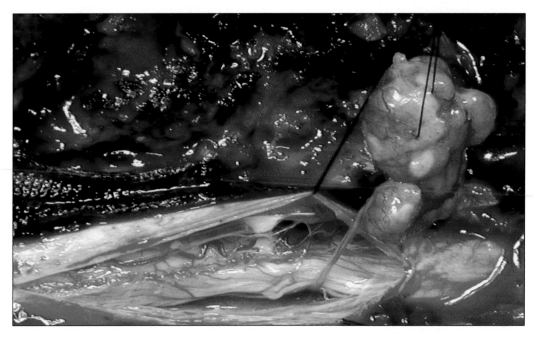

FIGURE 8

- Define gliotic planes and infold tumor into dissected region.
- Cavitation of the tumor with collapsing of the edges of the tumor's capsule into the cavitation defect affords minimal manipulation of the neural elements.

STEP 4

- After resection of the lesion, the wound is confirmed to have no active bleeding.
- Exploration of the surgical bed for residual neoplasm is necessary to confirm gross total resection.
- Dura is closed with nonabsorbable suture.
- Prior to completion of the dural closure, saline is injected into the subarachnoid space to confirm a watertight closure.
- The wound is closed in multiple layers.

Postoperative Care and Expected Outcomes

- MRI images of surgical resection should be obtained to confirm the extent of resection as well as serve as a basis for future comparisons.

Evidence

Brotchi J. Intrinsic spinal cord tumor resection. Neurosurgery. 2002;50:1059-66.

Burger PC, Scheithauer BW. Tumors of the central nervous system. In Rosai J, Sobin LH (eds). Atlas of Tumor Pathology, Ser. 3, Facs. 10. Washington, DC: Armed Forces Institute of Pathology, 1994.

Constantini S, Miller DC, Allen JC, et al. Radical excision of intramedullary spinal cord tumors: surgical morbidity and long-term follow-up evaluation in 164 children and young adults. J Neurosurg Spine. 2000;93:183-93.

Epstein FJ, Farmer JP, Freed D. Adult intramedullary astrocytomas of the spinal cord. J Neurosurg. 1992;77:355-9.

Mechtler L, Cohen ME. Clinical presentation and therapy of spinal tumors. In Bradley WG, Daroff RB, Fenchel GM, Marsden CD (eds). Neurology in Clinical Practice: The Neurological Disorders, ed 2. Boston: Butterworth-Heinemann, 1996.

Osborn AG. Diagnostic Neuroradiology. St. Louis: Mosby–Year Book, 1994.

Simeone FA. Intradural tumors. In Rothman RH, Simeone FA (eds). The Spine, ed 3. Philadelphia: WB Saunders, 1992.

Endoscopic Thoracic Diskectomy

Stepan Kasimian and J. Patrick Johnson

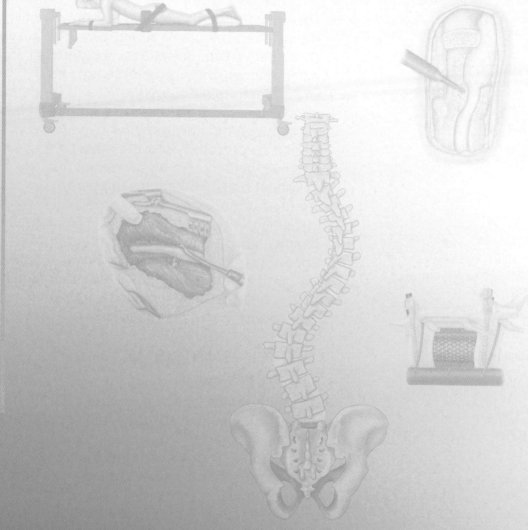

Figures in this chapter are courtesy of J. Patrick Johnson, MD; From Johnson JP, Rogers CD. Thoracoscopic diskectomy. *In* Kim DH, Fessler RG, Regan JJ (eds): Endoscopic Spine Surgery and Instrumentation. New York: Thieme, 2005.

Controversies

- Use of navigation systems has been shown to facilitate operation (Holly et al., 2001).
- Posterolateral approaches such as a transpedicular or costotransversectomy approach could address a ventral herniation; however, these approaches are ideal for paracentral lesions (Johnson et al., 2000).
- Multilevel procedure may be better undertaken with thoracotomy due to longer operative time with thoracoscopy.
- Preoperative angiogram has been recommended to determine location of the *artery of Adamkiewicz* (Di Chiro et al., 1970). However, for a thoracic diskectomy, ligation of a segmental artery is rarely necessary.
- Fusion may be necessary when excessive disk material is removed or the spine is otherwise destabilized.

Indications

- The indications for thoracoscopic diskectomy are similar to the indications for other procedures to treat central thoracic disk herniations.
  - Ventral herniated thoracic disk causing myelopathy, gait disturbance, lower extremity weakness, or loss of sphincter control
  - Thoracic disk herniation with axial back pain, thoracic radiculopathy, or leg pain that has failed conservative care (injections, nonsteroidal anti-inflammatory drugs, physiotherapy, etc.)
- Thoracoscopic spinal surgery may also be performed for nerve sheath tumor resection, anterior release for scoliosis, sympathectomy for hyperhidrosis, or vertebral corpectomy. Figure 1 shows a 55-year-old female patient with an incidental finding of a mediastinal mass on a chest radiograph. An axial computed tomography (CT) scan (Fig. 1A), as well as axial (Fig. 1B) and sagittal (Fig. 1C) magnetic resonance imaging (MRI), showed a dumbbell-shaped tumor (peripheral nerve sheath tumor) of a nerve root with expansion of the neuroforamen. The tumor was successfully removed with simultaneous posterior and thoracoscopic excision.

Examination/Imaging

- Symptoms of a thoracic herniated disk correlate with thoracic radiculopathy, thoracic back pain, myelopathy or vague leg pain (Anand and Regan, 2002).
- Selective thoracic nerve root blocks can be performed for therapeutic and diagnostic purposes.
- MRI has superior soft tissue detail and can demonstrate cord compression in multiple planes.
  - Figure 2 shows a patient who presented with myelopathy. Sagittal (Fig. 2A) and axial (Fig. 2B) T2-weighted MRI demonstrated a midline central disk herniation with severe cord compression. A ventral approach is required for safe decompression.

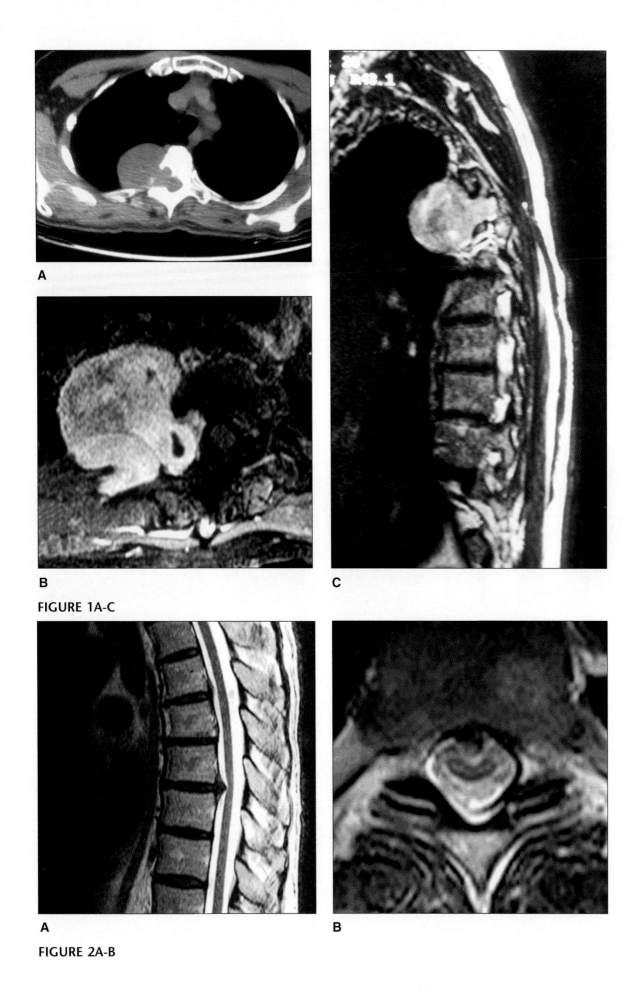

A

B

C

FIGURE 1A-C

A

B

FIGURE 2A-B

- Figure 3 shows an acute herniated soft disk with significant spinal cord compression on T2-weighted MRI.
- CT scans define the bony detail and a calcified disk better than MRI.
  - Figure 4 compares T1-weighted MRI (Fig. 4A) and CT (Fig. 4B) of a calcified paracentral disk herniation causing thoracic radiculopathy. Note the improved delineation of the calcified paracentral disk with CT.
  - In Figure 5, a large paracentral calcified disk herniation with progressive myelopathy is well demonstrated with CT (Fig. 5A) and sagittal reconstruction (Fig. 5B).
- High-quality plain radiographs are needed to confirm level. This can be important in patients with anomalous thoracic vertebrae (e.g., 13 thoracic vertebrae).

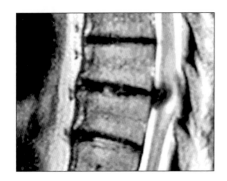

FIGURE 3

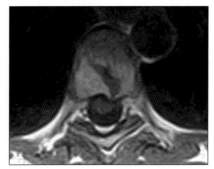

A

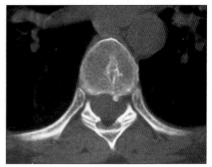

B

FIGURE 4A-B

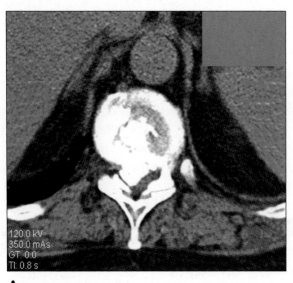

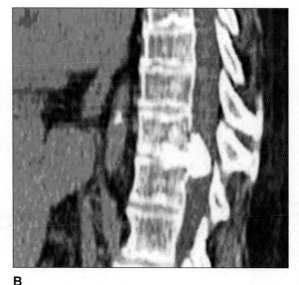

A

B

FIGURE 5A-B

Treatment Options

- Open thoracotomy and excision of central disk herniation through transthoracic approach (Fig. 6A)
- Posterolateral approach for lateral calcified disk herniation or central soft disk herniation: transpedicular or transfacet pedicle-sparing approaches (Fig. 6B)
- Other methods of treatment for ventral disk herniation include lateral extracavitary and costotransversectomy approaches (Bohlman and Zdeblick, 1988) (Fig. 6C).

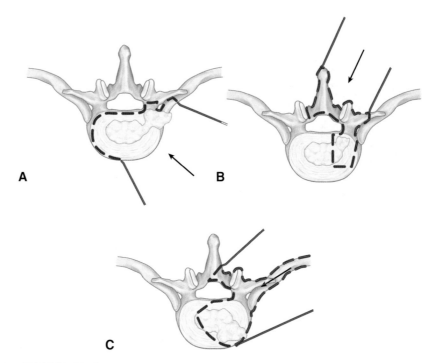

A

B

C

FIGURE 6A-C

Surgical Anatomy

- The neurovascular bundle runs on the inferior border of the rib. The rib heads are more cephalad (i.e., closer to the disk space) in the cephalad levels. Above T10, a complete rib head resection may be needed to expose the disk space (Johnson et al., 2000; Moro et al., 2004).

- *Use a bed with a break to allow lateral bending of the patient to open the rib interspaces in small patients.*

- *Position the patient parallel to the room architecture.*

- *Check fluoroscopy prior to incision to assure adequate imaging of appropriate level.*

- *Prepare ipsilateral iliac crest in case fusion procedure is necessary.*

- *Ensure that table can easily tilt anteriorly, to aid in lung retraction.*

- *Trendelenburg position can facilitate hemostasis.*

- *Poor positioning of monitors can hinder vision and flow of the operation.*

- *If there is a history of previous thoracic surgery, strongly consider entering the chest from the contralateral side to avoid adhesions and scar tissue.*

- *Vacuum sand bag, intraoperative monitoring wires, and bed attachments in line with the fluoroscope may hinder high-quality intraoperative images.*

Equipment

- A standard radiolucent table with a kidney rest; break table to open rib interspace, if necessary.
- Bolsters that attach to the table may assist with lateral positioning; however, pillows, straps, and tape are sufficient.

- For a T7/8 diskectomy, the T8 rib head should be resected.
- The disk space is cephalad to the pedicle.
- The artery of Adamkiewicz is usually on the left and between T9 and L3.
- Segmental vessels are located in the midportion of the vertebral body. For a diskectomy, these can be moved aside or coagulated, if necessary.
- The diaphragm can be injured if portal entry is below T7.

Positioning

- Give prophylactic antiobiotics for gram-positive organism coverage.
- The proper surgical team, anesthesiologist, and monitoring setup is crucial.
- Apply stockings and sequential pneumatic compression.
- A double-lumen endotracheal tube is placed for single-lung ventilation.
- The patient is placed in the lateral decubitus position with the ventilated lung down (Fig. 7). The arm is held in an "airplane"-type holder to expose the chest wall.
- Pad all bony prominences and superficial nerves (e.g., peroneal and ulnar nerves).
- Prepare patient for possible thoracotomy. Also, prepare the patient's back for a possible simultaneous posterior approach.
- The surgeon and assistant should stand on the abdominal side of the patient. A second assistant can

Endoscopic Equipment

- 15-mm soft portals.
- Endoscope with conventional 5- or 10-mm lenses with 0°, 30°, or 45° angles (Fig. 8A). The angled scopes prevent "fencing" within the chest (30° angled scope is ideal).
- Standard illumination source, camera attachment, and video monitor.
- Pneumatic drill with a long shaft (25 cm) and pistol grip for rotational control (Fig. 8B).
- Coarse diamond burr or large round burr (5 mm) (Fig. 8C).
- Long-shaft Kerrison rongeurs, Cobb elevators, pituitaries, and currettes (Fig. 8D).
- Endoscopic cotton-tipped applicators.
- Harmonic scalpel (Ethicon Endosurgery, Cincinnati, OH).
- Long-shaft Fraser suction.
- Endoscopic fan blade for retraction of the lung.

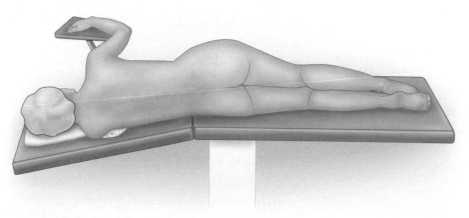

FIGURE 7

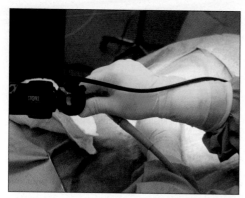

A

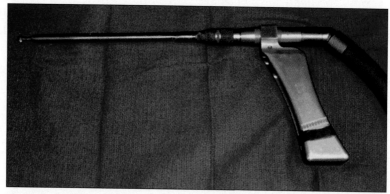

B

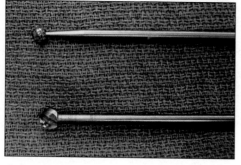

C

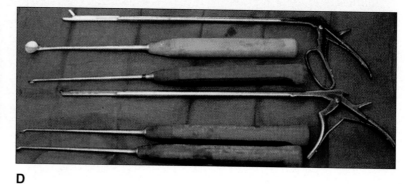

D

FIGURE 8A-D

Controversies

- Positioning the patient for either a left- or right-sided approach has been described.
- The thick and resilient aorta is less prone to injury on the left compared with the azygous system; however, in lower thoracic approaches the liver may interfere with exposure.

PEARLS

- *Prior to incision tape radiopaque markers (e.g., paperclips) on the patient's back and obtain a posteroanterior thoracic spine radiograph to mark the appropriate level. Then draw a line perpendicular to the side of the chest wall to localize the entry point of the portals.*

- *Use soft portals to prevent neuritis.*

- *Suture or staple the portals to the skin to prevent them from dislodging.*

- *A table attachment can be used to hold the endoscope within the chest once a diagnostic thoracoscopy is completed and the diskectomy is being performed.*

PITFALLS

- *The lung should be retracted cautiously to allow exposure to the spine.*

- *Portals not centered over the lesion will hinder adequate decompression.*

- *The diaphragm can be injured with portals below T7.*

stand on the back side of the patient in case extra instruments are necessary (Fig. 9).
- The monitors should be on both sides of the patient directly facing the surgeon, assistants, and operating room technician.

Portals/Exposures

- Three to four portals are usually sufficient to insert the endoscope, retractor, and suction-irrigation instrument and to perform the diskectomy.
- Portal placement should proceed with an incision centered on the rib and blunt dissection over the superior border (Fig. 10).
- The main working portal should be placed in the posterior axillary line, perpendicular to the

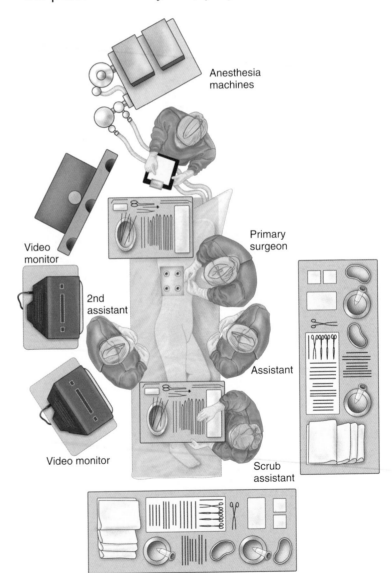

Anesthesia machines

Video monitor

2nd assistant

Video monitor

Primary surgeon

Assistant

Scrub assistant

FIGURE 9

Instrumentation

• *A trocar device is needed for penetrating the tough muscular abdominal wall (see Fig. 10).*

Controversies

• *Soft portals are less likely to cause thoracic neuritis, but hard portals are less likely to collapse and may facilitate introduction and withdrawal of instruments.*

PEARLS

• *The disk space and proximal rib head are co-linear and can keep the surgeon oriented.*

• *The neural foramen contains epidural fat that can be used to indicate proximity of the nerve root.*

• *To ensure the appropriate operative level, intraoperative fluoroscopy or radiograph of a metallic instrument overlying the disk space should be compared with preoperative radiographs and MRI scans.*

PITFALLS

• *A Steinmann pin can be inserted into the disk space for intraoperative radiographic localization; however, this may injure a normal disk if inserted at the wrong level.*

pathologic location (Fig. 11). However, the first portal should be above the sixth or seventh rib to avoid the diaphragm. Insert the other portals under direct visualization.

- Two to three other accessory portals can be placed in the anterior axillary line, cephalad and caudad to the main working portal, to triangulate within the chest (see Fig. 11).

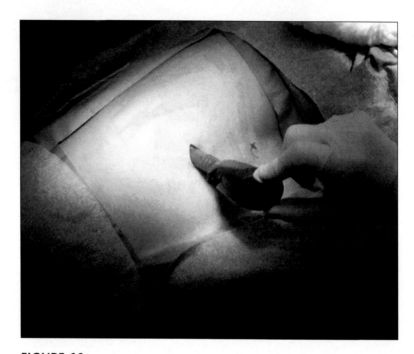

FIGURE 10

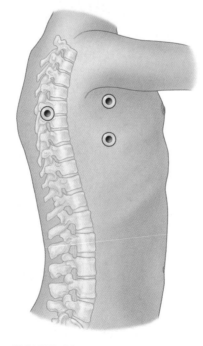
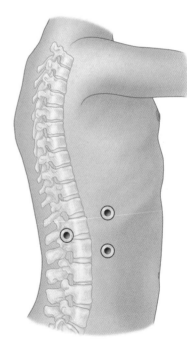

FIGURE 11

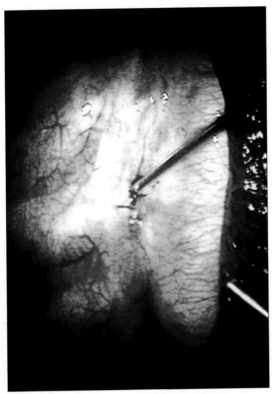

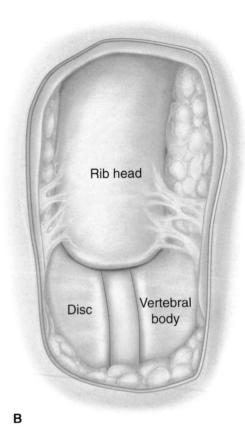

Rib head

Disc

Vertebral body

FIGURE 12A-B **A** **B**

- The perpendicular portal is usually where the drill and rongeurs are inserted, but all the portals can be used for passing various instruments to proceed with the diskectomy safely.

Procedure

STEP 1

- Once portals are made and the lung retracted anteriorly with a fan retractor, the disk space is located by tracing the rib to the spine.
- Fluoroscopy or an anteroposterior thoracic spine radiograph can be taken with a metallic instrument on the disk space to confirm appropriate level (Fig. 12).
- Adjacent segmental vessels can be retracted or cauterized depending on the extent of bony decompression.
- The parietal pleura is widely dissected off the rib head and disk space using a Harmonic scalpel (Ethicon Endosurgery, Cincinnati, OH) (Fig. 13).
- The proximal 2 cm of the rib are removed with a pneumatic drill to expose the lateral wall of the pedicle and neural foramen (Fig. 14).
- The pedicle is then drilled away to expose the dura of the spinal cord.

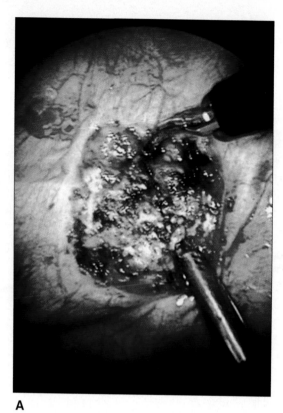

A

FIGURE 13A-B

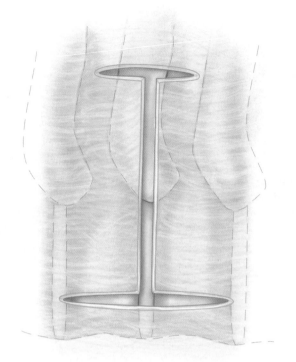

B

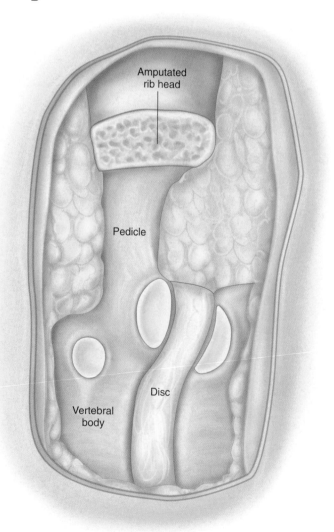

FIGURE 14

PEARLS

- *A 5-mm burr may be used for more aggressive decompression depending on surgeon preference.*

PITFALLS

- *Bleeding may be encountered during burring of the end plates and vertebral bodies. Control is obtained with bone wax on an endoscopic cotton-tipped applicator.*

STEP 2

- Subsequent to removal of the pedicle and exposure of the neural foramen and epidural fat, the posterior margin of the vertebral body is palpated and the superior and inferior end plates are drilled away (Fig. 15).
- Begin drilling from the posterior margin of the vertebral body to approximately one third of the sagittal distance, leaving a cortical shell posteriorly to protect the ventral aspect of the spinal cord.
- The anterior two thirds of the vertebral body should be left intact.
- The cephalad and caudad extension of the vertebral body decompression depends on the size and migration of the herniated disk fragment.

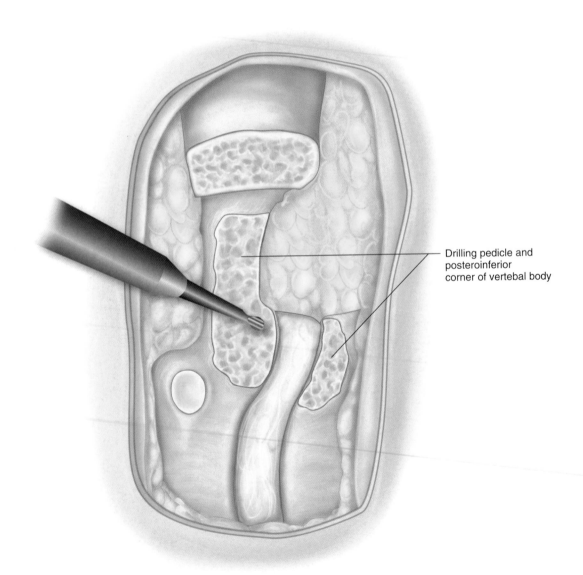

Drilling pedicle and posteroinferior corner of vertebal body

FIGURE 15

STEP 3

- Burr the tunnel to the opposite pedicle depending on the size of the disk herniation.
- Confirm location of the burr with anteroposterior fluoroscopy.
- Once burring is completed, the floor of the canal that is left as a cortical shell can be removed with fine currettes or Kerrison rongeurs.
- The portion of the disk that is not herniated and is between the vertebral bodies is removed.
- A rent is made in the posterior longitudinal ligament with a blunt probe or nerve hook and the ligament is subsequently resected with Kerrison rongeurs.
- The remaining herniated portion of the disk is subsequently pulled into the defect created by the bony decompression (Fig. 16).

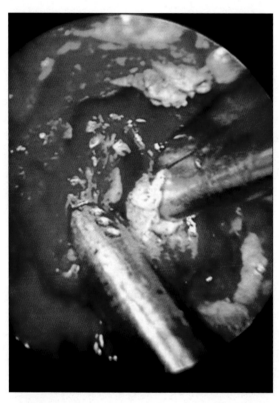

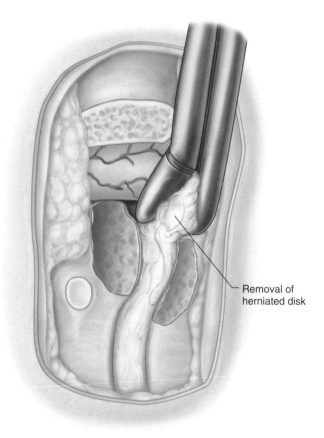

Removal of herniated disk

FIGURE 16

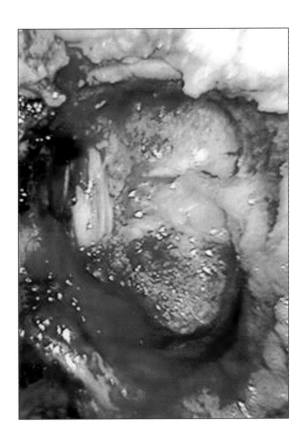

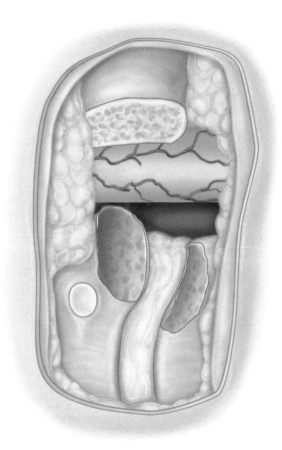

FIGURE 17

Controversies

- Extensive decompression could lead to increased mobility of the spinal segment. Potentially, this could lead to increased axial back pain and disability. Certain patients could benefit from a fusion after decompression (Anand and Regan, 2002). According to Broc et al. (1997), a cadaveric study showed slightly increased instability after endoscopic thoracic diskectomy without gross instability.

- A calcified disk can be cracked and pulled into the decompressed space. This allows complete decompression of the spinal cord without any manipulation (Fig. 17).

STEP 4

- A chest tube is placed through one of the portals or through a separate incision, tunneled through the subcutaneous tissue, and guided endoscopically to the apex of the chest cavity.
- Suction is applied at 20 cm H_2O, and the lung is reinflated.
- A chest radiograph is obtained after extubation to ensure that the lung is inflated.
- The fascia is sutured with 2-0 Vicryl and the skin with 3-0 Vicryl subcuticular interrupted sutures, followed by Steri-Strips over the incision.

Postoperative Care and Expected Outcomes

- The chest tube is removed when drainage is less than 100 ml/day; usually by postoperative day 2.
- The patient is ambulated on postoperative day 1.
- Oral analgesic medications are usually sufficient for adequate pain control.

SURGICAL OUTCOMES

- Patients with severe myelopathy or dense neurologic loss usually stabilize or slightly improve (Anand and Regan, 2002; Johnson et al., 2000; Oskouian and Johnson, 2005).
- Patients with milder forms of myelopathy generally have significant improvement (Johnson et al., 2000; Oskouian and Johnson, 2005). Figure 18A shows a preoperative T2-weighted MRI in a patient with acute ventral herniated nucleus pulposis causing myelopathy. The T1-weighted MRI in Figure 18B was taken after thoracoscopic decompression with complete resolution of symptoms. Note that the extent of the bony decompression should be large enough to reduce the herniated disk without manipulation of the spinal cord.
- Axial back pain or thoracic radiculopathy also improves after thoracoscopic diskectomy, albeit the results are more modest, paralleling treatment for mechanical lumbar back pain (Anand and Regan, 2002; Rosenthal and Dickman, 1998).

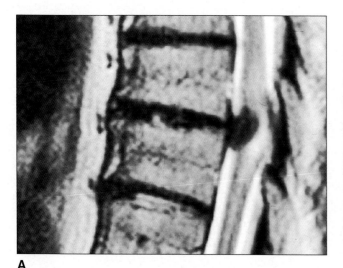

A

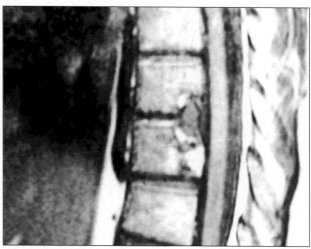

B

FIGURE 18A-B

COMPLICATIONS AND AVOIDANCE

- Intercostal neuralgia
  - Most common complication.
  - Usually due to stiff portals.
  - Most cases will subside (Le Huec et al., 2002).
- Atelectasis
  - Common after single-lung ventilation.
  - Aggressive pulmonary toilet postoperatively decreases complications from atelectasis.
  - Early in the learning curve, consider reinflating the lung for 5 minutes every hour of the procedure (Rosenthal and Dickman, 1998).
- Pneumonia: generally not as common in endoscopic cases compared to thoracotomy (Rosenthal and Dickman, 1998).
- Retained disk fragment:
  - Ensure preoperative location of disk fragment on imaging studies in case a fragment has migrated cephalad or caudad.
  - Palpate posterior to vertebral bodies with fine-angle curettes.
- Neurologic loss or paralysis:
  - Potentially due to retained disk fragment.
  - Could be caused by manipulation of cord.
  - Ensure that bony decompression is adequate before "reducing" herniated disk fragment into decompressed area.
- Dural tear:
  - Dura may have adhesions to disk fragment.
  - Usually primary repair or patching is important in chest cavity due to negative pressure.
  - In case of a persistent dural leak, place a lumbar drain and keep the chest tube on waterseal drainage.
- Persistent chest tube drainage: meticulous hemostasis during decompression with application of bone wax to bleeding surface of bone can avoid this.

Evidence

Anand N, Regan JJ. Video-assisted thoracoscopic surgery for thoracic disc disease: classification and outcome study of 100 consecutive cases with a 2-year minimum follow-up. Spine. 2002;27:871-9.

Grade B recommendation for decompressing thoracic spine with a herniated nucleus pulposus. A prospective study of 100 patients with thoracic disk herniations undergoing endoscopic excision showed safety and clinical improvement, especially in patients with myelopathy. (Level 2 evidence)

Bohlman, HH, Zdeblick, TA. Anterior excision of herniated thoracic discs. J Bone Joint Surg Am. 1988;70:1038-47.

Grade B recommendation for excision of herniated disk using costotransversectomy or transthoracic approach based on retrospective results of 22 patients.

Broc GG, Crawford NR, Sonntag VKH, Dickman CA. Biomechanical effects of transthoracic microdiscectomy. Spine. 1997;22:605-12.

Grade B recommendation for not fusing thoracic spine after diskectomy. This cadaver study showed that endoscopic or microscopic diskectomy did not significantly destabilize the thoracic spine despite slight increase in mobility.

Di Chiro G, Fried LC, Doppman JL. Experimental spinal cord angiography. Br J Radiol.1970;43:19-30.

Grade B recommendation for choosing a right-sided approach to the thoracolumbar spine due to the vascular supply. This is an anatomic study investigating spinal cord blood supply.

Holly LT, Bloch O, Obasi C, Johnson JP. Frameless stereotaxy for anterior spinal procedures. J Neurosurg Spine. 2001;95:196-201.

Grade B recommendation supporting the use of stereotactic guidance in spinal surgery to increase accuracy with instrumentation and decompression of the anterior spine.

Johnson JP, Filler AG, Mc Bride DQ. Endoscopic thoracic discectomy. Neurosurg Focus. 2000;9:Article 11.

Grade B recommendation for safely excising a thoracic disk herniation using the thoracoscopic approach. This is a prospective study of 36 patients who underwent thoracoscopic diskectomy and 8 patients who underwent diskectomy through an open thoracotomy.

Le Huec JC, Lesprite E, Touagliaro F, Hadidaner R, Magendie J, Husson JL. Complications of thoracoscopic spinal surgery: Analysis of a series of patients. J Bone Joint Surg Br. 2002;84:44.

Grade B recommendation for endoscopic treatment over open thoracotomy procedures for disk herniations, tumor, and fracture care.

Moro T, Kikuchi S, Konno S. Necessity of rib head resection for anterior discectomy in the thoracic spine. Spine. 2004;29:1703-05.

Grade B recommendation for complete rib head removal above T9 (cadaver study).

Oskouian RJ, Johnson JP. Endoscopic thoracic microdiscectomy. J Neurosurg Spine. 2005;99:459-64.

Grade B recommendation for treating thoracic disk herniation with endoscopic technique. Forty-six patients were followed prospectively after endoscopic thoracic diskectomy.

Rosenthal D, Dickman CA. Thoracoscopic microsurgical excision of herniated thoracic discs. J Neurosurg. 1998;89:224-35.

Grade B recommendation for endoscopic thoracic diskectomy over thoracotomy with respect to safety and outcome. Thirty-six patients were in the endoscopic group and 18 patients were in the thoracotomy group.

VEPTR Opening Wedge Thoracostomy for Congenital Spinal Deformities

Robert M. Campbell, Jr.

PITFALLS

- *Progressive thoracic insufficiency syndrome, the prime FDA indication for VEPTR treatment, is difficult to define. Thoracic insufficiency syndrome (TIS) is the inability of the thorax to support normal respiration or lung growth (Campbell et al., 2004), and the presence of either component enables the diagnosis of TIS. The disabled thorax, such as seen in a child with fused ribs, cannot expand the lung with chest wall motion on the involved side, so normal biomechanical respiration is not possible. The same thorax, if unable to grow properly because of the rib cage constriction due to rib fusion, also has the second component of TIS.*

- *TIS does not mean a child requires oxygen support. Pediatric patients needing oxygen, continuous positive airway pressure, or ventilator support have respiratory insufficiency, which means the respiratory mechanism is unable to provide physiologic oxygenation for the needs of the patient. Respiratory insufficiency may be due to intrinsic disease of the lungs and/or severe thoracic disability from volume depletion deformity (Campbell et al., 2003a) or abnormal thoracic function. Occult respiratory insufficiency syndrome in children with early TIS may be masked by an increase in respiratory rate, or adaptive behavior through reduction in activity levels for age. End-stage TIS almost always has associated respiratory insufficiency syndrome.*

Indications

- The titanium rib, or VEPTR (vertical expandable prosthetic titanium rib), is approved by the Food and Drug Administration (FDA) and available for use under the Humanitarian Device Exemption regulations. One approved use is for constrictive chest wall disorders, including fused ribs and scoliosis.
  - Progressive thoracic congenital scoliosis in patients age 6 months to skeletal maturity
  - Three or more fused ribs at the apex of the concave hemithorax
  - Greater than 10% reduction in space available for lung (Campbell et al., 2004)
  - Presence of progressive thoracic insufficiency syndrome (Campbell et al., 2004)

Examination/Imaging

- Patients are evaluated for curve flexibility, head decompensation, trunkal decompensation, and trunk rotation.

Controversies

- Patients with TIS and congenital scoliosis who are almost at the age of skeletal maturity: If thoracic height is near normal and thoracic volume and function adequate, then the growth-sparing aspect of VEPTR treatment on the spine deformity will have marginal impact on lung growth, so definitive spine fusion is preferable.
- Isolated hemivertebra of thoracolumbar congenital scoliosis with limited rib fusion: If the thoracic spine is near normal height for age and treatment with hemivertebrectomy or hemiarthrodesis/hemiepiphyseodesis would involve three segments or less, then these techniques are preferable to VEPTR treatment.
- Mobile chest wall on the concave side of the curve: Although invariably the chest wall on the concave side of the curve is stiff from rib fusion and the potential for VEPTR treatment to stiffen the concave chest wall is thus a moot point, if the thumb excursion test does show mobility with normal outward motion of the concave chest wall during respiration, then a growth-sparing treatment other than VEPTR should be considered.

Treatment Options

- Limited (one or two spinal segment) hemivertebrectomy or convex hemiarthrodesis/ hemiepiphyseodesis for isolated hemivertebra when the thoracic spine is of relatively normal length and the chest wall is mobile.
- Growing rod instrumentation of the spine when the congenital spine deformity is more extensive and the chest wall is mobile on the concave side of the curve.
- Posterior spine fusion for patients approaching skeletal maturity, when expansion of the chest will have no effect on growth of the underlying lungs.

- Resting respiratory rate is measured and compared to normative values. An elevated rate suggests the child has occult respiratory insufficiency. The lips are examined for cyanosis. The fingers are examined for clubbing, a sign of chronic respiratory insufficiency, and the percentile normal weight for age is determined. When the work of breathing is excessive, children are often underweight.
- Thoracic function due to chest wall expansion is assessed by the thumb excursion test (Campbell et al, 2004).
  - The examiner's hands are lightly placed on each side of the patient, around the lateral base of the thorax, with the thumbs in back pointing upward medially, equidistant from the spine (Fig. 1). The patient breathes spontaneously, and rib cage motion carries the thumbs outward away from the spine. Greater than 1 cm of thumb motion away from the spine is normal and is graded as a +3 thumb excursion test; 0.5–1 cm is a +2 thumb excursion test, less than 0.5 cm motion is +1, and no thumb excursion with respiration is graded +0.
  - Causes of abnormal thumb excursion test include extensive fused ribs or the distortion of rib hump. Absent chest wall motion is a sign of TIS since the rib cage cannot aid the diaphragm in expanding the lung during normal respiration.
- Radiographs should include anteroposterior (AP) and lateral films of the entire spine, including the entire rib cage and the pelvis. These are assessed for Cobb angle, space available for the lungs, and head and

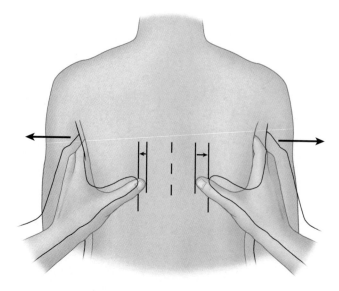

FIGURE 1

trunkal decompensation (Fig. 2). Space available for the lungs is determined by the ratio of the height of the concave lung from the middle of the most proximal rib to the top of the hemidiaphragm compared to the height of the convex lung measured in the same fashion. Head decompensation is measured from the center sacral line to the middle of C7, and truncal decompensation is measured from the midthorax at T6 to the center sacral line.

■ Supine lateral bending radiographs are used to determine curve flexibility and apex of rib cage constriction on the concave side of the curve (Fig. 3, *arrow*). In cases of thoracic kyphosis, a cross-table lateral radiograph of the spine with a bolster at the apex of the curve is included to assess for flexibility.

■ Cervical spine films, with flexion/extension laterals, are performed to assess for cervical spine abnormalities and instability.

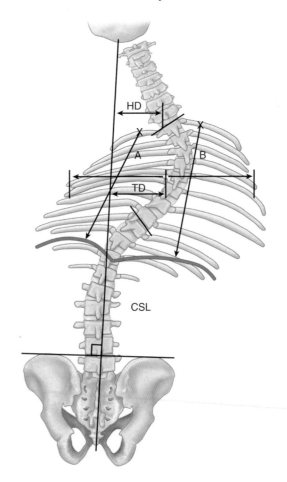

A/B = SAL
HD = Head decompensation
TD = Trunk decompensation

FIGURE 2

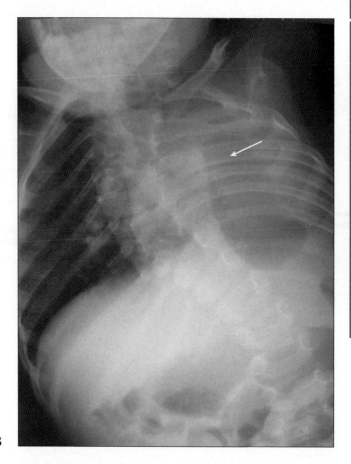

FIGURE 3

■ Computed tomography (CT) scans of the chest and spine are performed, unenhanced, at 0.5-cm intervals from T1 to the sacrum, to assess for three-dimensional spine and rib cage abnormality. Thoracic rotation from rotation of the spine into the convex hemithorax with loss of lung volume is the angle between the sagittal plane of the spine and the sternum (Fig. 4). To minimize radiation exposure, the scan should be performed at pediatric settings, with appropriate milliamperage and pitch angle.

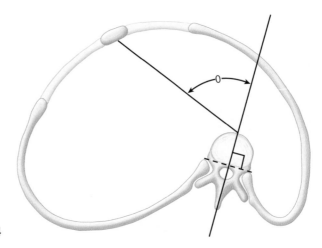

FIGURE 4

- Fluoroscopy of the diaphragm is performed to document normal function.
- Magnetic resonance imaging of the entire spinal cord is performed to assess for spinal cord abnormalities.

Surgical Anatomy

- Proximally, the common insertion of the middle and the posterior scalene muscle on the first and second ribs is identified. The brachial plexus and the artery lie immediately anterior to this (Fig. 5). It is an important landmark since the neurovascular bundle is just anterior. The safe zone for VEPTR proximal rib cradle attachment is posterior to the scalene muscles, extending from the second through the fourth ribs. Attachment anterior to the scalene muscles or posterior to the first rib endangers the neurovascular bundle.
- Absent ribs in the exposure are identified by palpating the flail area. These are commonly associated with dysraphism of the spine, and care should be taken to avoid violating the spinal canal in the dissection. The preoperative CT scan commonly identifies bony defects in the canal. Figure 6 shows the CT scan of an infant with a spinal dysraphism with the meningocele extending up to the medial border of the scapula that was poorly appreciated on radiographs. In surgery, the scapula was gently retracted upward and the rhomboid muscles dissected just adjacent to the edge of the scapula so that the dura was not injured.

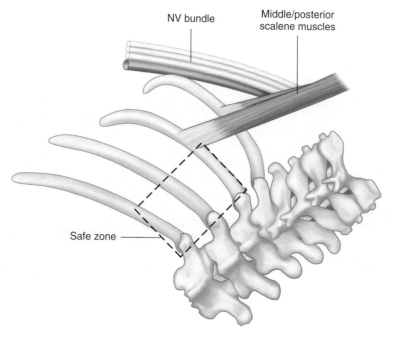

FIGURE 5

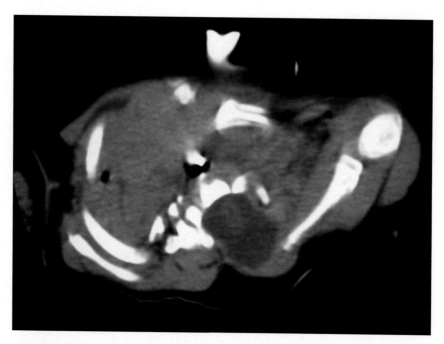

FIGURE 6

PEARLS

- *An axillary roll is used as well as a pad under the pelvis and the lower extremities. A soft bolster pad is placed under the apex of the thoracic deformity to help provide correction.*

- *A pulse oximeter is placed on the upward hand to monitor vascularity of the upper extremity. Both upper and lower extremities are monitored for spinal cord function with somatosensory evoked potentials and transcranial motor evoked potentials.*

PITFALLS

- *Do not allow the upper arms to extend beyond 90° because this puts tension on the brachial plexus.*

Controversies

- If a contralateral VEPTR device is also to be placed on the convex hemithorax, the patient is placed in the prone position, with care taken to drape the concave opening thoracostomy side low enough on the operating room table to allow adequate thoracotomy exposure.

Positioning

- The patient is placed in a modified lateral decubitus position with the torso tilted slightly forward (15°) (Fig. 7).
- The upper extremities are draped outside the exposure. They are positioned with the shoulders in 90° of flexion with the elbows also flexed. An axillary roll is placed, along with another soft bolster under the apex of the convex hemithorax. The extremities are immobilized by placing hand towels on the midcalf and the hips with a 2-inch cloth tape used to strap across the patient.
- Central venous line, arterial pressure monitoring line, urinary catheter, and spinal cord monitoring leads are placed.

Portals/Exposures

- To avoid skin slough, a long curvilinear incision is made, beginning proximally between the posterior spinous process of the spine at T1 and the medial edge of the scapula, extending distally down to the 10th rib, then anteriorly in a gentle curve along the rib to the posterior axillary line (Fig. 8).
- The trapezius, latissimus dorsi, and rhomboid muscles are divided by cautery in line with the skin incision.
- The scapula is gently retracted laterally.
- An interval is developed by blunt dissection between the chest wall and the overlying scapula, anteriorly to the costochondral junction, and superiorly up to the first rib. The middle and posterior scalene muscle insertion on the first and second rib is identified in order to protect the neurovascular bundle just anterior to the muscle.

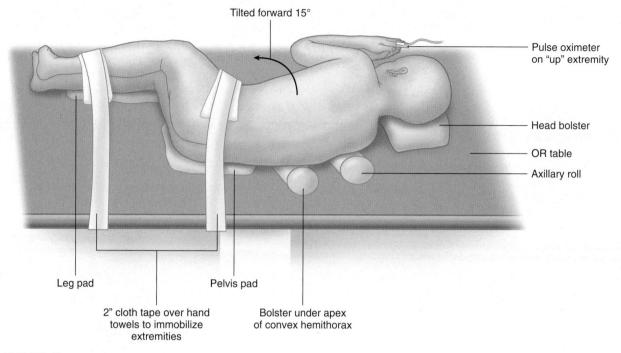

Tilted forward 15°

Pulse oximeter on "up" extremity

Head bolster

OR table

Axillary roll

Leg pad

Pelvis pad

2" cloth tape over hand towels to immobilize extremities

Bolster under apex of convex hemithorax

FIGURE 7

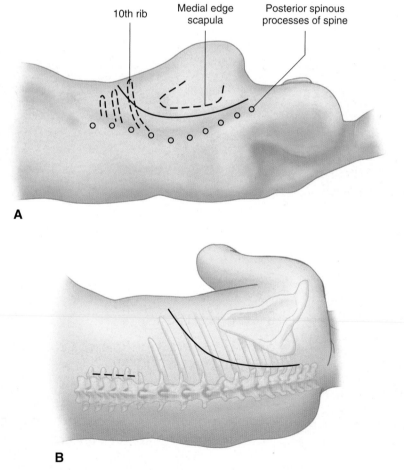

10th rib

Medial edge scapula

Posterior spinous processes of spine

A

B

FIGURE 8A-B

PEARLS

• *In congenital deformity of the thorax and spine, commonly the anatomy is very distorted with rib fusion and anomalous muscle insertion. The scalene muscles, however, are consistently present and, although anomalous in appearance, can often be palpated readily, thus providing a landmark for identification of the neurovascular bundle anteriorly.*

• *For purposes of identifying correct rib levels for insertion of devices, the first rib can usually be palpated posteriorly between the common insertion of the scalene muscles and the tips of the transverse processes, and levels then counted distally through palpation.*

PITFALLS

• *Care should be taken to avoid damaging the spinal cord in areas of dysraphic spine adjacent to rib absence.*

• *In Sprengel's deformity, associated with fused ribs and scoliosis, there is commonly a fibrous or bony connection between the spine and the upwardly displaced hypoplastic scapula, but if there is dysraphism, the medial edge of the scapula may actually be inside the spinal canal, adjacent to the spinal cord. In this anatomic variant, a regular thoracotomy approach may injure the spinal cord when the rhomboid muscles are released medially, so in these cases the scapula is gently retracted upward out of the canal by a small rake and the medial muscles carefully stripped off the scapula above the canal, with care taken not to enter the dura to avoid spinal cord injury (Fig. 10). A preoperative CT scan can define this variant.*

■ The separate incision for the hybrid laminar spinal hook is to be made one centimeter lateral to midline of the proximal lumbar spine posterior spinal processes.

■ The paraspinal muscles are reflected by cautery, laterally to medially, up to the tips of the transverse spinous processes, leaving a 1-mm thick layer of soft tissue overlying the ribs to avoid rib devacularization (Fig. 9). The spine is not uncovered in order to avoid in advertent fusion.

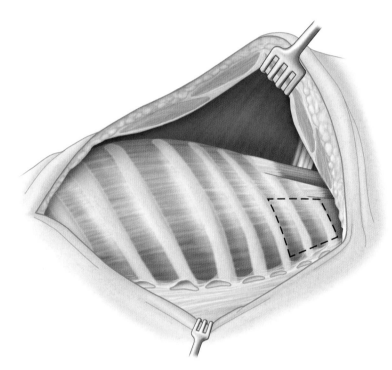

FIGURE 9

Procedure

STEP 1: INSERTION OF SUPERIOR RIB CRADLE FOR THE HYBRID VEPTR

■ After exposure is completed, the level of the insertion of the superior rib cradle is located. This is based on radiographic evidence and confirmed by locating the first rib by palpation and counting ribs downward. The superior cradle should be placed at the proximal end of the rib cage constriction, which is commonly proximal to the apex of the congenital spinal curve.

Instrumentation

- It is helpful to retract the scapula with an Israel retractor placed under the scapula, with two small towel clips clamped under the muscle tissue in the manner of M.D. Smith. The clips are then attached by Ray-tec sponges around the larger retractor. The Israel retractor is then attached by a Ray-tec sponge to a large towel clip attached to an ether screen bar at the head of the operating table (Fig. 11). This provides excellent self-retraction.

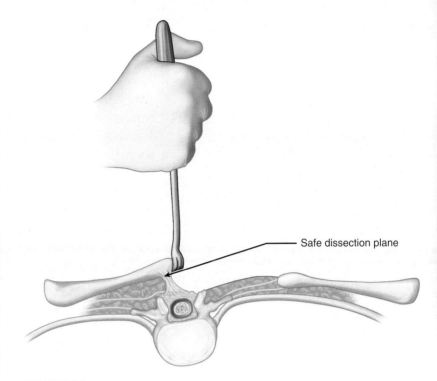

Safe dissection plane

FIGURE 10

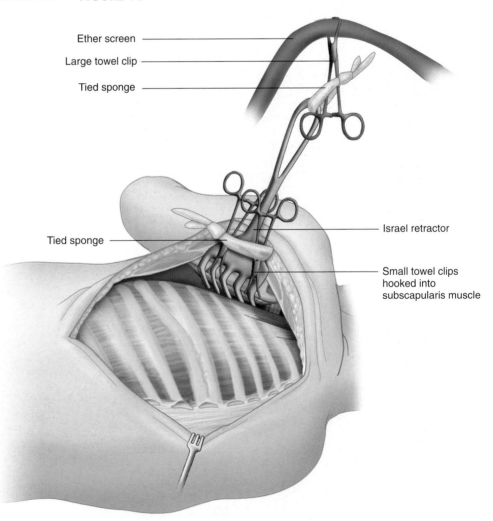

Ether screen

Large towel clip

Tied sponge

Tied sponge

Israel retractor

Small towel clips hooked into subscapularis muscle

FIGURE 11

Controversies

- The long, sweeping distal thoracotomy incision is performed for two reasons: a long thoracotomy flap is easier to stretch for closure after opening wedge thoracostomy and, in females, a more distal flap avoids cutting across breast tissue, which reduces risk of later breast growth disturbance in adolescents.

PEARLS

- *If the site of attachment chosen for the superior cradle is a thin rib, then two ribs can be encircled to increase strength of attachment, using an extended cradle cap.*

- *If the ribs of attachment are somewhat mobile, the site of attachment can be moved medially to encompass 5 mm of the transverse processes for increased strength.*

- *If either the superior or inferior attachment point of the rib cradle is within a sheet of solid bone of fused ribs, then a channel for insertion of the superior cradle, 5 mm by 1.5 cm, can be cut with a power burr, adjacent to the transverse process tip.*

PITFALLS

- *Take care not to insert the rib cradle above the thoracic constriction in a mobile proximal segment of spine. The distraction force of the VEPTR will overcorrect the proximal thoracic spine into a compensatory curve, without effect on either the primary thoracic constriction or the congenital scoliosis.*

The site is marked by cautery just lateral to the tips of the transverse processes.

- A 1-cm portal for insertion of the superior cradle is made by cautery at the correct level in the midportion of the intercostal muscle or the fibrous adhesion between ribs, just adjacent to the tip of the transverse processes.

- Another portal, 5 mm in width, is placed superiorly for the upper portion of the superior cradle, called the cradle cap. If a standard cradle cap is used, then approximately 1 cm of distance should separate the inferior and superior portals for the rib cradle. If an extended cradle is used to surround more bone or even two ribs, then a 1.5-cm distance is needed.

- A curved Freer elevator is then inserted through an intercostal incision into the inferior portal, pointed proximally, and is used to strip away the combined pleura/periosteum from the anterior surface of the rib, carefully creating a soft tissue tunnel up to the superior portal without damaging the neurovascular bundle. Next, a second Freer elevator is inserted into the superior portal and touched to the tip of the inferior Freer elevator in order to verify that a continuous soft tissue tunnel has been developed (Fig. 12).

- The trial for the device is then inserted into the inferior and the superior portals to enlarge the soft tissue tunnel.

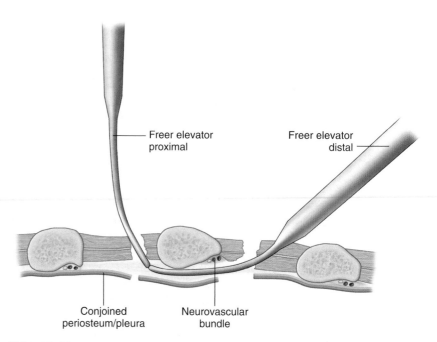

Freer elevator proximal

Freer elevator distal

Conjoined periosteum/pleura

Neurovascular bundle

FIGURE 12

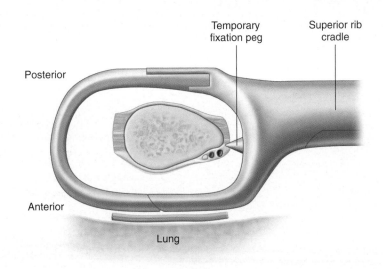

Controversies

- If, after placement of the superior cradle, the rib(s) of attachment are found to be too weak for effective distraction, then the superior cradle should be reinserted around a stable rib more distally.

Instrumentation/ Implantation

- The superior cradle cap is inserted by forceps into the superior portal, deep between the ribs, facing laterally to avoid the esophagus and the great vessels, and is then rotated downward into position.
- Next, the superior cradle is inserted into the inferior portal deeply, with the temporary fixation pegs anterior to the rib to hold the device in low profile (Fig. 13). The superior cap is mated to the superior cradle and the cradle cap lock is used to lock the two together.
- If there is inability to completely engage the rib cap into the rib cradle because of soft tissue, then spinal compression forceps are used to compress the superior cradle and the cradle cap together and a cradle cap lock is added.
- The forceps attached to the cradle cap are removed, and the forceps attached to the rib cradle are used to gently move it upward to verify stability.

Temporary fixation peg

Superior rib cradle

Posterior

Anterior

Lung

FIGURE 13

STEP 2: OPENING WEDGE THORACOSTOMY

- The opening wedge thoracostomy is then performed at the center of the thoracic constriction. This is identified on plain AP radiographs, especially on the bending films, where there is an area of frank constriction of fused ribs or narrowed intercostal spaces.
- In a rib fusion mass of three or four ribs, generally an opening wedge thoracostomy through the center is recommended.
- The line of the thoracostomy is first marked by cautery at the correct level along the groove between fused ribs.
- The opening wedge thoracostomy is begun anteriorly where the ribs begin to separate, where there is usually fibrous tissue or an intercostal muscle interval that gradually narrows to a groove in the fused bone posteriorly (Fig. 14).
- Once this fibrous tissue or muscle has been lysed by Bovie cautery, a no. 4 Penfield elevator is inserted, pointing posteriorly along the line of the thoracostomy to be created, to strip away the pleura and periosteum for distance of 2 cm. Then a Kerrison rongeur or Midas Rex bone cutter is used to cut medially along the groove through the bone, with the Penfield elevator protecting the underlying soft tissues. This step is repeated until the tip of the transverse processes is reached.

PEARLS

- *The superior cradle is tilted medially at insertion because of the oblique position of the rib of attachment, but with successful hemithorax deformity correction through thoracostomy, it gradually assumes a position parallel to the longitudinal axis of the body, with transverse orientation of its rib of attachment.*

- *If the area of rib fusion on the concave side of the curve is greater than four ribs, a second or even third thoracostomy must be performed to completely correct the deformity, with at least two rib thicknesses between thoracostomies.*

- *It is important to use a soft tissue–sparing technique in performing the thoracostomy and inserting rib cradles. Stripping the periosteum over the ribs to facilitate exposure may devascularize the ribs and result in later absorption.*

- *Small rents in the pleura (under 2 cm) are not serious and do not need repair. Larger tears are patched with Surgisis® bioabsorbable membrane.*

- *Chest tubes are usually placed only if there is a "leak" from a visceral pleural tear of the lung or large quantities of pleural fluid are expected postoperatively.*

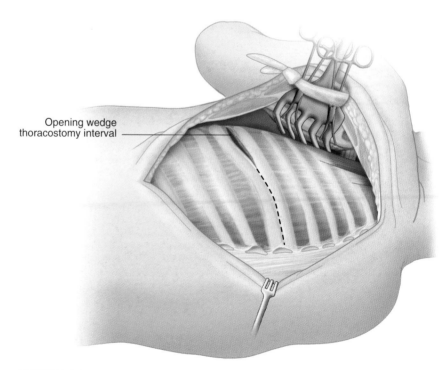

Opening wedge thoracostomy interval

FIGURE 14

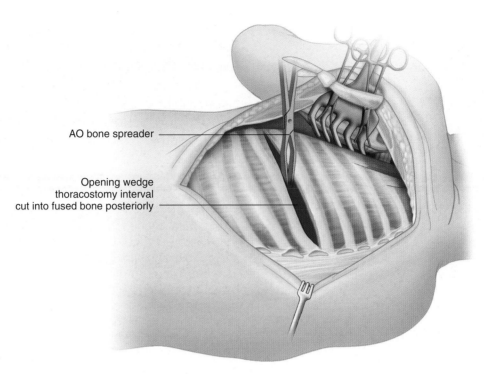

AO bone spreader

Opening wedge
thoracostomy interval
cut into fused bone posteriorly

FIGURE 15

■ The thoracostomy should also extend anteriorly to the costochondral junction.

■ If there is fibrous adhesion between ribs or intact intercostal muscle close to the center of the fused mass, the thoracostomy is preferentially placed there. In this case, the intercostal muscle or fibrous tissue is incised by cautery, with a right-angle clamp elevating the muscle to minimize damage to the underlying pleura.

■ Once the thoracostomy interval through bone, fibrous tissue, or intercostal muscle is complete, an AO bone spreader is inserted between the ribs to gradually widen the thoracostomy interval, with lengthening of the concave hemithorax and indirect correction of the scoliosis (Fig. 15).

■ The interval medial to the transverse processes should open easily, but if there is dense fibrous tissue, this is gently probed with a Freer elevator to lyse it, with care taken not to enter the spinal canal.

■ If bone is present medial to the tips of the transverse processes along the interval, it must be resected.

■ The fused rib is exposed carefully with a Freer elevator, with resection by a rongeur. A 1-cm wide channel is cut down to the vertebra. Care must be taken not to violate any anaomalous segmental arteries exiting through the rib fusion mass. Within 1 cm of the spine, the remaining bone is removed by a curved curette, using it to disarticulate the remaining medial portion of the fused rib.

- The AO bone spreader is removed, and a VEPTR rib retractor is placed to further enlarge the opening wedge thoracostomy.
- With a small moist sponge on a clamp, the pleura is then mobilized by rolling it down from the underlying periosteum of the ribs, both proximally and distally, from the line of the opening wedge.

Controversies

- The goal of VEPTR opening wedge thoracostomy is to create a lengthened hemithorax while indirectly correcting the scoliosis without spine fusion so that the thoracic spine can continue to grow and contribute to thoracic volume increase. There is no need to perform concurrent spine osteotomies, hemivertebrectomies, or convex hemiarthrodesis/hemiepiphyseodesis during VEPTR procedures. Unilateral segmented bars of the concave side of the curve increase in length, presumably from growth, with VEPTR treatment with effective growth of the thoracic spine (Campbell et al., 2003b). There is also risk of spine avulsion and severe neurologic injury if spine procedures are performed along with opening wedge thoracostomy because of the distraction power of the VEPTR device.

Step 3: The Hybrid VEPTR

- Once the proximal exposure for the hybrid VEPTR is complete, a lumbar spinal exposure is made distally to place a spinal hook for the hybrid VEPTR lumbar extension (Fig 8B).
- A 6-cm longitudinal skin incision is made just lateral to the proximal lumbar spine. Cautery is used to develop a flap extending medially to the midline. Only two vertebral levels are to be exposed.
- The apophysis of the two posterior spinous processes are split by cautery, and a Cobb elevator is used to strip the muscles laterally.
- The ligamentum flavum is resected.

Instrumentation

- The lamina hook is inserted into the interspace, pointing medially, then rotated distally.

Controversies

- Take care to place the hook well below any areas of junctional kyphosis to avoid progression of the deformity.

Pearls

- *Ensure that there is adequate room for hook insertion. Ligament flavum should be well resected for optimal position of the hook laterally. Partial laminotomy of the superior lamina may need to be performed to provide enough space for hook insertion.*

Pitfalls

- *Take care not to damage the cortex of the inferior lamina where the hook is to be placed. Once the cortex is violated, it becomes weakened. Partial laminotomies of the inferior lamina are also to be avoided for the same reason.*

- *Insert a no. 4 Penfield elevator distally between the dura and the lamina to free up any scarring so there is clearance for the hook.*

Instrumentation/ Implantation

- Once the device is in place, the chest tube is removed and the hybrid rod is threaded into the hook, and then the rib sleeve is then threaded into the superior cradle and locked with a distraction lock.
- The C-clamp is attached to the rod, the rod is distracted, the hook is tightened, and the clamp removed.
- When the rib distractor is then removed, the opening wedge thoracostomy should remain open from the distraction of the hybrid VEPTR if the device is properly tensioned (Fig. 17).

Controversies

- Although extremely rare, if there are changes is spinal cord monitoring of the lower extremities with distraction, then distraction is relaxed 0.5 cm and repeat tracings are performed.
- If changes persist, then distraction is further decreased until they cease.

STEP 4: IMPLANTATION OF THE HYBRID VEPTR

- The correct size of hybrid VEPTR device needed for implantation is determined by measuring the distance from the inferior part of the rib, attached to the superior rib cradle, to the inferior end plate of T12. The location of T12 can be estimated clinically by palpating the 12th rib. This distance in centimeters will correspond to numbers inscribed on the VEPTR rib sleeve and lumbar hybrid extension (Fig. 16).

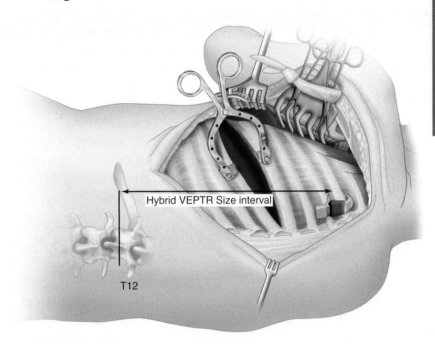

FIGURE 16

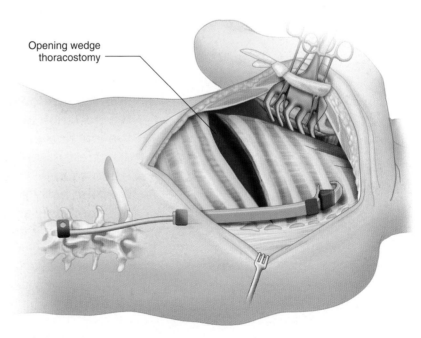

FIGURE 17

- The correctly sized device is placed into the operative field, and the end of the rod is marked 1.5 cm below the hook.
- The rod is cut, and the lumbar hybrid extension bent into mild lordosis and valgus to fit.
- An intramuscular tunnel is then created from the proximal to the distal incision for passage of the joined VEPTR rib sleeve and the lumbar hybrid extension. To safely accomplish this, a long Kelly clamp is first inserted through the proximal incision through the paraspinal muscles, distally toward the lumbar incision, with care taken not to penetrate the rib cage.
- Emerging in the distal incision just above the spinal hook, the clamp is attached to a no. 20 chest tube, which is pulled by the clamp into the proximal incision. The spinal rod end of the VEPTR rib sleeve and lumbar hybrid extension of correct length, locked with a distraction lock, is placed into the chest tube so the hybrid can be safely guided through muscle into the distal wound.

STEP 5: HYBRID VEPTR ATTACHMENT TO PELVIS BY DUNN-MCCARTHY HOOK OVER ILIAC CREST

- If there are inadequate posterior elements of the posterior spine for attachment of the VEPTR hybrid spine hook, such as in myelomeningocele or dysraphism in congenital scoliosis, distraction is achieved by bypassing the spine and attaching the VEPTR hybrid lumbar extension rod to the iliac crest through a Dunn-McCarthy hook placed on top of the iliac crest.
- A longitudinal 6-cm skin incision is made over the iliac crest on the side of the lumbar hybrid extension and carried down to the dorsal fascia, just lateral to the posterior superior iliac spine. The apophysis at the junction of the middle and posterior thirds of the iliac crest is exposed.
- Using cautery, the hip abductors are released over the bony part of the iliac crest just below the apophysis and reflected laterally with a Cobb elevator to create a pocket for the outer portion of the Dunn-McCarthy hook within the central third of the iliac crest (Fig. 18).

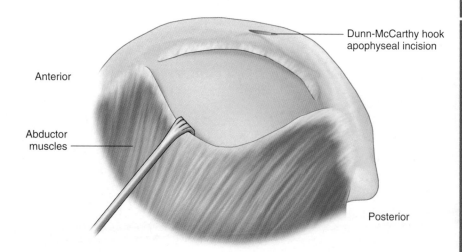

Anterior

Abductor
muscles

Dunn-McCarthy hook
apophyseal incision

Posterior

FIGURE 18

- A transverse incision is made in the middle of the apophysis with equal amounts of cartilage above and below. The interval is widened with Crigo elevators, and a tract is created over the anterior cortex of the iliac crest. The sacroiliac joint should be just medial to the tract. This is confirmed by placing a Crigo elevator through the apophyseal incision of the crest and then shifting the instrument to touch the lateral edge of the sacroiliac joint (Fig. 19). The Dunn-McCarthy hook is then inserted through the incision.

- Once the hook is in place, a 1 Prolene suture is placed through the apophysis and around the hook to help acutely immobilize the hook. A bone cap forms over the hook within 4 weeks of surgery.

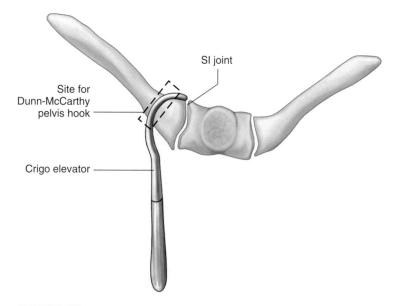

SI joint

Site for
Dunn-McCarthy
pelvis hook

Crigo elevator

FIGURE 19

Instrumentation

- After the Dunn-McCarthy hook is inserted, a 5- to 6-mm step-down domino coupling is placed over the hook with the 6-mm opening medial.
- A soft tissue channel from the proximal chest incision to the pelvic incision is made by a clamp and the chest tube is brought into the proximal wound.
- The lumbar hybrid extension and rib sleeve are sized to extend down to the bottom of T12. The rod is cut long enough to overlap the end of the Dunn-McCarthy hook by 2 cm and bent into mild lordosis. No valgus bending is necessary because the pelvis hook is directly in line with the proximal site of attachment of the device.
- The assembled rib sleeve, and lumbar hybrid extension, with distraction lock are threaded by the chest tube into the pelvic incision.
- The lumbar extension is first passed into the domino, then mated with the superior cradle, and locked to the superior cradle with the distraction lock.
- The device is distracted through the rod end, and the domino is tightened (Fig. 21).

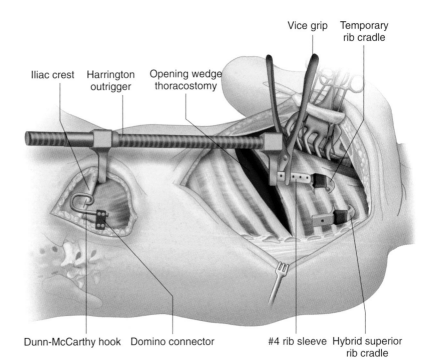

Vice grip   Temporary rib cradle

Iliac crest   Harrington outrigger   Opening wedge thoracostomy

Dunn-McCarthy hook   Domino connector   #4 rib sleeve   Hybrid superior rib cradle

FIGURE 20

Controversies

- The Dunn-McCarthy hooks will gradually migrate distally into the pelvis with time. This is generally not symptomatic, and they can migrate several centimeters into the crest without harm. The hook may require revision if symptomatic, or if the tip of the hook is within 5 mm of the acetabulum.
- The incision is reopened, and the abductor muscles are stripped off the hook and the domino coupling. The iliac crest usually has reformed and is often thicker than normal above the migrated hook. The domino is removed and a small curette is used to remove some of the bone just above the hook end penetrating the crest. The hook is then pulled free. The Dunn-McCarthy hook can be reinserted easily on top of the reformed iliac crest in its former position (Fig. 22).
- Avoid implanting the hook backward on the iliac crest. Reseating such hooks is difficult because the bulk of the hook and its domino will eventually migrate deep into the pelvis anterior to the iliac crest.

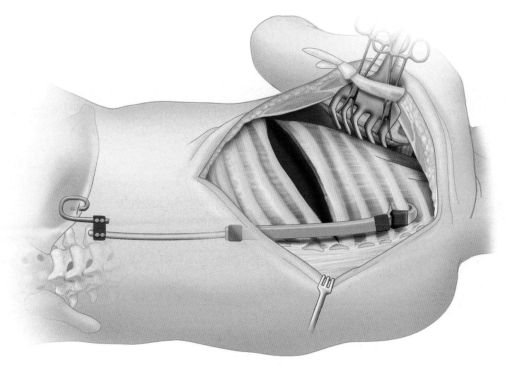

FIGURE 21

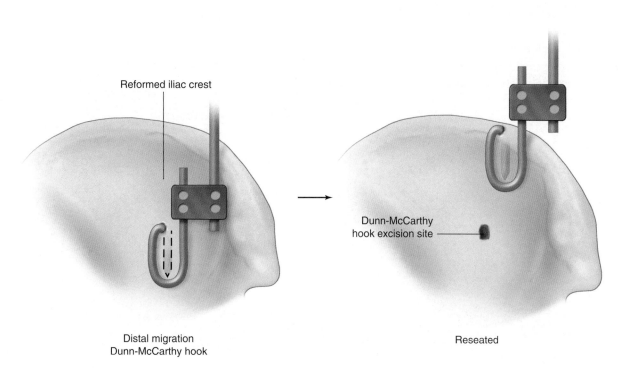

Reformed iliac crest

Dunn-McCarthy
hook excision site

Distal migration
Dunn-McCarthy hook

Reseated

FIGURE 22

Instrumentation

- With the superior cradle in place, the correctly sized rib cradle with the rib sleeve is then placed over the inferior rib of attachment and mated to the superior cradle.
- With forceps, the device is gently maneuvered into place, and then locked superiorly with a distraction lock. The device is then expanded 0.5 cm and a second distraction lock is added distally.
- The rib distractor is then removed.
- A no. 7 and a no. 10 Jackson-Pratt drain are placed beneath the muscle flaps.

Controversies

- Do not use the expandable nature of the device to adjust for correct size. The measured interval should match the number designated on both the VEPTR rib sleeve and the inferior cradle/hybrid lumbar extension used.
- For children under age 18 months, with inadequate spinal canal to accept a hook,

STEP 6: ADDITION OF SECOND RIB-TO-RIB VEPTR

- A second VEPTR, a rib-to-rib construct, is next placed in the posterior axillary line to aid the hybrid device in deformity correction. The rib-to-rib VEPTR is placed laterally to the hybrid device, either parallel to it or slightly tilted toward it to avoid distal lateral migration (Fig. 23).
- The second superior rib cradle is placed around the proximal ribs that are encircled by the superior cradle of the hybrid device.
- The site of inferior rib cradle attachment is then chosen, usually the 9th or 10th rib, and the cradle site is prepared in the same fashion as that for the superior cradle.
- The Synthes rib retractor is reinserted, and the thoracostomy interval is expanded.
- The distance from the bottom of the rib within the superior cradle to top of the rib of attachment inferiorly is measured in centimeters. The distance in centimeters corresponds to the number coded for the VEPTR rib-to-rib device needed.

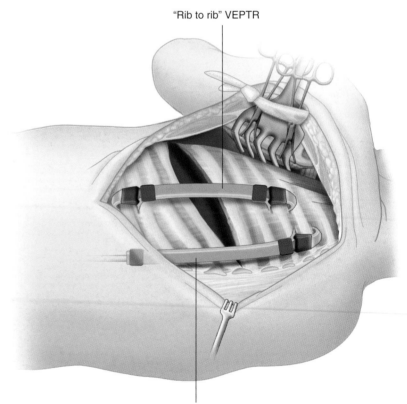

"Rib to rib" VEPTR

FIGURE 23   Hybrid VEPTR

a hybrid VEPTR generally should not be used. A sole VEPTR rib-to-rib construct is used instead. Once the child is older than 18 months, then the rib-to-rib construct can be replaced with a hybrid, if desired.

STEP 7: CLOSURE

- The paraspinous muscles are placed back laterally over the medial device.
- With a Kocher clamp, the muscle at the inferior tip of the scapula is next gently pulled distally and three separate 0 Vicryl figure-of-eight sutures are used to approximate the muscle flaps back together at the corner of the thoracotomy incision. The Kocher clamp is removed, and the remaining muscle layers are approximated in separate layers with running sutures of 0 Vicryl. Deep tissue and skin are closed with absorbable suture.

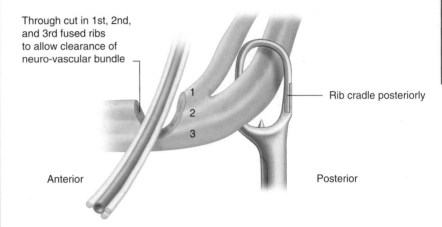

Through cut in 1st, 2nd, and 3rd fused ribs to allow clearance of neuro-vascular bundle

Rib cradle posteriorly

1
2
3

Anterior

Posterior

FIGURE 24

Controversies

- Chest tubes are seldom needed unless visceral lung pleura is violated. If there is a significant "leak" in the lung, then a no. 20 chest tube is also inserted in addition to the two Jackson-Pratt drains.
- Steri-Strips are placed over the wounds and a soft dressing is applied over the incisions. Surgical polyurethane foam is also added over the dressings to help pad the incisions and avoid skin slough.

Postoperative Care and Expected Outcomes

- Patients are kept in the intensive care unit for observation for approximately 3–5 days.
- Extubation is usually possible 48–72 hours after surgery.
- Pain control is addressed with intravenous morphine and oral codeine.
- Chest radiographs are taken on a daily basis for 3–4 days.
- Although minimal blood loss is usually encountered during the actual procedure, the risk of requiring transfusion is approximately 50% because of continued oozing beneath the flaps. The hematocrit and hemoglobin should be checked daily for several days. My institution transfuses children in order to maintain a hematocrit of 30% to maintain good oxygen-carrying capacity.
- Intensive pulmonary toilet, with percussion and nebulizer treatments, is performed for at least a week postoperatively.
- The patients are mobilized as soon as possible. They are allowed to sit in bed, have assisted sitting bedside, and ambulate with assistance.
- No spine braces are used because of concern regarding their constrictive effect on the chest.
- The Jackson-Pratt drains are removed when each one has an output of only 20 ml or less over a 24-hour period.
- Chest tubes are removed when drainage has decreased to 1 ml/kg/day.
- Postoperative radiographs and CT scans are performed after all drains are removed. This includes weight-bearing AP and lateral films of the entire spine, including the chest, and an unenhanced CT scan of the chest and lumbar spine, to include the pelvis, at 5-mm intervals. This verifies position of instrumentation.
- Usually a large pleural effusion is seen on CT scan; this is normal. This procedure acutely enlarges the thorax while the underlying lung remains of normal size, so the additional volume is filled by pleural effusion. This effusion will slowly be replaced by the enlarging lung over a period of 3–6 months after surgery.
- Prophylactic intravenous (IV) antibiotics are used for 7 days for implants, 3–5 days for replacement procedures, and 2 days for expansion procedures.

- Expected outcomes of treatment of fused ribs and congenital scoliosis include an average reduction in curvature of 25°, improvement in the space available for the lungs to an average of 80% (Campbell et al., 2003b), and an average 7% increase in length of unilateral unsegmented bars with growth in height of the thoracic spine (Campbell and Hell-Vocke, 2003). The percent normal vital capacity at follow-up is most favorable for those patients treated by VEPTR opening wedge thoracostomy at age 2 years or younger, and least favorable in those patients older than age 2 years at time of VEPTR surgery with history of prior spine fusion (Campbell et al., 2003b).

Expansion of the Devices

- Devices are expanded on schedule every 6 months.
- Under general anesthesia in an outpatient surgery setting, 3-cm incisions are made over the distraction locks of the devices, the locks are removed, and the devices are expanded with distraction pliers until the reactive force becomes large (about 5 to 10 mm) (Fig. 25). Distraction is continued at 2 mm every 3 minutes until the reactive force is too great to continue. Total expansion ranges from 0.5 to 1.5 cm

PEARLS

- *Distraction of the devices should be slow. When there is excessive reactive force within the first 5 mm of expansion, the distraction forceps are locked by the nut on the handles, and a relaxation period of 3 minutes is allowed to enable the chest wall tissues to accommodate the distraction and the reactive forces to dissipate. Another distraction of 2–3 mm is then performed. The cycle is repeated until the reactive force is consistently large, and then the distraction lock is placed.*

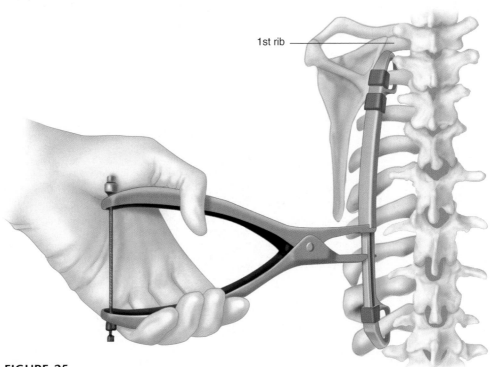

1st rib

FIGURE 25

on average. The devices are then locked with new distraction locks and the wounds are closed, with meticulous soft tissue handling.

■ The wounds are anesthesized with subcutaneous 0.5% Marcaine injection, and Steri-Strips are placed. Soft dressings are placed over the incision.

■ Intraoperative AP radiographs are taken to verify position of the devices.

Replacement Procedure

■ When devices are completely expanded and the patient is still growing, then a change to a longer size is warranted.

■ In an outpatient setting, under general anesthetic, limited skin incisions are made over key areas. For the hybrid devices, the rib sleeve–superior cradle junction, the distraction lock of the rib sleeve, and the hook are accessed through separate incisions. For rib-to-rib devices, the rib sleeve–superior cradle junction, the distraction lock of the rib sleeve, and the distal end of the inferior rib cradle are accessed. The devices are unlocked by removal of the distraction locks and the cradle end locks, and loosening of the hook. The old devices are removed through the inferior incisions. Longer devices, appropriate for the new length, are inserted and then distracted to tension the construct.

■ Wounds are closed in the usual fashion, and postoperative care is similar to that for the expansion procedure.

Evidence

Campbell RM, Hell-Vocke AK. Growth of the thoracic spine in congenital scoliosis after expansion thoracoplasty. J Bone Joint Surg Am. 2003;85:409-20.

Campbell RM Jr, Smith MD. Thoracic insufficiency syndrome and exotic scoliosis. J Bone Joint Surg Am. 2007;89(Suppl 1):108-22.

Campbell RM, Smith MD, Hell-Vocke AK. Expansion thoracoplasty: the surgical technique of opening-wedge thoracostomy. Surgical technique. J Bone Joint Surg Am. 2004;86(Suppl 1):51-64.

Campbell RM Jr, Smith MD, Mayes TC, Mangos JA, Willey-Courand DB, Kose N, Pinero RF, Alder ME, Duong HL, Surber JL. The characteristics of thoracic insufficiency syndrome associated with fused ribs and scoliosis. J Bone Joint Surg Am. 2003a;85:399-408.

Campbell RM, Smith MD, Mayes TC, Mangos JA, Willey-Courand DB, Kose N, Pinero RF, Alder M, Duong HL, Surber J. The effect of opening wedge thoracostomy on thoracic insufficiency syndrome associated with fused ribs and congenital scoliosis. J Bone Joint Surg Am. 2003b;85:1615-24.

Posterior Thoracolumbar Fusion Techniques for Scoliosis—Lenke Classification

Timothy R. Kuklo and Teresa M. Schroeder

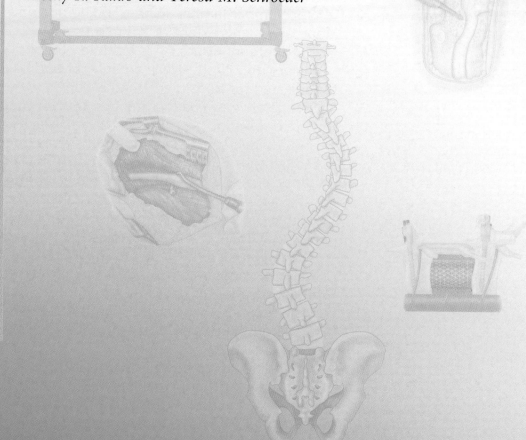

Controversies

- A selective thoracic fusion is possible for 1C or 2C curves if overall balance is maintained. The distal instrumentation should generally extend to the stable zone.

Indications

- Adolescent idiopathic scoliosis

UNDERSTANDING AND APPLYING THE LENKE CLASSIFICATION SYSTEM

- The Lenke system is a comprehensive classification system for adolescent idiopathic scoliosis based on three components (curve type, lumbar spine modifier, and sagittal thoracic modifier) that differentiates structural and nonstructural curves in the proximal thoracic, main thoracic, and thoracolumbar-lumbar spine to guide operative approaches and extent of arthrodesis.
  - The posterior approach is indicated for all six major curve types, while an anterior approach is indicated for both type 1 and 5 curves.
  - Preoperative evaluation requires 36-inch standing anteroposterior (AP) and lateral radiographs, and 36-inch supine left and right side-bending radiographs for proper classification.
- All three curves are measured by the Cobb method on the standing and side-bending radiographs: proximal thoracic, main thoracic, and thoracolumbar-lumbar (O'Brien et al., 2005) (Fig. 1).
  - The major curve is the largest measured curve, and the other curves are considered minor curves. The only exception to this is a type 3 curve (double major curve) in which the main thoracic curve is the largest curve, ≤5° less than the thoracolumbar-lumbar curve.
  - If the difference between the main thoracic and thoracolumbar-lumbar curves is less than 5°, then the curve should be classified as a type 3, 4, or 5.
  - By definition a curve is determined to be structural if the Cobb angle on the side-bending radiograph is determined to be at least 25°. A sagittal measurement of ≥20° as measured from T2 to T5 will classify the proximal thoracic curve as structural, whereas a sagittal measurement of ≥20° from T10 to L2 will classify the main thoracic or thoracolumbar-lumbar curve as structural.
  - These are important points, as the extent of arthrodesis should generally include the major curve and any structural minor curves.
- Six major curve types
  - Type 1: main thoracic
  - Type 2: double thoracic
  - Type 3: double major

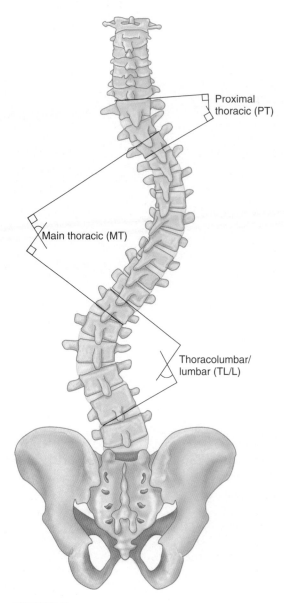

Proximal thoracic (PT)

Main thoracic (MT)

Thoracolumbar/ lumbar (TL/L)

FIGURE 1

- Type 4: triple major
- Type 5: thoracolumbar-lumbar
- Type 6: thoracolumbar-lumbar/main thoracic
■ Lumbar spine modifier
  - Assesses the degree of lumbar deformity by the relationship of the center sacral vertical line (CSVL) to the lumbar curve apex, which is the most horizontal and laterally placed vertebra on the standing AP radiograph.
  - Modifier A: the CSVL bisects, but does not touch, the pedicles of the lumbar apex. This is only used for types 1–4 curves.
  - Modifier B: the CSVL lies between the medial pedicle and the lateral margin of the apical vertebral body.

- Modifier C: the CSVL lies "outside" or medial to the lumbar apical vertebral body.
  - Sagittal thoracic modifier
    - Assesses the amount of thoracic kyphosis present on the standing lateral radiograph. Normal thoracic kyphosis is generally 10–40° as measured from T5 to T12.
    - (−) Identifies a thoracic sagittal curve of less than 10° (hypokyphosis)
    - (N) Identifies a normal thoracic sagittal curve of 10–40° (normal kyphosis)
    - (+) Identifies a thoracic sagittal curve of greater than 40° (hyperkyphosis)
  - Curve classification is then determined by combining the curve type with the modifiers. For example, a main thoracic curve (type 1) with the CSVL lying between the pedicles of the lumbar apex (A modifier) and a 23° thoracic kyphosis measured from T5 to T12 (N modifier) would be considered a type 1AN curve.

Treatment Options

- Alternatively, an anterior spinal fusion (ASF) may be considered for type 1 main thoracic curves, via an open or endoscopic approach.
- ASF may be ideal for type 5 thoracolumbar-lumbar curves with a nonstructural main thoracic curve. This is best performed with dual-rod instrumentation.

Examination/Imaging

- Both 36-inch standing AP and lateral radiographs and 36-inch supine left and right side-bending radiographs are required for proper classification. Here a Lenke type 1AN curve is shown. (Fig. 2A–2E).
- Optional 36-inch supine AP, push-prone, and/or traction radiographs may be obtained to further assess curve flexibility.
- Magnetic resonance imaging is not required for routine adolescent idiopathic scoliosis, but is indicated for an abnormal neurologic examination, congenital scoliosis, juvenile scoliosis, left main thoracic curves, or a rapidly progressing curve.
- Close clinical observation for shoulder imbalance and trunk shift is necessary to achieve optimal clinical results.

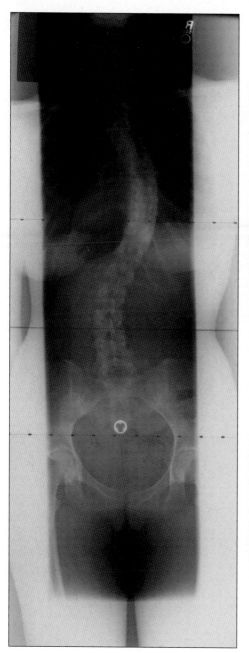

A

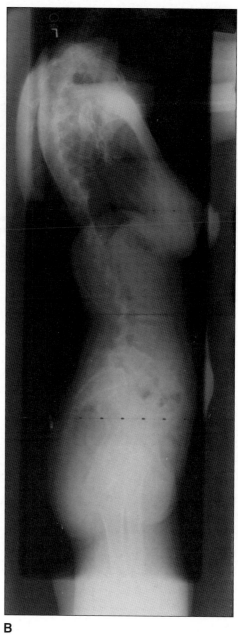

B

FIGURE 2A-B   *Continued*

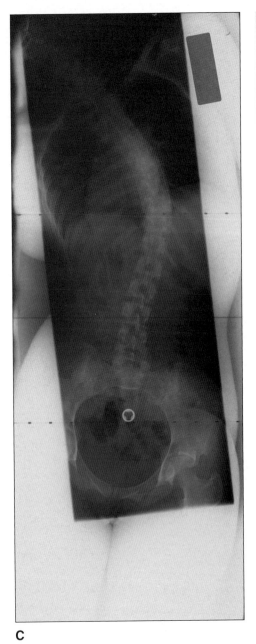

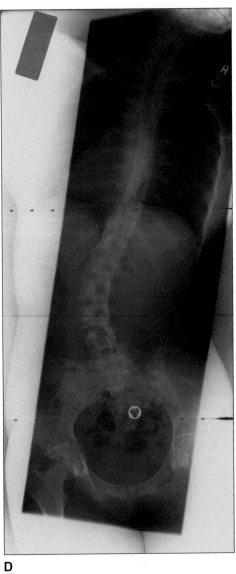

C

D

FIGURE 2C-D   *Continued*

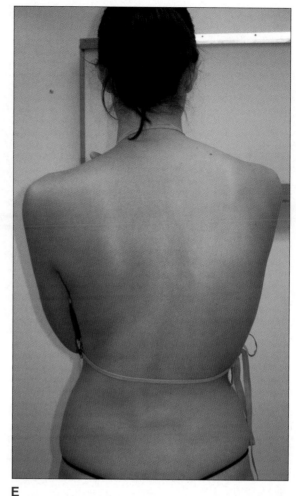

E

FIGURE 2E   *Continued*

Surgical Anatomy

- The standard midline posterior approach with subperiosteal dissection of the thoracic and/or thoracolumbar spine is utilized. Care should be taken to preserve the interspinous ligament at the cephalad and caudad levels of instrumentation, and to minimize disruption of the facet joints proximally to prevent adjacent segment/junctional kyphosis.
- Facetectomies should be performed to decorticate and expose these joints for arthrodesis, and to fully visualize the starting points for thoracic pedicle screw insertion.
- The interspinous ligament, and occasionally the ligamentum flavum, should be removed to increase curve flexibility. The spinous processes are preserved whenever possible to minimize instrumentation prominence.

PEARLS

- *The arms are placed with the shoulders and elbows at 90° of flexion to minimize stretch of the brachial plexus.*
- *The abdomen is free to reduce potential compression on the inferior vena cava, which will reduce epidural venous engorgement.*

PITFALLS

- *The upper thoracic spine can be somewhat difficult to image fluoroscopically, specifically in the lateral view, secondary to positioning on the Jackson frame and the position of the arms.*

Equipment

- Halo-femoral traction can easily be applied with the Jackson frame if required.

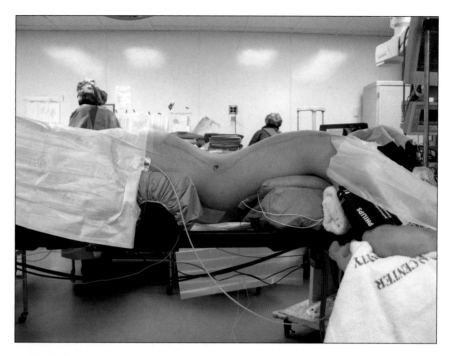

FIGURE 3

Positioning

- The patient is placed supine on an open Jackson frame with the hips extended (Fig. 3). This includes four large pads distally (two for the anterior superior iliac spines and two for the thighs), and two additional pads for the thorax (or alternatively a single chest pad). The arms are positioned in 90° shoulder and elbow flexion.

Procedure

STEP 1

- After positioning, the proximal and distal extent of the incision is marked, and a longitudinal midline incision is made.
- Dissection is carried down to the spinous processes, and then the spine is exposed subperiosteally out to the transverse processes bilaterally (Fig. 4).
- Instrumentation levels are confirmed with fluoroscopy or intraoperative radiographs.

STEP 2

- Pedicle screws are then sequentially placed by fluoroscopic or image guidance, or a freehand technique. Each of these techniques has its advantages; nonetheless, a detailed understanding of the surgical anatomy is required.

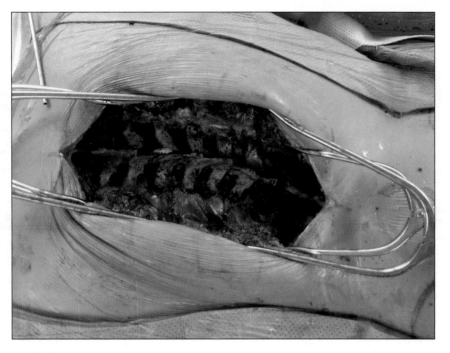

FIGURE 4

PEARLS

• *Supplemental sublaminar wires provide excellent coronal correction, especially at the curve apex.*

Instrumentation/ Implantation

• Monaxial screws also have a smaller sagittal profile than multiaxial screws.
• Insertion of thoracic pedicle screws in a straightforward trajectory provides improved pullout strength over placement via the anatomic trajectory.

■ In general, the lumbar pedicle screw starting point is at the intersection of the pars interarticularis, a line extended along the midpoint of the transverse process and the mammary process. The thoracic pedicle screw starting point varies slightly by level and technique; however, it is generally at the intersection of the pars interarticularis and the proximal third of the transverse process just lateral to the midpoint of the facet.

STEP 3

- After the starting point is identified, the dorsal cortex is removed with a burr or rongeur.
- After "feeling" the projected pedicle screw tract with a fine-tipped probe to ensure accurate screw placement, the hole is tapped (undertapping by 1.0 mm is preferred to improve pedicle screw pullout strength). The hole is then probed again, and then the screw is placed. Usually a screw is placed at each level on the correcting side (usually the curve concavity) (Fig. 5A).
- On the convexity, two screws are preferred at both the distal and proximal construct ends, and additional screws are placed intermittently in between. As well, a screw is usually placed at the curve apex on the convexity to improve apical derotation.
- Monaxial pedicle screws are preferred over multiaxial screws to improve rotational correction via a direct vertebral rotation technique.

STEP 4

- The concave rod is then measured, cut, and contoured to the expected correction. This is then set in place by bringing the screws to the rod, and the set screws are loosely applied.
- A surgical assistant then applies a posterior-anterior and lateral-medial force on the apical convex screws, and the concave rod is then locked in place. This adjustment can be repeated several times. Derotation can also be accomplished with pedicle tube extenders (Fig. 5B).
- Following this, further rod bending/contouring is performed with in situ coronal and sagittal benders. Care is taken to note overall coronal balance and to ensure that proper tilt is approximated in the lowest instrumented vertebra.

STEP 5

- The convex rod is then cut and contoured, and locked in position (Fig. 5C).

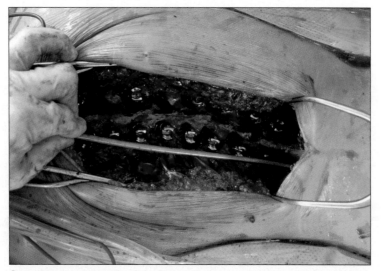

A

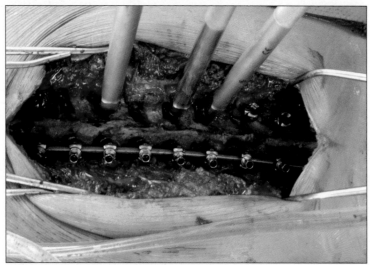

B

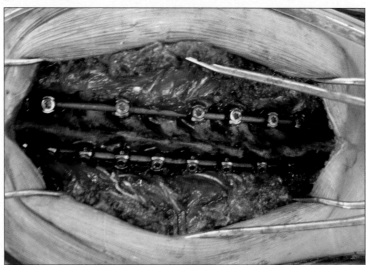

C

FIGURE 5A-C

- Anteroposterior and lateral radiographs can be obtained at this point to assess overall correction, as well as coronal and sagittal balance (Fig. 6A and 6B).
- Shoulder balance can be improved by compressing proximal screws to "lower" an elevated shoulder.
- Overall rotational correction can be approximated by assessing the apical vertebral body–rib ratio and the apical rib spread or symmetry.
- A cross-link is also preferred as this adds construct torsional stability. Torsional instability is pronounced in long constructs in which torsional loads are transmitted throughout the entire length of the rod, which in turn generates cumulative displacements and loss of correction. The cross-link is placed after decortication and bone grafting.

Postoperative Care and Expected Outcomes

- Patients are mobilized on postoperative day 1, and discharged when discontinued from intravenous medications, and when cleared by physical therapy to negotiate stairs.
- Postoperative bracing is not routinely utilized, unless bone quality is compromised by an underlying medical condition.
- With pedicle screw constructs, patients are returned to school and activities as tolerated, with no artificial restrictions.
- Loss of correction is negligible with pedicle screw constructs.

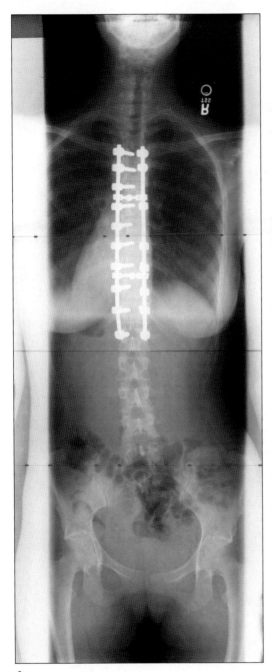 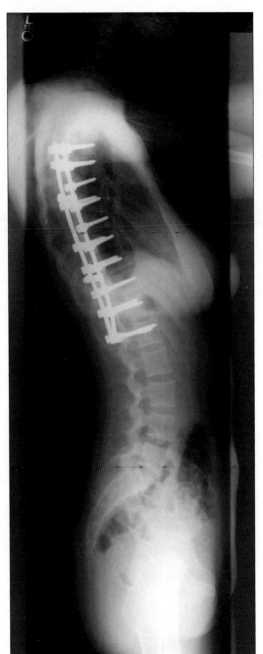

A   B

FIGURE 6A-B

Evidence

Hackenburg L, Link T, Liljenqvist U. Axial and tangential fixation strength of pedicle screws versus hooks in the thoracic spine in relation to bone mineral density. Spine. 2002;27:937-42.

The article found the correlation of bone mineral density and pullout strength was significant for pedicle screws and pedicle hooks, while the resistance of pedicle screws on axial and tangential loading was significantly higher compared to pedicle and laminar hooks.

Kim YJ, Lenke LG, Bridwell KH, et al. Free hand pedicle screw placement in the thoracic spine: is it safe? Spine. 2004;29:333-42.

This article finds the free hand technique of thoracic pedicle screw placement performed in a step-wise, consistent and compulsive manner as an accurate, reliable, and safe method of insertion to treat a variety of spinal disorders, including spinal deformity.

Kuklo TR, Lehman RA. Effect of various tapping diameters on insertion of thoracic pedicle screws: a biomechanical analysis. Spine. 2003;28:2066-71.

This article describes the values of undertapping the thoracic pedicle screw pathway. By undertapping 1-mm, this increases the Maximum Insertional Torque (MIT) by 93% (P > 0.0005) when compared with tapping line-to-line.

Kuklo TR, Potter BK, Polly DW, Lenke LG. Monaxial versus multiaxial thoracic pedicle screws in the correction of adolescent idiopathic scoliosis. Spine. 2005;30:2113-20.

This article developed several new measures to test the correctional capacity of monaxial and multiaxial thoracic pedicle screws in the treatment of Lenke 1 AIS patients. The authors found that monaxial screw constructs provide better correction of the rotational deformity as assessed by thoracic torsion and symmetry.

Lenke LG, Betz RR, Bridwell KH, et al. Spontaneous lumbar curve coronal correction after selective anterior and posterior thoracic fusion in adolescent idiopathic scoliosis. Spine. 1999;24:1663-72.

The article compared anterior thoracic fusion to posterior thoracic fusion and found that the anterior approach appears to have a distinct advantage in allowing improved thoracic correction with corresponding improved lumbar spontaneous correction, especially for lumbar curve modifier C (true King Type II curves).

Lenke LG, Betz RR, Harms J, et al. Adolescent idiopathic scoliosis: a new classification to determine extent of spinal arthrodesis. J Bone Joint Surg Am. 2001;83:1169-81.

This is a comprehensive classification system of AIS which analyzes the structural nature of the proximal, main thoracic and thorocolumbar-lumbar curves. Surgical approach guidelines are also directed at various curve classifications.

O'Brien et al. Spinal deformity study group radiographic measurement model. Medtronic Sotamar Danck Inc. 2005.

Parent S, Labelle H, Skalli W, et al. Thoracic pedicle morphometry in vertebrae from scoliotic spines. Spine. 2004;29:239-48.

The author found that the pedicle width on the concave side of the thoracic curve of a scoliotic patient to be significantly diminished and that caution should be used when using pedicle screws.

Potter BK, Kuklo TR, Lenke LG. Radiographic outcomes of anterior spinal fusion versus posterior spinal fusion with thoracic pedicle screws for treatment of Lenke type 1 adolescent idiopathic scoliosis curves. Spine. 2005;30:1859-66.

The authors compared curve correction in Lenke Type I curves using anterior spinal fusion (ASF) and posterior spinal fusion (PSF) with thoracic pedicle screws (TPS). The PSF technique with TPS provided superior instrumented correction of main thoracic curves and spontaneous correction of TL/L curves, as well as improved correction of thoracic torsion and rotation when compared to ASF.

Suk SI, Kim WJ, Kim JH, et al. Indications of proximal thoracic curve fusion in thoracic adolescent idiopathic scoliosis. Spine. 2000;25:2342-9.

This was a retrospective study on idiopathic thoracic scoliosis. The authors concluded that all patients with a proximal thoracic curve of more than 25° and level or elevated left shoulder should be considered a double thoracic curve pattern and should be treated by fusing both the proximal and the distal curves when using segmental instrumentation.

Suk SI, Kim WJ, Lee SM, et al. Thoracic pedicle screw fixations in spinal deformities: are they really safe? Spine. 2001;26:2049-57.

This was a retrospective study on thoracic deformity. The authors found that thoracic pedicle screw fixation is a reliable method of treating spinal deformities with excellent deformity correction and a high margin of safety.

Suk SI, Lee CK, Kim WJ, et al. Segmental pedicle screw fixation in the treatment of thoracic idiopathic scoliosis. Spine. 1995;20:1399-405.

This is the first article to directly compare all hook, hybrid and all pedicles screw constructs in terms of initial correction and loss of correction at follow-up. All pedicle screw constructs were found to have superior correction and maintenance of correction.

Thoracoplasty for Rib Deformity

Suken A. Shah and Mohan Belthur

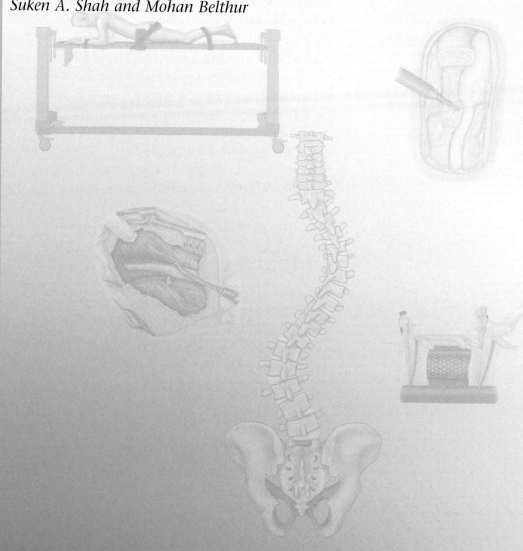

Controversies

- Use of thoracoplasty seems to be on the wane because:
  - Early detection and treatment of scoliosis is common.
  - Segmental spinal instrumentation with pedicle screws allows three-dimensional realignment of the spine and derotation, reducing the rib prominence.
  - Objective data demonstrating ongoing long-term benefit of this procedure are lacking.
  - Patients who would benefit most from thoracoplasty due to severe rib prominence may sometimes be unable to tolerate the procedure (syndromic patients/juvenile-onset scoliosis).

Treatment Options

- Posterior/extrapleural thoracoplasty
- Anterior/internal thoracoplasty

Indications

- Adolescent/adult scoliosis: rib prominence associated with rigid, rotated, decompensated thoracic and double major curves. In these patients a convex thoracoplasty may be necessary if it is not possible to fully derotate the curves during posterior instrumented spinal fusion. An example would be a rib hump greater than 4 cm, rib angle greater than 15°, and curve flexibility less than 50%.
- Rib prominence associated with a compensated curve where posterior spinal fusion is not necessary or a previously fused curve. The indication may be poor appearance or discomfort when sitting in a chair or leaning against a wall.
- To increase flexibility of the curve: concave rib osteotomies and elevation of the concavity dorsally out of the chest.
- To procure autologous bone graft for fusion.

Examination/Imaging

- Measurement of angle of thoracic rotation by inclinometer
- Pulmonary function testing
- Whole-spine posteroanterior, lateral, bending, and Stagnara views
- Clinical photos of the patient

Surgical Anatomy

- Ribs/transverse process: parts of the ribs corresponding to vertebrae in the structural curve are resected
- Thoracolumbar fascia
- Serratus posterior
- Latissimus dorsi
- Intercostal neurovascular bundle
- Pleura

Positioning

- The patient is positioned in prone on a Jackson spinal table in the standard manner for a posterior spinal fusion and prepped and draped in the standard fashion.

Portals/Exposures

- Single incision technique
  - An incision is drawn with a marking pen using the electrocautery cord. The top of the cord is placed at C7 and the bottom at the midgluteal crease and a straight line is drawn down the spine.
  - For a selective right thoracic spinal fusion with thoracoplasty, it is necessary to extend the skin incision distally by $1/2$–1 inch to retract the thoracolumbar fascia adequately from the midline.
  - After skin incision, the spinous processes are outlined and the thoracolumbar fascia incised.
  - The thoracolumbar fascia is picked up with a forceps or retracted with a rake, and the interval between the paravertebral muscle and fascia is developed with a combination of sharp and blunt dissection, working laterally (Fig. 1). The fascia is retracted dorsally and laterally towards the convexity of the curve over the rib deformity. An assistant is required to hold retractors for proper visualization.
- For concave rib osteotomies to increase scoliotic curve flexibility, the steps are similar.

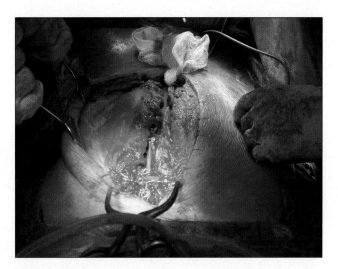

FIGURE 1

PEARLS

- *The fascial plane interval should be developed properly with minimal blood loss and trauma to the muscle tissue.*

- *The incision needs to be carried slightly distal to the lowest vertebra to be fused to allow adequate exposure of all ribs to be resected.*

PITFALLS

- *Avoid any dissection in the high thoracic area around the scapula, as painful scarring may result.*

Instrumentation

- Cobb elevators
- Weitlaner retractors
- Rake
- Forceps
- Bovie electrocautery

Controversies

- Alternatively, an incision may be made directly over the rib prominence, lateral to the midline, for direct access to the ribs to be addressed; however, this is cosmetically undesirable.

PEARLS

- *It is important to pull the periosteum off the rib and not push as with ordinary periosteal stripping, to prevent slipping off the rib inadvertently and plunging through the pleura.*

Instrumentation/ Implantation

- Bovie electrocautery
- Alexander elevator
- Cobb and Doyen elevators

Controversies

- Some surgeons differ on the timing of the rib resection: before the instrumentation and correction, or after the spinal procedure. We favor the rib resection prior to curve correction in order to obtain additional flexibility of the spinal deformity and achieve superior correction of the spine.

PEARLS

- *The rib is grabbed with a towel clip to prevent its sharp edge from plunging through the pleura when it is cut.*

- *One can always return after the spinal correction and instrumentation portion of the procedure is completed to take more rib out, but it cannot be put back. Taking too much rib and creating a concavity is worse than leaving a residual rib deformity.*

- *The apex of the curve will translate to the midline of the spine, ultimately leaving a much larger gap than apparent at the time of rib resection.*

Procedure

STEP 1

- The ribs that are to be resected are palpated, and a subperiosteal exposure of the rib 2–3 cm lateral to the transverse process, or as close to the apical portion of the rib as possible, is started with Bovie electrocautery in its midline (Fig. 2).
- A Freer elevator, a small Cobb elevator, or an Alexander elevator is used to subperiosteally expose each rib on its dorsal surface over the entire length of the resection (usually 2 cm is needed).
  - A small elevator or curved hemostat is gently passed underneath (ventrally) the rib subperiosteally; care is taken to avoid injury to the pleura underneath (Figs. 3 and 4).

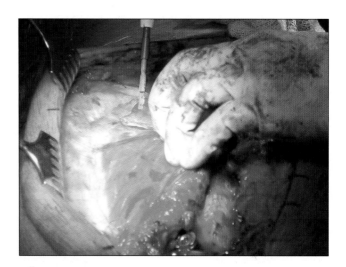

FIGURE 2

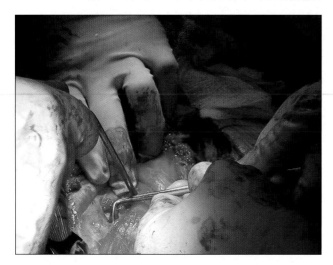

FIGURE 3

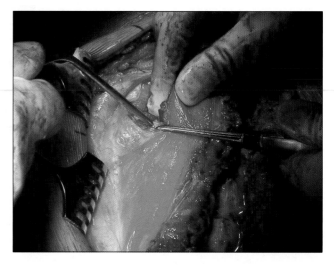

FIGURE 4

PITFALLS

- *Pleural violation should be recognized and immediately repaired with 2-0 absorbable suture.*

- *It is important to resect the medial portion of the ribs as well, since failure to do so will create a ridge.*

Instrumentation/ Implantion

- Cobb elevator
- Right-angle retractors
- Rib cutter
- Towel clip

- A Doyen elevator is passed circumferentially and passed medially and laterally to extend the exposure for a short distance and confirm adequate subperiosteal release of the rib (Figs. 5 and 6).

STEP 2

- Two right-angle retractors are placed on the medial side of the rib, pulling back the paraspinal muscle.
- A Cobb elevator is used to strip the periosteum further to expose the medial-most attachment of the rib to the transverse process (Fig. 7).
- A rib cutter is then passed around the rib and pushed as far medially as possible, right up against the transverse process (Fig. 8). The rib is then cut medially, with the plane of the cut as parallel to the floor as possible.

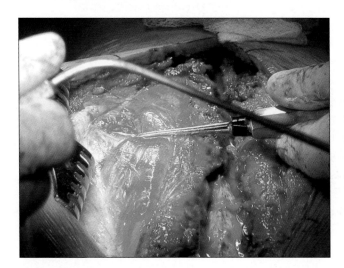

FIGURE 5

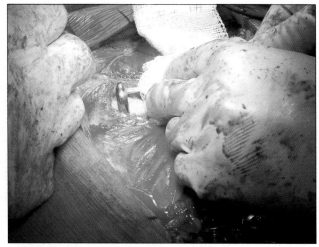

FIGURE 6

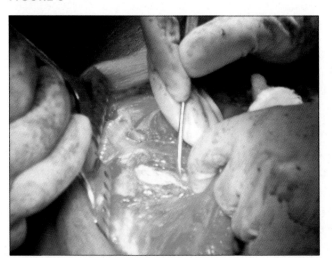

FIGURE 7

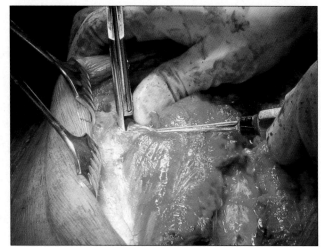

FIGURE 8

- The rib cutter is moved laterally and about 2 cm of the rib should be cut to start (Fig. 9). Starting at the apical levels, a symmetric resection of the ribs is made both proximal and distal to the apex. Generally as one goes proximally and distally, less rib is cut. The most important part of the procedure is to decide how much rib deformity to resect (Fig. 10).
- Bone wax is applied to the ends of the ribs (lightly) and Gelfoam is packed into the periosteal bed to assist with hemostasis (Fig. 11).

Step 3

- The portions of the ribs that are resected can be morselized and used for autologous bone graft for fusion.
- After the spinal instrumentation, correction, and bone grafting, the ribs may be brought together with heavy absorbable suture through small drill holes in the rib ends. This provides additional correction of the rib hump and stability of the rib ends to facilitate healing and patient comfort. The rib periosteum is approximated.
- A water test is performed to make absolutely certain the pleura is intact. Using a small pitcher, saline is poured into the wound carefully so as not to create any additional air bubbles. The anesthesiologist performs a Valsalva maneuver three times to look for a leak in the pleura. Any pleural leaks are repaired with 2-0 absorbable suture.
- The intercostal muscle layer is approximated with suture, and a medium Hemovac drain is placed over the resected rib bed and brought out lateral to the spine. The thoracolumbar fascia is closed with a running long-acting absorbable suture starting at the distal end of the wound.

Postoperative Care and Expected Outcomes

- A small protective shell is applied over the rib resection area if desired. This shell helps avoid a postoperative flail chest and minimizes motion of the cut ribs over the pleura, and may decrease the accumulation of a pleural effusion. (This is optional.)
- Thoracoplasty may increase pain or mildly prolong the postoperative course following spinal fusion with instrumentation.

PEARLS

- *The drain assists with hematoma formation and subsequent leakage into the chest.*

PEARLS

- *A postoperative chest radiograph may rule out pnuemothorax or pleural effusion.*

- *Chest physiotherapy postoperatively.*

PITFALLS

- *Unrecognized pleural effusion or hemothorax*

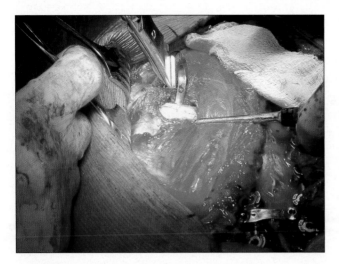

FIGURE 9

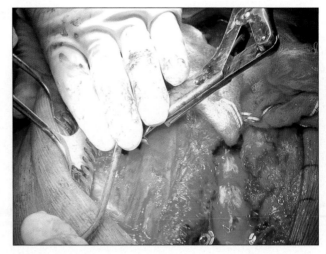

FIGURE 10

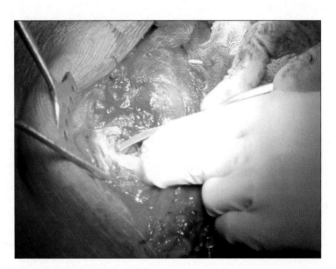

FIGURE 11

- Aggressive pulmonary toileting and chest physiotherapy is necessary with adequate pain control to allow mobilization.
- Patients with moderate or severe pulmonary symptoms are monitored with semierect radiographs for 2–3 days. If a significant amount of pleural fluid accumulates and the patient is symptomatic, a thoracocentesis is performed; if fluid accumulation occurs a second time, a chest tube is considered.
- For small pleural effusions, oral or intravenous furosemide may be used to diurese the patient.
- A consistent decrease in pulmonary function is observed in the early postoperative period, which mandates proper patient selection. A decline of forced vital capacity of 22%, forced expiratory volume in 1 second of 24%, and total lung

capacity of 25% were found in the first 6 months. Gradual improvement occurs over the next 3 years. Patients with less than 60% of predicted values should be cautiously approached as candidates for thoracoplasty.

■ Thoracoplasty does improve appearance and patient satisfaction in those patients undergoing surgery for scoliosis, but at a cost to pulmonary function and patient comfort.

Evidence

Barnes J. Rib resection in infantile idiopathic scoliosis. J Bone Joint Surg Br. 1979;61: 31-5.

Barret DS, Maclean JG, Betany J, et al. Costoplasty in adolescent idiopathic scoliosis: objective results in 55 patients. J Bone Joint Surg Br. 1993;75:881-4.

Flinchum D. Rib resection in the treatment of scoliosis. South Med J., 1979;36:1378-80.

Geissele AE, Ogilvie JW, Cohen M, et al. Thoracoplasty for treatment of rib prominence in thoracic scoliosis. Spine. 1994;19:1636-39.

Harvey CJ Jr., Betz RR, Clements DH, Huss GK, Clancy M. Are there indications for partial rib resection in patients with adolescent scoliosis treated with Cotrel-Dubboset instrumentation? Spine. 1993;18:1593-8.

Manning CW, Prime FJ, Zorab PA. Partial costectomy as a cosmetic operation in scoliosis. J Bone Joint Surg Br. 1973;55:521-7.

Owen R, Turner A, Banforth JSG, Taylor JF, Jones RS. Costectomy as the first stage of surgery for scoliosis. J Bone Joint Surg Br. 1986;68:91-5.

Shufflebarger HL, Smiley K, Roth HJ. Internal thoracoplasty: a new procedure. Spine. 1994;19:840-4.

Steel HH. Rib resection and spine fusion in correction of convex deformity in scoliosis. J Bone Joint Surg Am. 1983;65:920-5.

Thulburne T, Gillespie R. The rib hump in idiopathic scoliosis: measurement, analysis and response to treatment. J Bone Joint Surg Br. 1976;56:64-71.

Westgate HD, Moe JH. Pulmonary function in kyphoscoliosis before and after correction by Harrington instrumentation method. J Bone Joint Surg Am. 1969;51:935-46.

Complete Vertebral Resection for Primary Spinal Tumors

Rick C. Sasso and Gregory D. Dikos

Pitfalls

- *Complete vertebral resection is contraindicated in tumors with multiple skip lesions.*

- *Contiguous involvement of more than three vertebrae is a relative contraindication for complete vertebral resection.*

Treatment Options

- Preoperative embolization of bilateral segmental arteries at the affected level as well as the levels cephalad and caudal reduce blood flow to the involved vertebra by 75% without influencing spinal cord evoked potentials, thus decreasing intraoperative hemorrhage.

Indications

- Malignant or locally aggressive benign primary spinal tumors
- Intracompartmental lesions involving the vertebral body and extending into the pedicles and posterior elements (Weinstein-Boriani-Biagnini [WBB] Surgical Staging System: zones 1-12, layers B and C)
- Extracompartmental lesions with only epidural or paravertebral extension (WBB system: zones 1–12, layers A and D)
- Lesions without spread to or invasion of adjacent viscera with only minimal adhesion to the vena cava or aorta
- Solitary metastatic lesions without extension to the paraspinal area

Examination/Imaging

- Preoperative magnetic resonance imaging (MRI) is needed for proper tumor staging.
- MRI is also crucial for identification of vulnerable vascular anatomy and appropriate preoperative planning.

Surgical Anatomy

- The thoracic aorta is in intimate contact with the anterior vertebral column distal to T5 and must be carefully dissected and retracted anteriorly prior to resection of the involved vertebra. The aorta is less likely to be damaged from T1 to T4.
- The thoracic segmental arteries surrounding the involved vertebra must be identified and ligated. Variability has been reported in the anatomy of the segmental vasculature. Four percent of thoracic segmental arteries do not originate directly from the aorta. These arteries may arise from the intercostal arteries. Additionally, 8% of vertebrae in the mid- to lower thoracic spine lack a segmental artery. Therefore, careful dissection is crucial.
- The nerve root exiting cephalad to and crossing the body of the involved vertebra must be identified and ligated to facilitate the en bloc corpectomy (Fig. 1A and 1B).

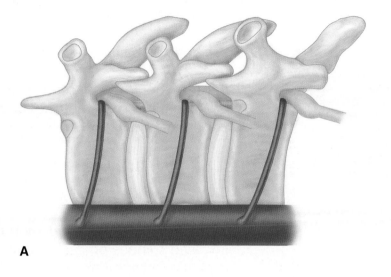

A

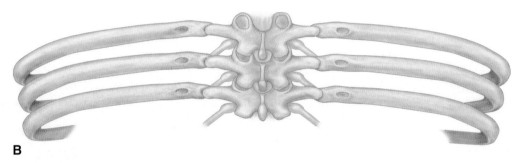

B

FIGURE 1A-B

PEARLS

- *Suspending the anterior chest wall above the table allows the chest to expand freely and facilitates adequate ventilation.*

- *Suspending the abdominal wall above the table reduces venous plexus filling around the spinal cord and reduces intraoperative blood loss.*

Equipment

- A specialized table such as a Jackson spinal surgery table can be used to allow freedom of the chest and abdominal walls.

PEARLS

- *Dissection must be wide enough to expose the transverse processes bilaterally.*

Positioning

- Position the patient prone on the operating table (Fig. 2).
- Bolsters should be placed longitudinally on each side of the patient such that the anterior chest wall and abdominal wall clear the operating table.

Portals/Exposures

- This procedure is ideally performed through a single, posterior approach.
- Make a vertical midline incision centered over the involved spinous process and extending one vertebra caudal and cephalad.
- Dissect the paraspinal muscles from the spinous processes and lamina at all three levels and retract laterally.

PITFALLS

- *If the patient underwent percutaneous biopsy, the biopsy tracts must be débrided at this time to prevent tumor contamination.*

Controversies

- Some authors recommend a second, anterolateral approach and thoracotomy to facilitate the ventral release in tumors with soft tissue extension.
- Alternatively, thoracoscopy has been used to facilitate ventral release and anterior column reconstruction with less morbidity than traditional thoracotomy.

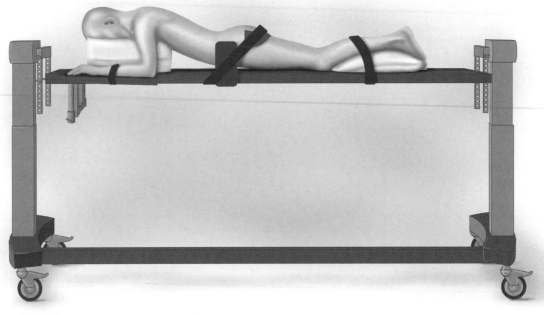

FIGURE 2

Procedure

STEP 1: EN BLOC LAMINECTOMY

- Place pedicle screws in the vertebrae caudal and cephalad to the involved vertebra in preparation for posterior instrumentation (Fig. 3).
- Transect the ribs of the involved vertebra 3–4 cm lateral to the costotransverse joint and bluntly dissect the pleura from the vertebra.
- Remove the spinous process and inferior articular processes of the cephalad vertebra to expose the superior articular process of the involved vertebra.
- Pass a thread-wire saw from the medial cortex of the lamina through the intervertebral foramen in a cephalocaudal direction (Fig. 4A).

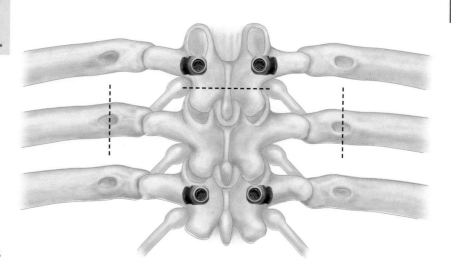

FIGURE 3

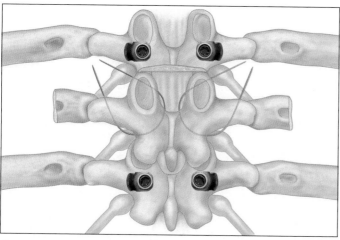

A

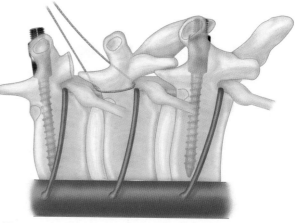

B

FIGURE 4A-B

Instrumentation/ Implantation

• The rods used for provisional fixation should have a large lateral bend so as not to obstruct the operative field.

■ Place the lateral end of the thread-wire saw beneath the superior articular process and the transverse process to wrap the saw around the pedicle.

■ While applying force in a cephalad direction, use a reciprocating motion of the saw to cut the pedicle from caudal to cephalad (Fig. 4B).

■ Repeat this process to cut the contralateral pedicle, and remove the posterior elements (spinous process, superior articular processes, inferior articular processes, transverse processes, and pedicles) as a single unit (Fig. 5).

■ Apply provisional posterior fixation.

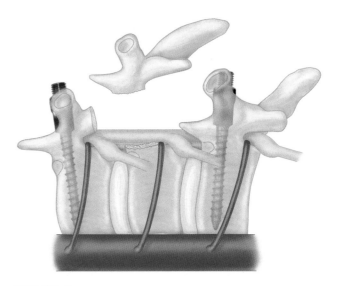

FIGURE 5

PITFALLS

• *Because the vertebral body cuts are made directed at the spinal cord, it is imperative to protect the spinal cord with instruments such as spatulas or malleable retractors.*

STEP 2: EN BLOC CORPECTOMY

■ Bluntly dissect around the vertebral body, identifying the segmental arteries bilaterally.

■ Ligate and divide the spinal branch of the segmental artery of the involved vertebra (Fig. 6).

■ Cut the nerve root crossing the involved vertebral body on the side from which the vertebral body will be removed.

■ Bluntly dissect laterally and anteriorly to develop the plane between the vertebral body and the pleura.

■ Dissect the aorta from the anterior aspect of the vertebral body.

■ Pass thread-wire saws anterior to the vertebral body.

■ Mobilize the spinal cord by blunt dissection.

■ Make vertebral body cuts with the thread-wire saws through the inferior end plate of the cephalad vertebra and the superior end plate of the caudal vertebra (Fig. 7).

■ Rotate the vertebral body around the spinal cord and remove it intact (Fig. 8).

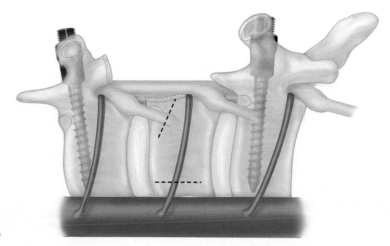

FIGURE 6

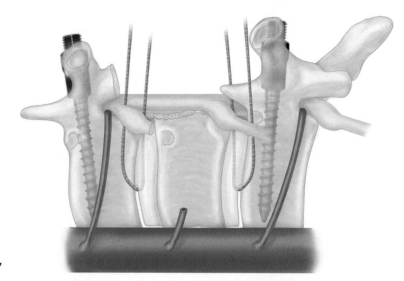

FIGURE 7

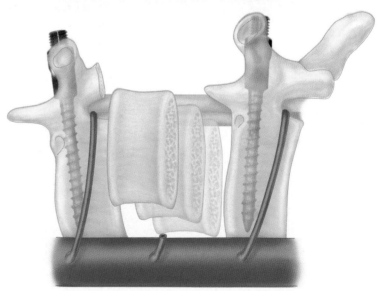

FIGURE 8

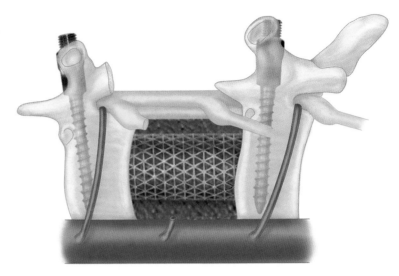

FIGURE 9

STEP 3: ANTERIOR RECONSTRUCTION AND POSTERIOR STABILIZATION

- Insert cage to reconstruct the anterior column (Fig. 9).
- Remove rods used for provisional fixation and apply rods to previously inserted pedicle screws for final fixation.

Postoperative Care and Expected Outcomes

- Insert deep drains and apply suction for 2–3 days.
- Keep patient non–weight bearing for 1 week.
- Patient should be fitted for and wear a thoracolumbosacral orthosis for 2–3 months.

Evidence

Boriani S, Weinstein JN, Biagini R. Primary bone tumors of the spine: terminology and surgical staging. Spine. 1997;22:1036-44.

This review article describes the Weinstein-Boriani-Biagnini (WBB) Surgical Staging System for primary spinal tumors. The WBB system provides a consistent method for classifying and planning the resection of tumors involving the unique three-dimensional anatomy of the vertebra.

Kawahara N, Tomita K, Baba H, Toribatake Y, Fujita T, Mizuno K, Tanaka S. Cadaveric vascular anatomy for total en bloc spondylectomy in malignant vertebral tumors. Spine. 1996;21:1401-7.

This cadaveric study characterized the vascular anatomy about the spine. The thoracic aorta is in direct contact with the anterior vertebral column. Furthermore, variability in the segmental arteries has been reported. Therefore, familiarity with the vascular anatomy around the involved level as well as careful dissection is critical when performing complete vertebral resection.

Nambu K, Kawahara N, Kobayashi T, Murakami H, Ueda Y, Tomita K. Interruption of the bilateral segmental arteries at several levels: influence on vertebral blood flow. Spine. 2004;29:1530-4.

This Level I study using a dog model demonstrated that embolization of bilateral segmental arteries at the affected level as well as the levels cephalad and caudal reduces blood flow to the involved vertebra by 75% without influencing spinal cord evoked potentials. Therefore, preoperative embolization may be a safe and effective means of decreasing intraoperative hemorrhage.

Tomita K, Kawahara N, Baba H, Tsuchiya H, Fujita T, Toribatake Y. Total en bloc spondylectomy: a new surgical technique for primary malignant vertebral tumors. Spine. 1997;22:324-33.

This Level IV study describes the surgical technique of complete vertebral resection used by Tomita et al. The study reports the results of this technique in seven patients. Primary spinal tumors are relatively rare; therefore, higher quality evidence is unavailable.

Van Dijk M, Cuesta MA, Wuisman PIJM. Thoracoscopically assisted total en bloc spondylectomy: two case reports. Surg Endosc. 2000;14:849-52.

This Level IV study describes thoracoscopically assisted ventral release and anterior column reconstruction as a safer alternative to traditional thoracotomy. The small number of subjects limits the quality of this study.

LUMBAR SPINE

Sacropelvic Fixation

Tapan Daftari, Alexander R. Vaccaro, and Jeff Fischgrund

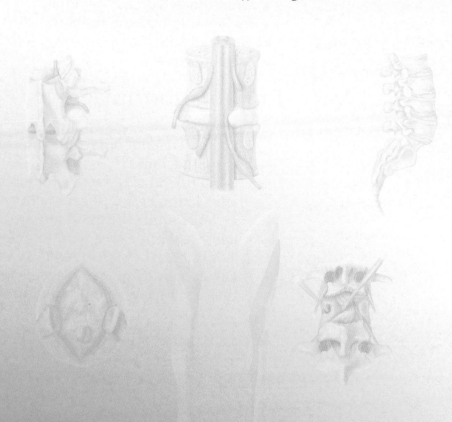

Controversies

- The particular choice of sacral and/or pelvic fixation is dependent on the particular anatomy of the patient and the training and familiarity of the surgeon with the particular options (Fig. 1).

Indications

- Fracture of lower lumbar vertebrae requiring lumbosacral fixation
- High-grade lumbar spondylolisthesis
- Adult thoracolumbar deformity
- Revision lumbosacral fixation
- Metastatic disease of the lower lumbar vertebrae
- Sacral fracture

Examination/Imaging

- Radiology
  - Spot lateral film of sacrum and true anteroposterior film of sacrum
  - Useful to visualize sacral promontory, superior articular process (SAP), sacral foramina, and S1-3 vertebral bodies (Figs. 2 and 3)
  - Inlet view is the best view to determine if screw length breaches the anterior S1 vertebral body. Outlet view is the best view to determine if the sacral screws are directed toward the sacral foramen.

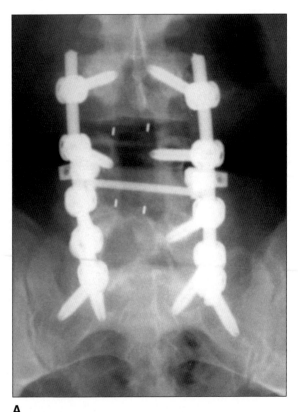

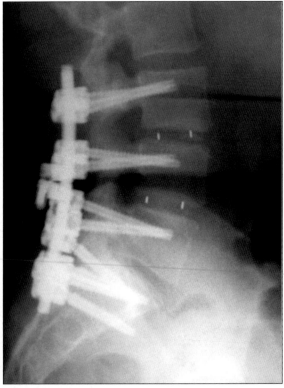

A **B**

FIGURE 1A-B

Treatment Options

- S1 pedicle screw
- S1 alar
- S2 screw
- Iliac screws
- Intrasacral rod (Jackson technique)

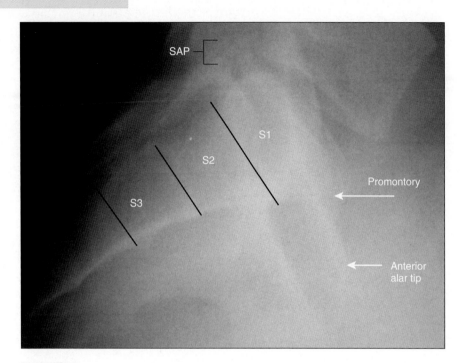

FIGURE 2

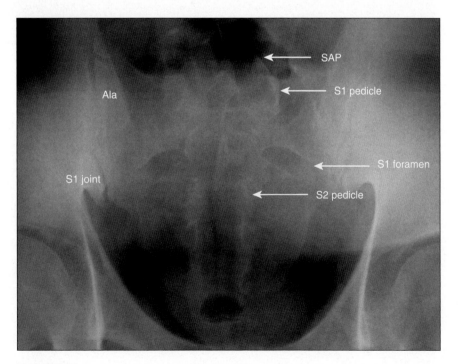

FIGURE 3

- Computed tomography (CT)
  - Gantry parallel to S1 vertebral body
  - Useful to visualize sacral body, sacral ala, sacral pedicle medial and lateral border, superior articular process of S1, S1 and S2 dorsal foramina, posterior ileum and overhang, posterior sacroiliac spine, sacroiliac joint, and position of anterior vascular and anterior neural structures (Figs. 4 and 5).
- Magnetic resonance imaging: usefulness similar to CT with added benefit of soft tissue visualization, especially of neural elements (Fig. 6).

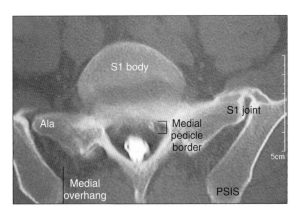

FIGURE 4

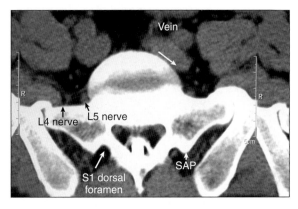

FIGURE 5

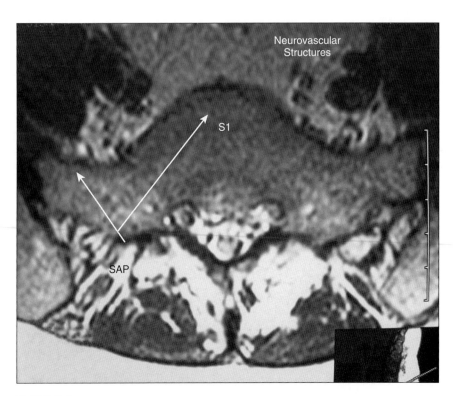

FIGURE 6

Surgical Anatomy

- Important anatomic features include the following (Figs. 7 and 8):
  - Spina bifida
  - Spinal canal
  - Medial border of sacral pedicle
  - S1 nerve root
  - Superior articular process (SAP)
  - Median sacral crest
  - Superior sacral notch
  - S1 dorsal foramina
  - S2 sacral foramina
  - Lateral sacral crest
  - Transverse sacral tubercles

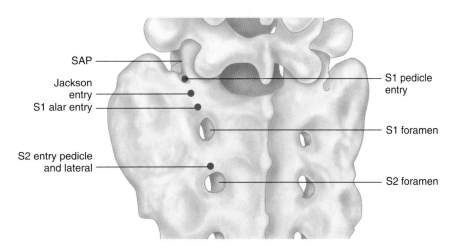

FIGURE 7

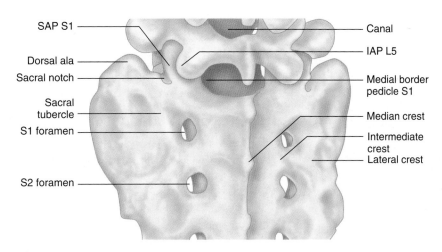

FIGURE 8

- The complete anatomy of the dorsal sacrum should be identified. The spinous processes of the sacrum are shallow and consist mostly of a prominent tip, otherwise known as the median crest. The sacral spinal canal is considerably more narrow than the lumbar spine. There is no segmentation between the sacral lamina. A continuous bony surface exists dorsally. However, care must be taken when dissecting in the midline as there may be an associated incomplete arch of the sacral lamina.
- The L5-S1 facet joint is made up of the inferior articular process of L5 and the superior articular process of S1. Lateral to the L5-S1 facet joint is the sacral ala. There is usually a notch called the superior sacral notch, which is a natural down-sloping area located between the superior articular process of S1 and the ala.
- There are four pairs of sacral foramina—S1, S2, S3, and S4—of which only the upper two (S1 and S2) are identified for instrumentation placement. The sacral pedicle heights at S1 measure on average 20 mm, those at S2 11 mm, and those at S3 7 mm. Inferior to the superior articular process of S1 is the dorsal S1 sacral foramen. There is a ridge or shelf of bone that connects the first and second dorsal foramina, otherwise known as the intermediate crest. The position and shape of the dorsal foramen are variable from one patient to the next. Lateral to the foramen is another shelf of bone known as the lateral crest.
- Care must be taken in exposing the dorsal foramen because within the foramen there is an exiting vein that may bleed excessively if violated. Bipolar cautery or Gelfoam is useful to gain hemostasis.
- When an S1 nerve root decompression is performed, the medial border of the S1 pedicle is easily identified.

Positioning

- The patient is positioned prone. Lumbar lordosis is maintained by pads placed to support the chest, iliac crests, and thighs. The abdomen is left hanging free, decreasing intra-abdominal pressure. This decreases epidural bleeding.

Equipment

- A radiolucent table is recommended, usually a Jackson table.
- Intraoperative fluoroscopy aids in instrument and implant placement.
- Image guidance may be helpful in selected patients, but is not commonly used.

Portals/Exposures

■ A posterior midline approach is made. Dissection is carried down on either side of the spinous processes. The dissection is carried inferiorly to expose at least the upper one third of the sacrum. Usually the S1 and S2 dorsal foramina are exposed.

■ When the iliac crest needs to be exposed, it is exposed medially as a continuation of the sacral exposure by elevating the erector spinae muscles. Care should be taken not to disrupt the distal muscular attachments to the sacropelvis to avoid muscular death and wound complications. The iliac crest is also exposed superficial to the deep fascia by dissecting between the subcutaneous fat and deep fascia from the midline out to the prominence of the posterior superior iliac crest. Dissection can be performed along the lateral outer surface of the iliac crest in a subperiosteal manner to expose the sciatic notch in anticipation of iliac screw placement.

■ Care must be exercised to avoid possible injury to the superior gluteal artery, which, if transected, may retract and result in significant blood loss.

Procedure: S1 Anteromedial (Pedicle) Screw

■ The starting point of the S1 pedicle screw is just inferior and lateral to the base of the superior articular process of S1 (Figs. 9 and 10).

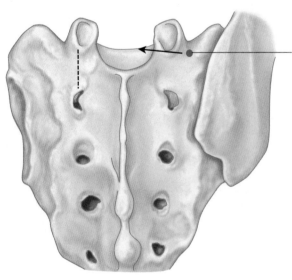

FIGURE 9

S1 screw pedicle anteromedial entry point trajectory

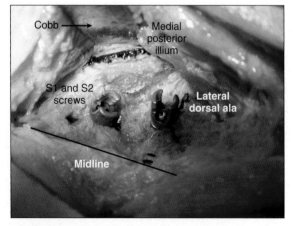

FIGURE 10

PITFALLS

- *Caution must be taken with insertion of the left S1 pedicle screw as the left internal iliac vein is at risk of injury with overpenetration of the anterior sacral cortex. If the screw is directed into the S1 body, or medial to the junction of the body and slope of the ala medially, then risk to neurovascular structures is avoided (Fig. 13).*

- The S1 foramen should be located, and the distance between the foramen and the superior articular process should be estimated. The starting point should about 2–5 mm lateral and no more inferior than one third of this distance. The starting point can be made with an awl, burr, or drill tip (Fig. 11A and 11B).

- A straight or slightly curved gearshift-type probe is used to sound the cancellous bone. The path of the screw should be directed anteromedially approximately 30–40° and superiorly toward the anterior tip of the promontory (Fig. 12). This is usually 15° cephalad in the frontal plane or 5–10° superior in the horizontal plane. The direction toward the anterior tip of the promontory can be estimated from preoperative CT scans or plain radiographs or intraoperatively with lateral fluoroscopy. Directing the screw parallel to the S1 end plate on the lateral view is also acceptable. Screw depth is then measured.

- If bicortical fixation is desired, perforation of the anterior sacral cortex can be performed with a Steinmann pin, drill bit, or dull sacral perforator.

- The range of screw length is approximately 35–50 mm, with the average being 40 mm.

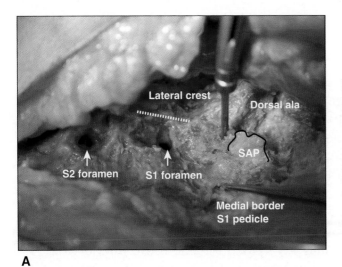

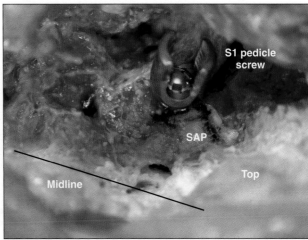

A

B

FIGURE 11A-B

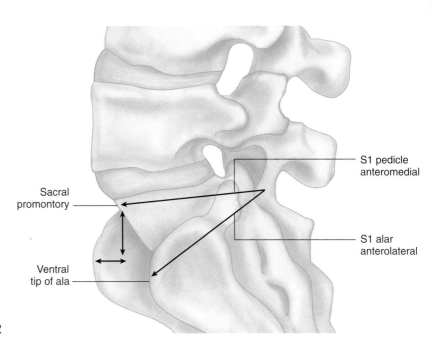

FIGURE 12

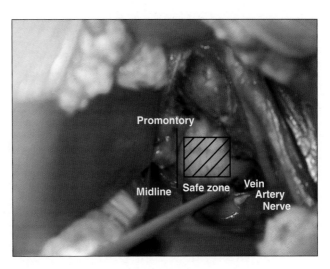

FIGURE 13

Procedure: S1 Anterolateral Screw (Alar)

- The starting point of the S1 alar screw is the intermediate crest, which is found lateral to a vertical line between the middle of the S1 foramen and the lateral border of the superior articular process (Fig. 14). This starting point in the transverse plain is halfway between the bottom of the superior articular process and the S1 foramen, usually at least 5 mm cephalad from the S1 foramen.
- The screw is angled laterally between 30° and 40° and caudally 25° (Fig. 15). The more inferior the screw starting point, the less caudal the screw angulation.
- The anterolateral screw should not be placed bicortically.
- The length of the anterolateral screw averages 35 mm.

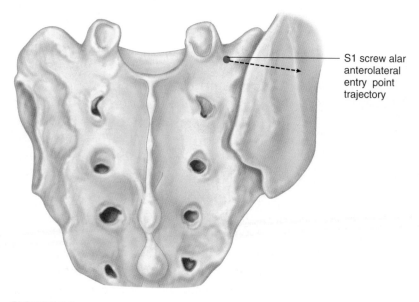

S1 screw alar
anterolateral
entry point
trajectory

FIGURE 14

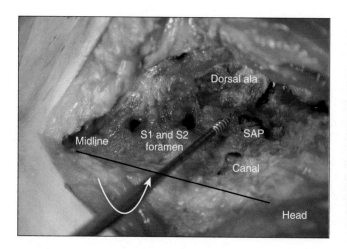

FIGURE 15

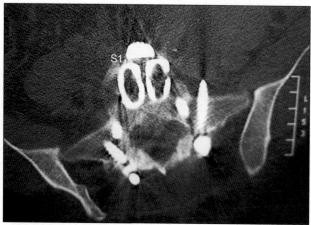

FIGURE 16

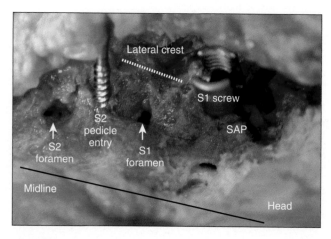

FIGURE 17

PEARLS

- *S2 screws are often used as an adjunct to S1 screws and usually never as a sole means of fixation to the sacrum.*

PITFALLS

- *The sigmoid colon on the left may be at risk for iatrogenic injury. The S1 nerve root can be at risk if the screw is angled too far laterally.*

Procedure: S2 Screw

- The starting point for an S2 pedicle screw in the vertical plain is halfway between the intermediate crest and the lateral crest. In the transverse plane, it is one third to one half the way between a line joining the borders of the S1 and S2 dorsal foramina, beginning at S1. The direction of screw insertion is 20° caudal. On a lateral intraoperative radiograph, this appears to be parallel to the S1 end plate.
- The screw in the transverse plain may be directed 20–30° medially or 30° laterally toward the ala (Figs. 18 and 19).
- The screw length averages 25–30 mm.
- Bicortical purchase may be necessary as unicortical S2 screws have poor resistance to pullout.

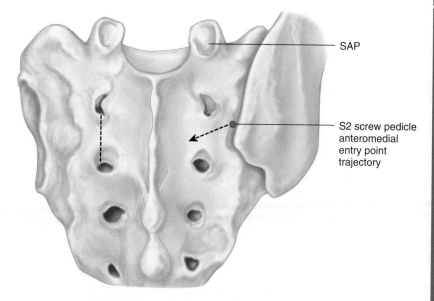

SAP

S2 screw pedicle anteromedial entry point trajectory

FIGURE 18

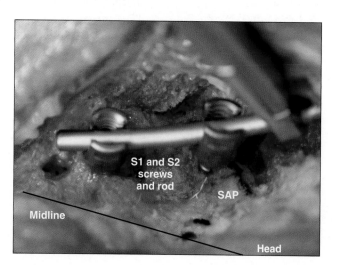

FIGURE 19

Procedure: Iliac Screws

- Iliac screws have supplanted in popularity the technique of rod insertion into the iliac wings (Luque-Galveston) because of the difficulties in rod contouring required in that technique (Fig. 20).
- A notch is made into the dorsal aspect of the iliac wing to expose the cancellous bone (Fig. 21A).
- The location and morphometry of the lateral surface of the iliac wing can be estimated by subperiosteal dissection and using a blunt Cobb elevator. This provides an estimation for screw trajectory within the iliac wing (Fig. 21B).
- A gearshift-type probe is then used to follow a path between the inner and outer iliac cortex (Fig. 22). The screw should be aimed toward the dense bone above the sciatic notch.
- The length of the iliac screws is generally 60–70 mm with a diameter of 7-8 mm.

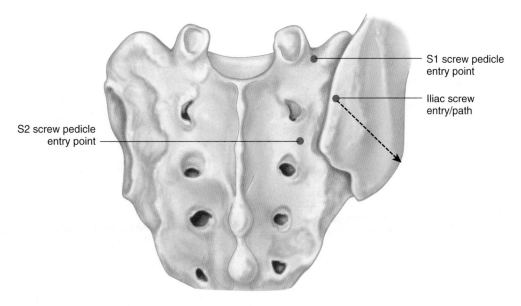

S1 screw pedicle
entry point

Iliac screw
entry/path

S2 screw pedicle
entry point

FIGURE 20

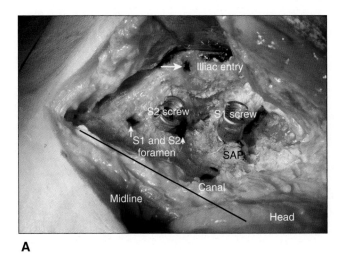

Iliac entry

S2 screw

S1 screw

S1 and S2
foramen

SAP

Canal

Midline

Head

A

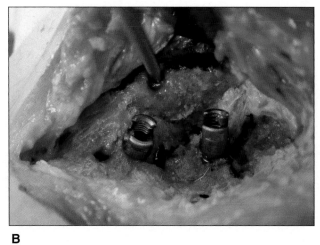

B

FIGURE 21A-B

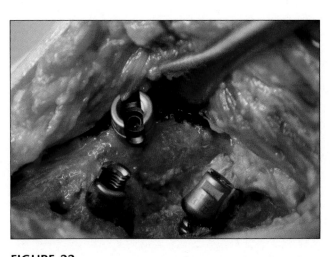

FIGURE 22

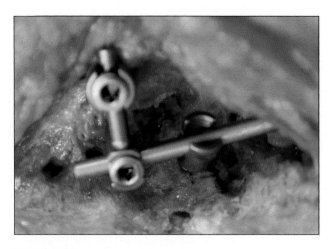

FIGURE 23

Procedure: Jackson Technique

- The Jackson "intrasacral" technique utilizes placement of the spinal rod within the dorsal and ventral tables of bone of the lateral sacrum from S1 to S3 (Fig. 24).
- The S1 screw is inserted within the lateral sacral crest at least 5 mm lateral and 10 mm inferior to the superior articular process of S1 (Fig. 25). This area is often raised in the sacrum and is known as the first sacral lateral tubercle. The screw is medially directed but angulated cephalad so that it actually breaches the anterior S1 end plate into the L5-S1 disk space.
- After the screw is placed, an angled perforator is used to open the dorsal cortex of the lateral sacrum. The rod follows the path of the lateral crest, aimed approximately 25° laterally down to the level of S3 (Fig. 26).
- The rod is placed lateral to the dorsal foramen.

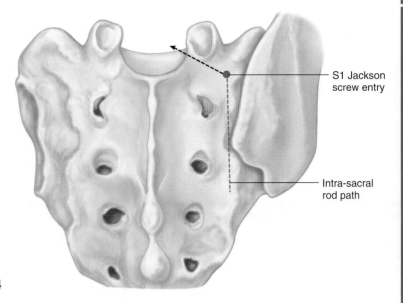

S1 Jackson
screw entry

Intra-sacral
rod path

FIGURE 24

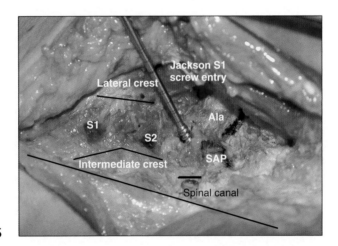

FIGURE 25

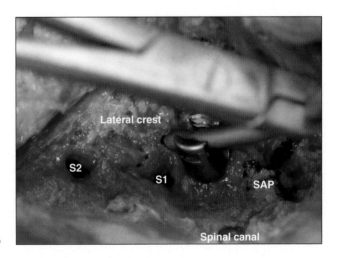

FIGURE 26

Evidence

Asher MA, Strippgen WE. Anthropometric studies of the human sacrum relating to dorsal transsacral implant designs. Clin Orthop. 1986;203:59-62.

Baldwin NG, Benzel EC. Sacral fixation using iliac instrumentation and a variable-angle screw device. J Neurosurg. 1994;81:313-6.

Ebraheim NA, Harman SP, Xu R, Stanescu S, Yeasting RA. The lumbosacral nerves in relation to dorsal S1 screw placement and their location on plain radiographs. Orthopedics. 2000;23:245-7.

Ebraheim NA, Lu J, Biyani A, Galluch D, Yang H, Yeasting RA. Location of the first and second sacral nerve roots in relation to pedicle screw placement. Am J Orthop. 2000;29:873-7.

Ebraheim NA, Lu J, Yang H, Heck BE, Yeasting RA. Anatomic considerations of the second sacral vertebra and dorsal screw placement. Surg Radiol Anat. 1997;19: 353-7.

Ebraheim NA, Mermer M, Xu R, Yeastling RA. Radiological evaluation of S1 dorsal screw placement. J Spinal Disord. 1996;9:527-35.

Ebraheim NA, Xu R, Li J, Yeasting RA. computed tomographic considerations of dorsal sacral screw placement. J Spinal Disord. 1998;11:71-4.

Esses SJ, Botsford DJ, Huler RJ, Rauschning W. Surgical anatomy of the sacrum—a guide for rational screw fixation. Spine. 1991;16:S283-8.

Jackson RP, McManus AC. The iliac buttress—a computed tomographic study of sacral anatomy. Spine. 1993;18:1318-28.

Kostuik JP, Valdevit A, Chang HG, Kanzaki K. Biomechanical testing of the lumbosacral spine. Spine. 1998;23:1721-8.

Licht NJ, Rowe DE, Ross LM. Pitfalls of pedicle screw fixation in the sacrum: a cadaver model. Spine. 1992;17:892-6.

Mazda K, Khairouni A, Pennecot G, Bloch J. The ideal position of sacral transpedicular endplate screws in jackson's intrasacral fixation: an anatomic study of 50 sacral specimens. Spine. 1998;23:2123-6.

McCord DH, Cunningham BW, Shono Y, Myers JJ, McAfee PC. Biomechanical analysis of lumbosacral fixation. Spine. 1992;17:S235-43.

Mirkovic S, Abitbol JJ, Steinman J, Edwards CC, Schaffler M, Massie J, Garfin SR. Anatomic consideration for sacral screw placement. Spine. 1991;16:S289-94.

Morse BJ, Ebraheim NA, Jackson WT. Preoperative CT determination of angles for sacral screw placement. Spine. 1994;19:604-7.

von Strempel A, Trenkmann S, Kronauer, Kirsch L, Sukopp C. The stability of bone screws in the os sacrum. Eur Spine J. 1998;7:313-20.

Templeman D, Schmidt A, Freese J, Weisman I. Proximity of iliosacral screws to neurovascular strutures after internal fixation. Clin Orthop. 1996;329:194-8.

Tsuchiya K, Bridwell KH, Kulko TR, Lenke LG, Baldus C. Minimum 5-year analysis of L5-S1 fusion using sacropelvic fixation (bilateral S1 and iliac screws) for spinal deformity. Spine. 2006;31:303-8.

Posterior Far Lateral Disk Herniation

Chadi Tannoury, D. Greg Anderson, Alexander R. Vaccaro, and Todd J. Albert

PITFALLS

- *Radiographic findings with no clinical correlation*

- *Diagnosis can be hard to make and is often overlooked.*

Controversies

- Presence of far lateral disk herniation with concomitant stenosis at the level above

Treatment Options

- Conservative
- Infiltration (local anesthetics, corticosteroids)—preferably done with fluoroscopic guidance
- Surgical
  - Intertransverse muscle-splitting approach (Fig. 1, arrow C)
  - Intertransverse transmuscular approach (Fig. 1, arrow B)
  - Midline interlaminar approach (partial/complete facetectomy, or removal of the pars interarticularis) (Fig. 1, arrow A)
  - Transforaminal percutaneous approach

Indications

- Unilateral, single-level disk herniation
- Far lateral herniation confirmed by computed tomography (CT) scan or magnetic resonance imaging (MRI): the disk herniation is completely out of the intervertebral foramen, or at least two thirds lateral to the pedicle (Papavero and Caspar, 1993).
- Absence of additional pathology such as spinal stenosis, or an associated central disk herniation
- Signs and symptoms consistent with symptomatic involvement of the exiting nerve root in relation to the disk herniation
- Failure of appropriate conservative management

Examination/Imaging

PRESENTATION

- Upper lumbar root syndrome (e.g., anterior thigh pain)
- Mostly in elderly
- More common in males

PHYSICAL EXAMINATION

- Antalgic gait, listing, limitation of lumbar movement
- Neurologic deficits (sensory, motor, or both)
- Decrease or loss of deep tendon reflex
- Positive nerve tension tests: straight leg raise and femoral nerve stretch test
- Muscular atrophy
- Paravertebral point tenderness (intertransverse membrane level)
- Absence of bowel or bladder dysfunction

IMAGING

- Plain radiography is performed to rule out other conditions (spondylolisthesis, spondylolysis, canal stenosis, etc.).
- MRI (axial and sagittal views) and CT scan are the most sensitive imaging studies. However, one third of extraforaminal disk herniations are overlooked on the CT/MRI (Osborn et al., 1988). Slices must be performed from L2 through S1.
- Seventy-five percent of far lateral disk herniations occur at L4-5 and above (O'Hara and Marshall, 1997).
- Diskography CT provides the most accurate diagnosis (Jackson and Glah, 1987).
- Other imaging studies include myelography, diskography, and selective radiculography.

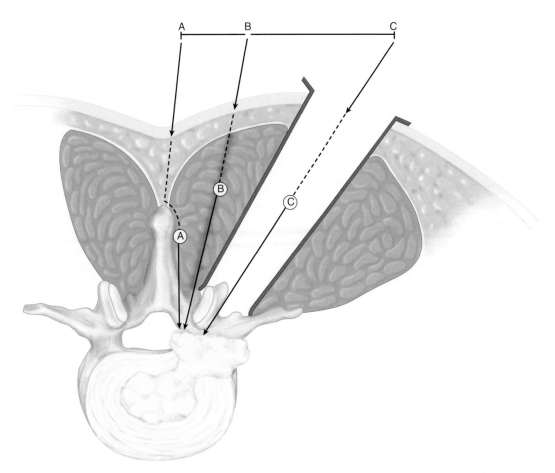

FIGURE 1

- Radiologic findings that should be sought include
  - Disk material lateral to the neural foramen
  - Displacement of paraspinal fat
- Imaging studies should include L2-3 and L3-4 levels as 46% of far lateral disk herniations occur at these levels.

Equipment

• Different positioning equipment has been recommended, such as a Wilson frame, an Andrews frame, a Montreal mattress, and others.

Instrumentation

• Preoperative and generous intraoperative use of C-arm fluoroscopy or plain radiography
• Modified Caspar lumbar speculum-retractor can be very helpful.

Surgical Anatomy

■ Anatomic definition: Far lateral or extreme lateral disk herniation primarily indicates that disk herniation is beyond the lateral intervertebral space, outside of the facet (Fig. 2). The spinal nerve is usually found displaced superiorly and laterally under tension from the herniated disk fragment.

■ The anatomic characteristic of the far lateral disk herniation is that it affects the exiting nerve root at the same level (Fig. 3A), in contrast to classic posterolateral disk herniation, which compresses the traversing nerve root (Fig. 3B).

■ The "operative window" (Fig. 4) for the intertransverse lateral approach is
  • Medial boundary: pars interarticularis
  • Inferior boundary: facet joint and superior border of the inferior transverse process
  • Superior boundary: lower edge of the pedicle and the superior transverse process

Positioning

■ Most surgeons favor the prone position with the abdomen decompressed.

■ Either general or local (Reulen et al., 1996) anesthesia can be used. However, general anesthesia with endotracheal intubation is preferred for safe control of the patient's airway and hemodynamics, and for the possibility of prolonged operation time in difficult cases.

Portals/Exposures

■ Accurate skin incision placement is possible with the assistance of plain radiographs; fluoroscopy is helpful to better localize the initial skin incision.

■ Using anteroposterior and lateral fluoroscopy, two horizontal lines are drawn: the lower line marking the lower border of the affected disk space, and the upper line marking the lower border of the transverse process above the affected disk.

■ Two vertical lines are also drawn: one marking the midline overlying the row of the spinous processes, and the second 4–5 cm lateral to the midline marking the lateral boundary of the pedicle "eye" above and below the affected disk level.

■ These horizontal and vertical lines help defining the site of skin incision, which is about 3–4 cm in length and 4–5 cm paramedian.

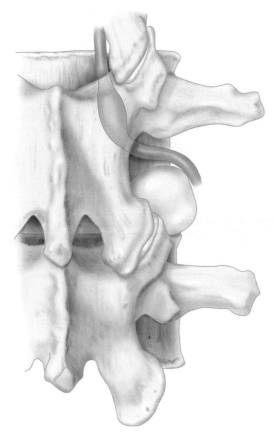

FIGURE 2

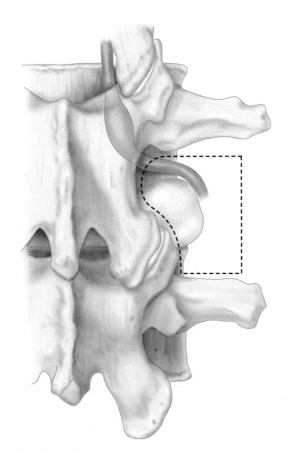

FIGURE 4

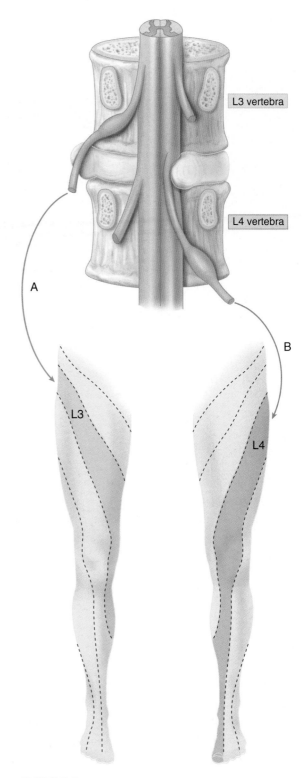

L3 vertebra

L4 vertebra

A

B

L3

L4

FIGURE 3

Controversies

- Intertransverse muscle-splitting versus transmuscular approach
- At L5-S1, the local anatomy can limit the working zone and a larger incision or a more midline incision may be required.
- Also, to accomplish the lateral diskectomy at L5-S1, removal of the L5 transverse process is usually necessary.

PEARLS

- *If using fluoroscopy, make sure you acquire true anterior-posterior and lateral views.*

Instrumentation/ Implantation

- A McCoullough or a Gelpi retractor might be helpful.

PEARLS

- *No. 2 curettes and an angled 3-0 curette are extremely helpful in clearing soft tissue off the bony and soft tissue anatomy and especially the intertransverse membrane.*

Instrumentation/ Implantion

- High-speed bone burr: long and angled drill handpiece
- Nos. 2 and 3-0 angled curette
- Blunt dissector
- A microscope is helpful for delineating the anatomy of the area.

- Muscle-splitting technique: Following skin incision, a second cut is made through the thoracolumbar fascia. Then the erector spinae aponeurosis is incised longitudinally and the cleavage between the multifidus and longissimus muscles is bluntly dissected. A self-retaining retractor of choice is then placed.
- The working zone is bounded medially by the lateral surface of the pars interarticularis, laterally by the tips of the transverse processes, superiorly by the lower surface of the superior transverse process, and inferiorly by the superior surface of the inferior transverse process (see Fig. 3).

Procedure

STEP 1

- Skin marking, incision, and soft tissue dissection (see Portals/Exposures)

STEP 2

- Exposure of transverse process, facet joint, and isthmus
- Bone drilling is rarely needed at the upper lumbar levels; however, it becomes more helpful in cases of significant facet joint hypertrophy and at the L5-S1 level. Partial excision of the lateral aspect of the pars may be required in order to improve exposure.

STEP 3

- The medial half of the intertransverse muscle is incised and reflected laterally, exposing the intertransverse ligament, also known as the "intertransverse membrane."
- Using a binocular loop magnification and a fiberoptic headlight versus a microscope, identification is made, if possible, of the posterior primary ramus as it passes through the medial aspect of the intertransverse membrane and before it distributes its branches to the dorsal musculature.
- The posterior primary ramus is used as a reference to locate the spinal nerve and dorsal root ganglion, which are embedded in extraforaminal fat and connective tissue beneath the intertransverse membrane.
- Gentle and careful superior and lateral retraction of the spinal nerve allows further access to the disk material.

Controversies

- Visualization: microscope versus loupe magnification
- Approach: open versus endoscopic

PEARLS

- *Tilting the operating table away from the surgeon by 15-20° gives a better view of the area lateral to the pedicles.*

- *The spinal nerve is usually found displaced superiorly and laterally under tension from the freely herniated, and often sequestrated (50% of cases), disk fragment (see Fig. 2).*

PITFALLS

- *Excessive retraction of the dorsal ganglion during dissection may result in postoperative burning dysesthesia; however, this usually resolves within several days.*

Instrumentation/ Implantation

- Loupe magnification and fiberoptic headlight source
- The use of the microscope can offer a three-dimensional view.
- Bayoneted instruments for lumbar microdiskectomy

Controversies

- Anatomic keys and landmarks:
- Posterior ramus of the spinal nerve (Fankhauser and de Tribolet, 1991)
- Lateral branch of posterior primary ramus (O'Brien et al., 1995)
- Medial branch of the posterior primary ramus (O'Hara and Marshall, 1997)

- Alternatively, the pedicle below can be identified, and slipping proximally allows identification of the disk. Sliding dorsally allows delineation of the nerve root, and it can then be protected.
- The nerve branches are in close proximity to the accompanying vessels and extruded disk herniation. Branches of the lumbar artery should be dissected carefully and spared whenever possible. However, accompanying veins can be cauterized if they hinder access to the herniated disk fragment.

STEP 4

- Microscopic decompression: a pituitary forceps is used to remove the herniated disk material.
- Removal of the fragment alone is usually sufficient for neural decompression.
- Further exploration, by probing the root canal with a double-angled blunt hook, may be required for the removal of any residual sequestrated disk material. After such exploration, the nerve may be covered with steroid-soaked Gelfoam.

STEP 5

- Placing a drain is seldom necessary.
- Wound closure: musculature reapproximation requires no suturing. However, fascia and aponeurosis are closed using absorbable stitches
- Marcaine without epinephrine is injected generously into the soft tissues for analgesia. Care should be taken to avoid anesthetizing the exiting nerve root.

Postoperative Care and Expected Outcomes

POSTOPERATIVE CARE

- Ambulation and activity as tolerated
- Physical therapy: often indicated to allow progressive mobilization
- Return to work: when tolerated. No heavy lifting or bending for 6 weeks following surgery in order to decrease the risk of recurrent herniations

EXPECTED OUTCOMES

- Good (30–35%) and excellent (41–60%) results are frequently reported (Darden et al., 1995; O'Hara and Marshall, 1997; Papvero and Caspar, 1993). Overall neurologic improvement is achieved in 89% of patients.
- There is 78% complete resolution of motor weakness.
- There is 50% complete resolution of sensory deficit.

COMPLICATIONS

- Exploration of the wrong level, necessitating a revision surgery: avoided by use of intraoperative radiography/fluoroscopy.
- Spondylodiskitis: usually resolves with antibiotics and immobilization
- Spinal instability, when there is excessive pars excision, may lead to accelerated degeneration and/or spinal instability.
- Unsatisfactory relief: due to inadequate decompression, battered nerve root syndrome, or wrong diagnosis (20% of cases)
- Facet distress syndrome: low back pain with pseudoradicular symptoms more often following L5-S1 decompression. However, its incidence rate in patients operated with a muscle-splitting technique is half that of patients operated with the conventional interlaminar approach.

Evidence

Darden BV 2nd, Wade JF, Alexander R, Wood KE, Rhyne AL 3rd, Hicks JR. Far lateral disc herniations treated by microscopic fragment excision: techniques and results. Spine. 1995;20:1500-5.

A series of patients who had been treated with microscopic facet-sparing paraspinal muscle-splitting approach for far lateral disk herniation were evaluated retrospectively using parameters such as history, physical examination, pain questionnaires, visual analog scales, and plain radiographs. The overall clinical results were encouraging, and no radiographic signs of instability were noted. In addition, the paraspinal muscle-splitting approach is thought to minimize manipulation of the dorsal root ganglion, which is responsible for postoperative dysesthesia.

Fankhauser H, de Tribolet N. Extraforaminal approach for extreme lateral lumbar disc herniation. In Torrens MJ, RA Dickinson (eds). Operative Spinal Sugery (Practice of Surgery Series). Edinburgh: Churchill Livingstone, 1991:145-60.

Using the transmuscular approach for far lateral disk herniation, the authors observed the posterior primary ramus of the spinal nerve during operative dissection. However, its usefulness as an anatomic landmark has been argued because of difficult identification of its branches and time consumption.

Jackson RP, Glah JJ. Foraminal and extraforaminal lumbar disc herniation: diagnosis and treatment. Spine. 1987;12:577-85.

In this study, 10% of patients undergoing lumbar diskectomy for herniated nucleus pulposus were found to have far lateral foraminal or extraforaminal disk herniation. Different diagnostic radiographic evaluations have been proposed; however, diskography-enhanced computed tomgraphy proved accuracy in more than 90% of cases. In terms of surgical approach, the authors opted for bilateral hemilaminectomy with partial medial facetectomy and partial internal foraminotomy as most effective for diskectomy and nerve root decompression.

O'Brien MF, Peterson D, Crockard HA. A posterolateral microsurgical approach to extreme-lateral lumbar disc herniation. J Neurosurg. 1995;83:636-40.

O'Brien et al. have adopted the posterolateral approach of Watkins for patients with a far lateral disk herniation. The authors recommend the use of the lateral branch of the posterior primary ramus as a key anatomic landmark to direct them to the spinal nerve and the intervertebral foramen.

O'Hara LJ, Marshall RW. Far lateral lumbar disc herniation: the key to the intertransverse approach. J Bone Joint Surg Br. 1997;79:943-7.

In a series of patients with far lateral lumbar disk herniation, an intertransverse muscle-splitting approach has been adopted with encouraging outcomes. A cadaver study describing the anatomic course of the posterior primary ramus within the intertransverse membrane has also been reported. The authors recommend the use of a muscle-splitting intertransverse approach to far lateral herniation, refering to the posterior primary ramus as the anatomic key to safe dissection.

Osborn AG, Hood RS, Sherry RG, Smoker WRK, Harnsberger HR. CT/MRI spectrum of far lateral and anterior lumbosacral disc herniations. AJNR Am J Neuroradiol. 1988;9:775-8.

A radiologic assessment of patients with extraforaminal disk herniations (EFDHs) using CT and/or MRI reported that the most commonly affected level was L4-5; however, 46% of EFDHs were overlooked and located at L2-3 or L3-4 levels. EFDHs can be readily diagnosed on both CT and MRI if appropriate scans are obtained from L2 through S1 and if the neural foramina and paravertebral spaces are carefully examined. Overlooked EFDHs are an important preventable cause of failed intraspinal diskectomy.

Papavero L, Caspar W. The lumbar microdiscectomy. Acta Orthop Scand Suppl. 1993;64:34-7.

Reulen HJ, Muller A, Ebeling U. Microsurgical anatomy of the lateral approach to extraforaminal lumbar disc herniations. Neurosurgery. 1996;39:345-50; discussion 350-1.

In lumbar spine specimens taken from human cadavers, the relevant distances and proportions of the operative window were measured at the levels L1-2 to L5-S1. The anatomic findings led to important conclusions regarding the microsurgical approach to extraforaminal lumbar disk herniations; at levels L1-2 to L3-4, the midline approach with lateral retraction of the paraspinal muscles allows for efficient exposure of the lateral neural foramen and avoidance of trauma to the facet joint. Often at level L4-5, and nearly always at level L5-S1, a tangential route through a paramedian transmuscular approach offers many advantages.

The Lateral Extracavitary Approach for Vertebrectomy

Kene T. Ugokwe and Edward C. Benzel

PITFALLS

- *The degree of difficulty of the operation requires experience, expertise, and a working knowledge of retroperitoneal surgical anatomy.*

- *It requires a moderate amount of endurance. The operative procedure, including placement of instrumentation devices, may last from 4 to 6 hours.*

- *A unilateral approach does not allow for access beyond the contralateral pedicle.*

- *This approach does not allow direct access to adjacent ventral intracavitary structures (e.g., aorta and vena cava), which may be involved with pathology or may be inadvertently injured.*

Controversies

- It is a difficult and complex operation, and the decision to subject a patient with metastases to this operation requires knowledge of the extent of systemic disease and treatability of the pathology.

Treatment Options

- Alternate approaches to the ventral thoracic and thoracolumbar spine include the retropleural and transpleural thoracotomy.
- Anterolateral transthoracic approach
- Posterolateral costotransversectomy
- Staged transthoracic and dorsal combined approach

Indications

- The lateral extracavitary approach popularized by Larson et al. in 1976 allows access to the anterior vertebral bodies, as well as the posterior elements of the spine, through a single incision, thereby providing a means of ventral decompression and dorsal fixation of the spine during a single procedure. It is a derivative of the lateral costotransversectomy.
- This approach was developed for treating tuberculous spondylitis with neurologic involvement (Alexander, 1946; Capener, 1954; Bohlman and Eismont, 1981).
- Spinal cord decompression surgery has undergone many transformations in the last 40 years (Clark, 1981; Schneider, 1962; Morgan et al., 1970; Wagner and Chehrazi, 1980).
- The lateral extracavitary approach may be used to address pathology anywhere from T3 to S1. This pathology may include tumors, infections (Capener, 1954; Larson et al., 1976), herniated disks, and fractures (Capener, 1954; Erickson, Leider, and Brown, 1977; Larson, 1980).
- This approach does not involve entry into the abdominal or thoracic cavities. It may also be used to approach the upper thoracic vertebrae without sternotomy or thoracotomy.
- The lateral extracavitary approach allows the surgeon to simultaneously decompress the ventral spinal cord and to place instrumentation devices dorsally through the same incision and under the same anesthetic.
- The approach may be performed on either the left or the right side depending on the location of the pathology.
- In cases of complete spondylectomy, a bilateral approach may be considered.

Examination/Imaging

- Spinal angiography can be used to identify and determine the course of the artery of Adamkiewicz. Spinal tumors, depending on the region of the pathology, can also be embolized 24–36 hours before resection.
- In the preoperative planning stage for a lateral extracavitary approach, the surgeon must have adequate radiographic imaging of the pathologic region.
- Magnetic resonance imaging (MRI) with gadolinium is very helpful in assessing the integrity of the thecal

sac and spinal cord. It can also be used to delineate the extent of tumor spread and areas of infection. The T_2-weighted sequence on MRI is also useful in determining soft tissue and ligamentous injury.

■ Computed tomography (CT) scans are also very useful in elucidating bony anatomy.

■ Plain radiographs in combination with CT scans can also help to determine bone quality and the ability of the spine to hold an implant.

■ Imaging should also be adequate to look at the position of adjacent ventral structures in relation to the pathology (e.g., is the tumor exophytic and encasing the aorta?).

Surgical Anatomy

■ The posterior musculature of the thoracic spine, which may be encountered during this operation depending on the level of the incision, is grouped into the superficial, intermediate, and deep layers.

■ Superficial muscles include the trapezius, latissimus dorsi, and rhomboids.

■ Intermediate muscles are the serratus posterior superior and inferior.

■ The deep layer includes the erector spinae muscles and the transversospinalis muscles.

■ The thoracic segmental vessels are located at the waist of the thoracic vertebral body and divide laterally into a dorsal and ventral division.

■ The thoracic nerve root exits the neural foramen beneath the pedicle and divides into a dorsal and ventral ramus. The dorsal ramus runs into the erector spinae muscle and is accompanied by the dorsal branches of the posterior intercostal vessels. These should be ligated to prevent bleeding.

■ The sympathetic trunk should be identified and protected.

Positioning

■ When general anesthesia is induced, the patient is placed in the three-quarter prone position.

■ It is important to note that the patient is intubated and prepared for surgery while on his or her bed in the supine position. After all lines and tubes are secured, the patient is slid to the edge of the bed and rolled to the lateral decubitus position on the operating table.

Equipment

- If the patient is placed in the prone position, the Jackson frame may be used, which allows the table to be rotated away from the surgeon to facilitate visualization.

Controversies

- Spinal cord monitoring, including somatosensory evoked potentials, motor evoked potentials, and electromyelography, is not routinely used because it is frequently unreliable and conflicting. Spinal cord monitoring may, however, be helpful during surgery for severe deformity correction.

PEARLS

- *Complete exposure of the vertebral elements above and below the pathologic level ensures adequate ventral exposure.*

- *Meticulous hemostasis during the initial exposure will help reduce blood loss.*

PITFALLS

- *Unrecognized pneumothorax from pleural violation*

- Four or five assistants help to move the patient, which minimizes the chance for inadvertent spinal manipulation that might cause neural injury.
- A generous axillary roll is placed with the "down arm" extended laterally in a position 10° above the perpendicular axis of the patient's body. The patient is then rolled further into a three-quarter prone position and secured in this position with 3-inch adhesive tape and rolls formed from sheets and blankets (Fig. 1).
- The patient's abdomen is freed of all compression. The upper arm may be placed on a well-padded Mayo stand or pillow. The operative table can be tilted from side to side in order to facilitate the view of the operative site by both the operating surgeon and the assistant.

Portals/Exposures

- An intraoperative radiograph after positioning and before draping also is helpful in localization as the skin incision should be centered over the lesion. It is important to prepare and drape a wide area to allow for maximal exposure.
- The approach may be performed on either the left or the right side depending on the location of the pathology. However, in cases of complete spondylectomy, a bilateral approach may be considered.
- A hockey stick–shaped incision is generally used, with the lateral limb curving off 8-10 cm toward the side of the pathology and the vertical limb running along the midline (Fig. 2). A gentle angle should be used in order to prevent ischemic injury to the skin flap. In certain cases, an L-shaped incision may be used, but this may lead to necrosis of a devascularized corner.
- The vertical limb of the incision can be taken down through the subcutaneous tissue and the thoracodorsal fascia to the spinous processes with monopolar cauterization.
- The thoracodorsal fascia is incised in the shape of a T. A subperiosteal dissection using a Cobb dissector or periosteal elevator also helps decrease bleeding and thermal injury to the muscle.

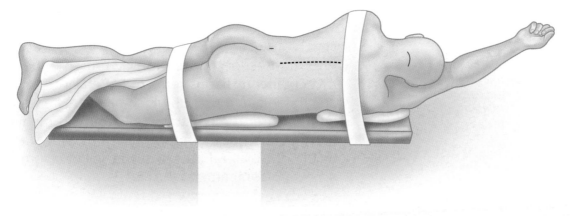

FIGURE 1

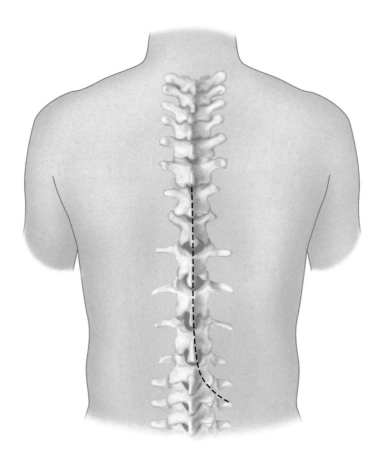

FIGURE 2

Procedure

STEP 1

■ After transection of the thoracic muscles, the myocutaneous flap is retracted laterally to expose the erector spinae muscles, which are retracted medially. Retraction of the erector spinae muscles medially and resection of the appropriate ribs allows access to the dorsolateral aspect of the spinal column via an extrapleural approach (Fig. 3).

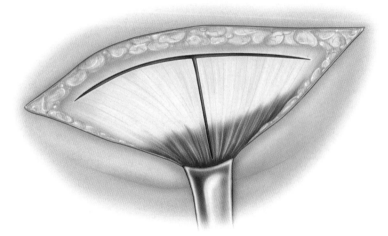

A

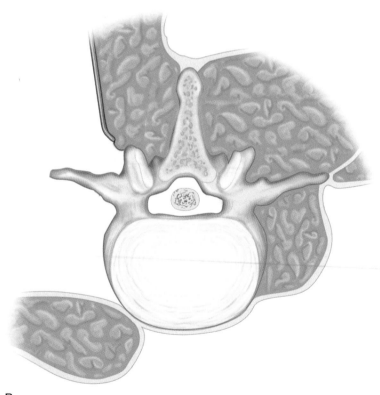

B

FIGURE 3A-B

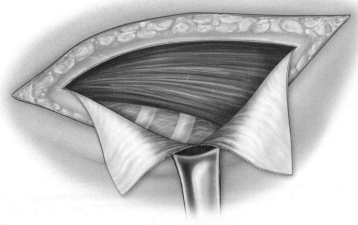

C

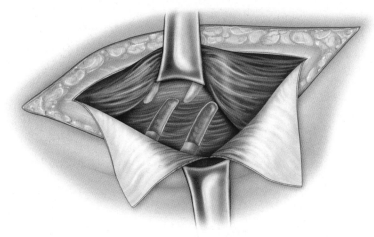

D

FIGURE 3C-D *Continued*

■ A Doyen rib dissector is used to remove the soft tissue on the undersurface or ventral aspect of the ribs. The ribs are dissected out to the costovertebral joints.

■ The next step involves resecting the rib using a rib cutter. Approximately 8-10 cm of rib is resected from the costovertebral joint for tumor surgery, and this is also adequate for vertebrectomy. For disk surgery, a rib resection of 3 cm is adequate. The resected rib should be saved to use as a bone graft for fusion.

PEARLS

- *Dural tears should be repaired primarily when possible. Another option is patching the dura with a substitute such as bovine pericardium or other dural substitutes.*

PITFALLS

- *Care must be taken during decompression to avoid pushing a fractured piece of bone into the spinal canal.*

- *Nerve root damage during decompression must be avoided.*

- *Preoperative angiography to identify the artery of Adamkiewicz will help determine which segmentals may be ligated.*

STEP 2

- When the neurovascular bundle is identified, it may be followed into the foramen. The neural foramina above and below the vertebrectomy site are enlarged, and an intraoperative radiograph may again be helpful for localization if the pathology is not clearly evident.
- The disk space immediately superior and inferior to the vertebrectomy site should be removed with a scalpel. The vertebral body can be removed with either a high-speed drill or a rongeur under direct visualization (Fig. 4). The dura can be further exposed using a high-speed burr, rongeurs, and curettes.
- The vertebral body resection should be carried out to the distal pedicle. It is imperative to completely decompress the spinal canal. This may be difficult, however, because visualization of all bony fragments is not always possible. The superior disk space should be explored for any bony fragments. The posterior longitudinal ligament may also be opened to explore the epidural space.

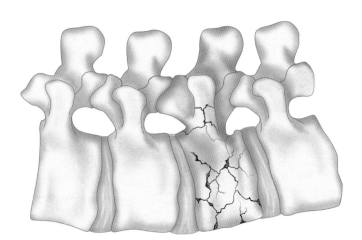

FIGURE 4

PEARLS

- *In the upper thoracic spine, the parietal pleura should be inspected for leaks. Small leaks may be repaired primarily and larger leaks may require chest tube placement.*

PITFALLS

- *Certain patients suffer significant morbidity from iliac crest graft harvest, and this should be avoided if possible.*

- *Placement of grafts too close to the spinal cord can lead to graft migration and spinal cord injury.*

Controversies

- Some surgeons are hesitant to place a surgical drain in the presence of a cerebrospinal fluid leak. If a drain is placed in this situation, it is important to ensure that the leak is repaired first and that the drain output is monitored closely.

STEP 3

- It is important after a vertebrectomy to maintain the integrity of the spinal column by reconstructing it. A midline subperiosteal exposure is performed along the spinous processes and laminae over the appropriate levels for placement of dorsal instrumentation. Freedom of movement at the level of the involved disk interspaces, which is gained by the vertebrectomy, allows optimal spine reduction.

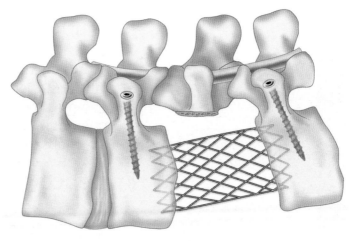

FIGURE 5

- Following placement of the dorsal instrumentation, the original operative site is re-exposed.
- An appropriately fashioned rib or iliac crest graft may be positioned with an impactor and a hammer. The iliac crest can be exposed through the lower lateral aspect of the operative field in the lumbar and low thoracic approaches in order to harvest tricortical iliac bone. In the thoracic and thoracolumbar region, appropriately fashioned rib segments may be used as strut grafts.
- Tibial allograft struts or titanium cages packed with bone from resected rib or vertebral body may also be used for a fusion (Fig. 5).
- When an interbody bone graft is to be placed, curettes are used to make troughs in the vertebral body above and below the decompressed area. Ventral plating followed by dorsal instrumentation may be inserted as deemed appropriate.
- The wound is closed in layers, and a surgical drain may be placed adjacent to the surgical site.

Postoperative Care and Expected Outcomes

- Most patients are kept intubated in the intensive care unit for the first night after surgery as a result of increased facial swelling.
- Patients are mobilized in an orthosis usually by postoperative day 2, and they are evaluated by physical therapy.
- Surgical drains are also usually removed by the second postoperative day.

PEARLS

- *Patients should be mobilized fairly quickly.*

- *If patients are not rapidly mobilized, they should be on prophylaxis for deep venous thrombi.*

PITFALLS

- *When removing surgical drains or epidural pain catheters, care must be taken to ensure that no part of the catheter is retained in the body.*

- Upright films are obtained.
- Patients may require patient-controlled analgesia devices.
- Most patients are ready for discharge by the third to fifth postoperative day.
- The most common complications include pneumothorax, pleural effusions, pneumonia, wound infections, and cerebrospinal fluid leaks.

Evidence

Alexander GL. Neurological complications of spinal tuberculosis. Proc R Soc Med. 1946;39:730-4.

Bohlman HH, Eismont FJ. Surgical techniques of anterior decompression and fusion for spinal cord injuries. Clin Orthop. 1981;154:57-67.

Capener N. The evolution of lateral rhacotomy. J Bone Joint Surg Br. 1954;36:173-9.

Clark WK. Spinal cord decompression in spinal cord injury. Clin Orthop. 1981;154:9-13.

Erickson DL, Leider LL, Brown WE. One stage decompression-stabilization for thoracolumbar fractures. Spine. 1977;2:53-6.

Larson SJ. Unstable thoracic fractures: treatment alternatives and the role of the neurosurgeon. Clin Neurosurg. 1980;27:624-40.

Larson SJ, Holst RA, Hemmy DC, et al. Lateral extracavitary approach to traumatic lesions of the thoracic and lumbar spine. J Neurosurg. 1976;45:628-37.

Morgan TH, Wharton GW, Austin GN, et al. The results of laminectomy in patients with incomplete spinal cord injuries. Paraplegia. 1970;9:14-21.

Schneider RC. Surgical indications and contraindications in spine and spinal cord trauma. Clin Neurosurg. 1962;8:157-84.

Wagner FC Jr, Chehrazi B. Spinal cord injury: indications for operative intervention. Surg Clin North Am. 1980;60:1049-54.

Osteotomy Techniques (Smith-Petersen and Pedicle Subtraction) for Fixed Sagittal Imbalance

Keith H. Bridwell

PITFALLS

- *Smith-Petersen osteotomies can lead to coronal imbalance, pitching the patient toward the concavity.*

- *Pedicle subtraction osteotomies can lead to neurologic deficits, subluxations, and substantial intraoperative blood loss.*

Controversies

- For most fixed sagittal and coronal deformities, the options are either multiple Smith-Petersen osteotomies or one pedicle subtraction procedure.

Indications

- Fixed sagittal and coronal imbalance
- Smith-Petersen osteotomies are reserved for lesser sagittal deformities that are long, smooth, and rounded (Fig. 1A and 1B). They can be safely performed in the thoracic and lumbar spine. No retraction of the thecal sac is needed.
- Pedicle subtraction procedures are indicated in sharp, angular deformities, and for a more marked sagittal deformity. They are best performed at L2 or L3 below the conus. They can be performed in the thoracic spine, but a costotransversectomy approach is then needed as the thecal sac should not be retracted in cord territory.

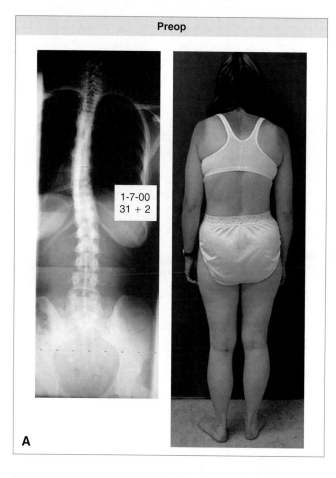

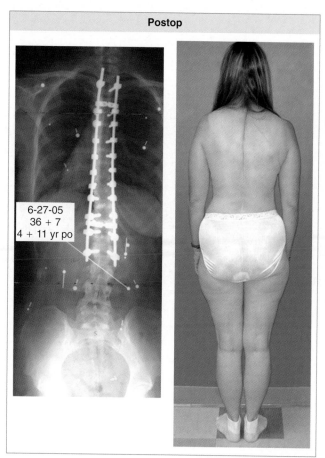

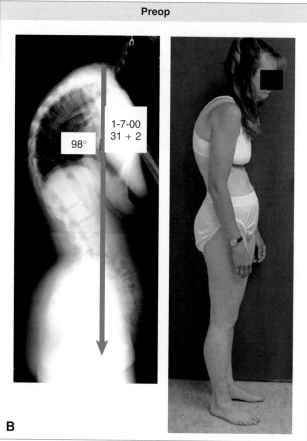

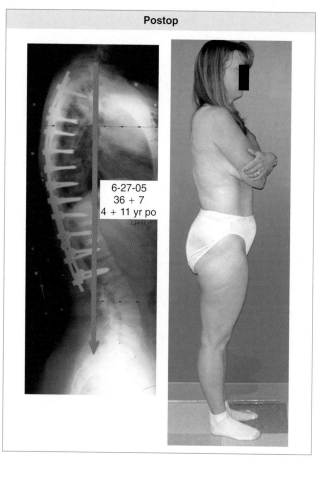

FIGURE 1A-B

Treatment Options

- Either multiple Smith-Petersen osteotomies or one pedicle subtraction procedure for fixed sagittal imbalance
- If the fixed sagittal deformity is associated with a coronal deformity such that shortening of the convex side will rebalance the patient, options are either multiple asymmetric Smith-Petersen osteotomies or one asymmetric pedicle subtraction procedure (Fig. 2).

Examination/Imaging

- Plain long cassette standing anteroposterior (AP) and lateral radiographs, preferably with the patient's knees fully extended
- Oblique AP and lateral radiographs to determine if there is pseudarthrosis from prior surgery
- Magnetic resonance imaging and computed tomography–myelogram to investigate areas of spinal stenosis
- Supine long cassette lateral radiograph to assess flexibility in the sagittal plane

Preop	Postop

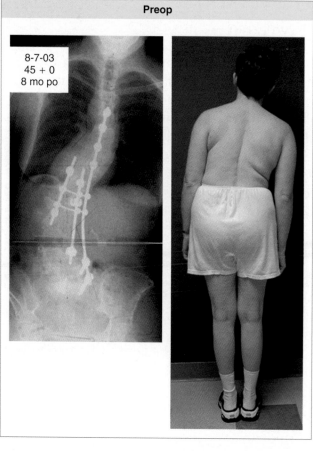

8-7-03
45 + 0
8 mo po

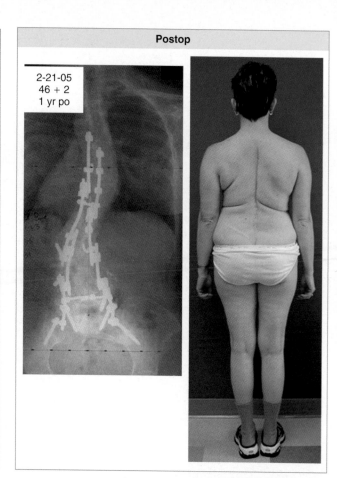

2-21-05
46 + 2
1 yr po

Preop	Postop

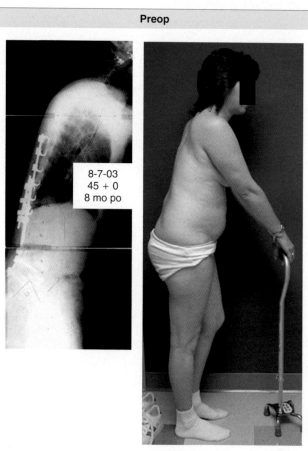

8-7-03
45 + 0
8 mo po

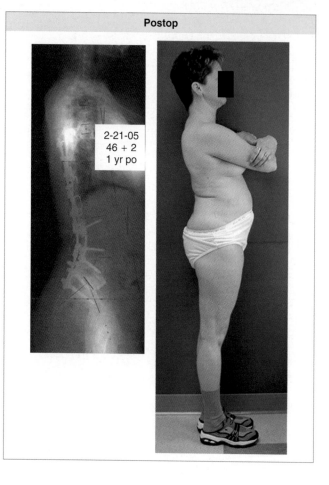

2-21-05
46 + 2
1 yr po

FIGURE 2

Surgical Anatomy

- Smith-Petersen osteotomies involve resecting of the posterior elements through the facet joints and pars intra-articularis. Then the posterior column is closed and the anterior column spontaneously opens through the disk space (Fig. 3).
- The pedicle subtraction procedure involves taking a V-shaped wedge out of the vertebral segment. This involves resection of the posterior elements, the pedicles, and the vertebral body (Fig. 4).

Positioning

- For both the procedures, the patient is placed prone.
- Have the abdomen free to reduce epidural bleeders.
- If the sagittal deformity is marked and fixed, position the patient with some flexion of the hips and knees. Closure of the osteotomies is facilitated by extending the hips under the drapes.

Portals/Exposures

- A standard midline exposure is performed out to the tips of the transverse processes of all the segments above and below the osteotomies.

Smith-Petersen Osteotomy

Preop	Postop
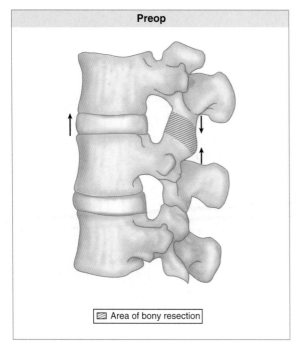	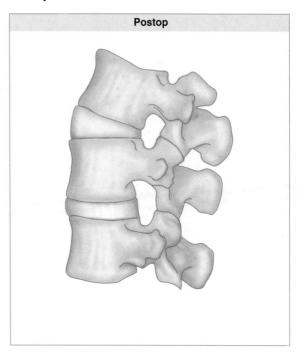

☒ Area of bony resection

FIGURE 3

Three Column Pedicle Subtraction Osteotomy

Preop	Postop
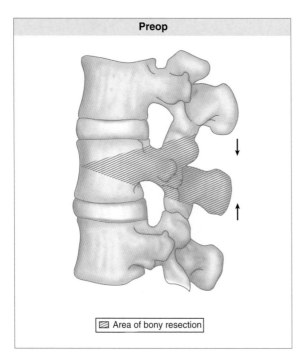	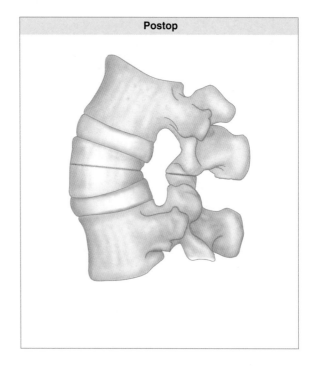

☒ Area of bony resection

FIGURE 4

Instrumentation/ Implantation

• Instrumentation should extend the entire length of the fusion area.

Procedure

STEP 1

■ Pedicle subtraction osteotomy
  • Resect all the posterior elements around the pedicles (Fig. 5).
■ Smith-Petersen osteotomy
  • Identify the pedicles at all levels where Smith-Petersen osteotomies are planned by placing pedicle screws (Fig. 6).

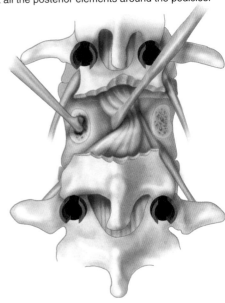

Resect all the posterior elements around the pedicles.

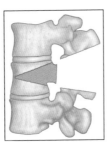

FIGURE 5

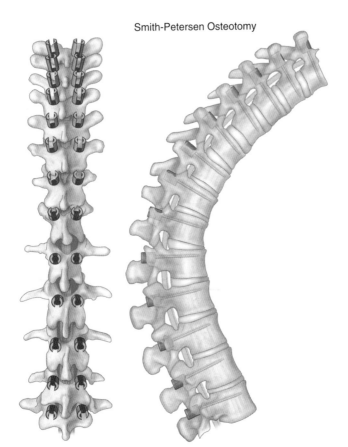

Smith-Petersen Osteotomy

FIGURE 6

PEARLS

- *With Smith-Petersen osteotomies, it is advisable to undercut as much as possible and to remove all ligamentum flavum.*

STEP 2

- Pedicle subtraction osteotomy
  - Decancellate the pedicles and the vertebral body (Fig. 7).
- Smith-Petersen osteotomy
  - Resect a V of bone that starts centrally and works out laterally through the facet joints and pars (Fig. 8).

Decancellate the pedicles and the vertebral body.

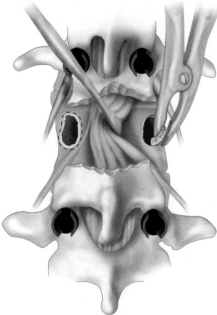
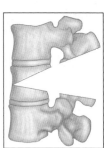

FIGURE 7

Smith-Petersen Osteotomy

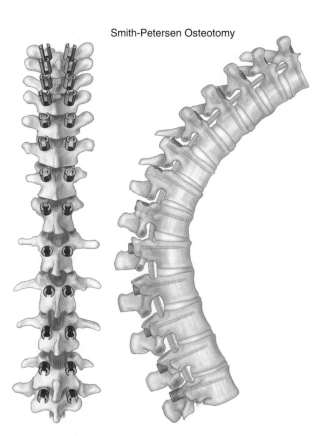

FIGURE 8

Instrumentation/ Implantation

• The rods should be strong, but not "too" stiff. The author prefers 5.5-mm stainless steel.

STEP 3

■ Pedicle subtraction osteotomy
  • Greenstick the posterior vertebral cortex with a Woodson elevator or reserve angled curette (Fig. 9).
■ Smith-Petersen osteotomy
  • Close the osteotomies by a combination of compression and cantilevering (Fig. 10).

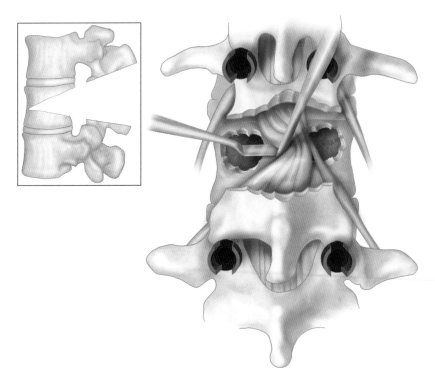

Greenstick the posterior vertebral cortex with a Woodson elevator or reversed angled curet.

FIGURE 9

Smith-Petersen Osteotomy

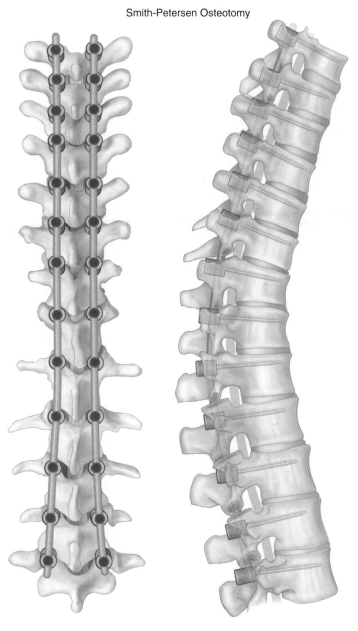

FIGURE 10

PITFALLS

- *With pedicle subtraction procedures, there is some risk of dural buckling and the posterior elements imploding on the dura. The author's preference is to enlarge the field centrally to observe dural buckling (Fig. 13A and B) and to "feel" the dorsal canal with nerve hooks/Woodson elevators.*

- *Watch carefully for subluxation.*

STEP 4

- Pedicle subtraction osteotomy: resect the lateral vertebral cortex with a Leksell rongeur bilaterally (Fig. 11).

STEP 5

- Pedicle subtraction osteotomy: close the osteotomy by compression/cantilever/extension of chest and lower extremities (Fig. 12)

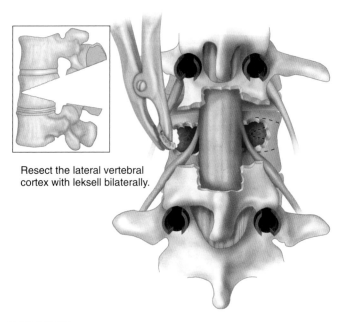

Resect the lateral vertebral cortex with leksell bilaterally.

FIGURE 11

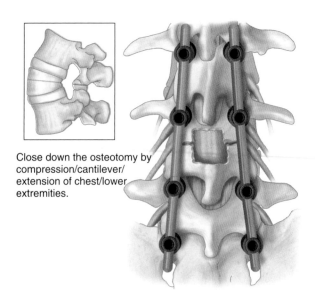

Close down the osteotomy by compression/cantilever/ extension of chest/lower extremities.

FIGURE 12

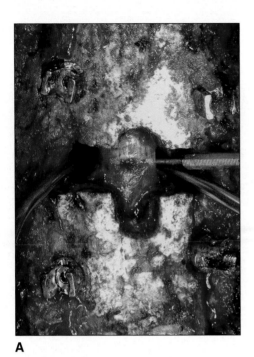 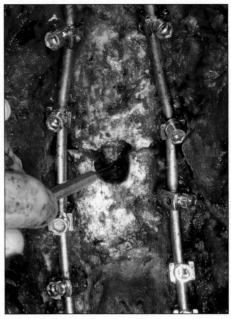

A   B

FIGURE 13A-B

Controversies

- There is some potential for the patient to add on to the kyphosis, either proximally or distally. There is also potential for pullout of the fixation points above and below, and therein additional deformity.

Postoperative Care and Expected Outcomes

- Improvement (20-30%) in SRS-30 and Oswestry Quality of Health (QOL) scores in most patients at 2 and 5 year follow-up per our publications.
- Stand the patient the morning after surgery and walk in place
- Walk three miles a day by 2 months postoperatively
- Avoid flexion and axial loading of the spine for at least 4 months postoperatively
- No cast or brace
- Off all pain medicines by 2 months postoperatively
- No non-steroidal anti-inflammatory drugs (NSAIDs) for 6 months postoperatively

Evidence

Berven SH, Deviren V, Smith JA, Emami A, Hu SH, Bradford DS. Management of fixed sagittal plane deformity: results of the transpedicular wedge resection osteotomy. Spine. 2001;26:2036-43.

Substantial correction can be obtained by performing a pedicle subtraction osteotomy. The procedure is not risk-free.

Bridwell KH, Lewis S, Edwards C, Lenke LG, Iffrig TM, Berra A, Baldus C, Blanke K. Complications and outcomes of pedicle subtraction osteotomies for fixed sagittal imbalance. Spine. 2003;28:2093-101.

Substantial complications associated with pedicle subtraction osteotomies include neurologic deficit, substantial blood loss, and adding on to the sagittal deformity if the entire thoracic and lumbar spine is not fused.

Bridwell KH, Lewis SJ, Lenke LG, Baldus C, Blanke K. Pedicle subtraction osteotomy for the treatment of fixed sagittal imbalance. J Bone Joint Surg Am. 2003;85:454-63.

Pedicle subtraction osteotomies have a role in patients with fixed sagittal imbalance following idioapthic scoliosis surgery, following distal degenerative lumbar spine surgery, and also for posttraumatic kyphosis and ankylosing spondylitis patients. Most patients receive substantial benefit from the procedures.

Cho K, Bridwell KH, Lenke LG, Berra A, Baldus C. Comparison of Smith-Petersen versus pedicle subtraction osteotomy for the correction of fixed sagittal imbalance. Spine. 2005;30:2030-37.

Three Smith-Petersen osteotomies accomplish approximately what is accomplished with one pedicle subtraction procedure. The blood loss is greater with a pedicle subtraction procedure.

Hehne HJ, Zielke K, Bohm H. Polysegmental lumbar osteotomies and transpedicled fixation for correction of long-curved kyphotic deformities in ankylosing spondylitis: report on 177 cases. Clin Orthop. 1990;258:49-55.

Ankylosing spondylitis sagittal deformities can be corrected through the use of transpedicular fixation and multiple Smith-Petersen osteotomies from T10 to the sacrum.

Lagrone MO, Bradford DS, Moe JH, Lonstein JE, Winter RB, Ogilvie JW. Treatment of symptomatic flatback after spinal fusion. J Bone Joint Surg Am. 1988;70:569-80.

Smith-Petersen osteotomies are useful in treating fixed sagittal imbalance syndromes occurring after idiopathic scoliosis surgeries performed many years prior.

McMaster MJ. A technique for lumbar spinal osteotomy in ankylosing spondylitis. J Bone Joint Surg Br. 1985;67:204-10.

Smith-Petersen osteotomy is a useful procedure for ankylosing spondylitis.

Smith-Petersen MN, Larson CB, Aufranc OE. Osteotomy of the spine for correction of flexion deformity in rheumatoid arthritis. J Bone Joint Surg Am. 1945;27:1-11.

This is the first description of a Smith-Petersen osteotomy. It is described for ankylosing spondylitis.

Thomasen E. Vertebral osteotomy for correction of kyphosis in ankylosing spondylitis. Clin Orthop. 1985;194:142-52.

This is the first peer-reviewed article describing a pedicle subtraction procedure. The initial description in a series of ankylosing spondylitis patients.

Voos K, Boachie-Adjei O, Rawlins BA. Multiple vertebral osteotomies in the treatment of rigid adult spine deformities. Spine. 2001;26:526-33.

Multiple Smith-Petersen osteotomies are useful in treating rigid adult deformities. Frequently, both anterior and posterior surgeries are required.

Spondylolysis Repair

Brian Walsh, Ernest Found, and Vincent C. Traynelis

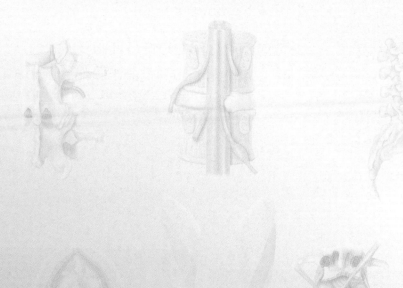

Treatment Options

- Arthrodesis with or without instrumentation
- Direct screw fixation of defect

Indications

- Pars defect must be source of pain
- No instability on imaging
- Minimal disk degeneration present
- Patient 30 years of age or younger
- Nonsmoker

Examination/Imaging

- Anteroposterior and lateral lumbar radiographs
- Flexion and extension lateral lumbar radiographs (Fig. 1A and 1B)

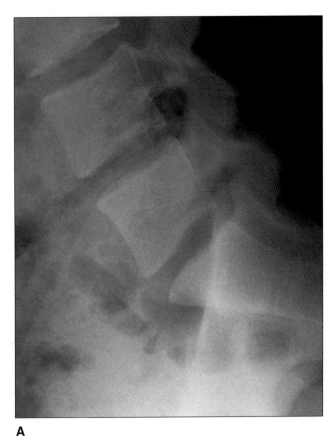

A

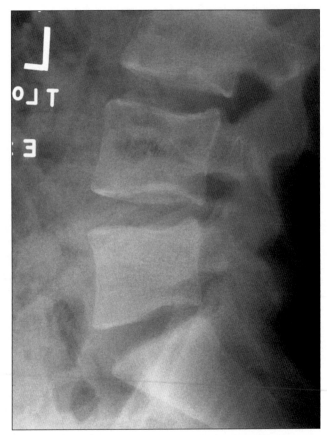

B

FIGURE 1A-B

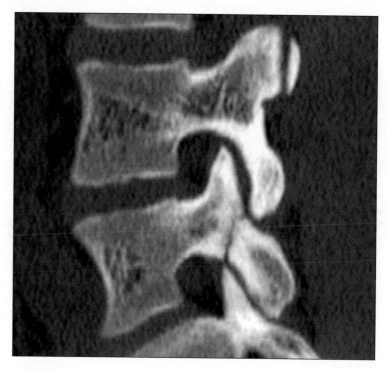

FIGURE 2

- Lumbosacral computed tomography (Fig. 2)
- Bone scan

Surgical Anatomy

- The affected lamina
- The affected pars interarticularis
- The pedicle of the affected vertebra

Positioning

- Prone on Wilson frame, laminectomy rolls, or Jackson table

Portals/Exposures

- A standard posterior lumbar exposure is used to access the affected vertebra. The lamina, facets, and proximal transverse process should be exposed.

Procedure

STEP 1

- Curettage of the pars defect is performed.
- A burr is utilized to freshen fracture surfaces (Fig. 3). Note that the burr and exposure of the defect margins are enlarged in Figure 3 to illustrate the technique. The actual débridement should disrupt as little bone as possible.
- The soft tissue between the fracture surfaces is removed (Fig. 4).

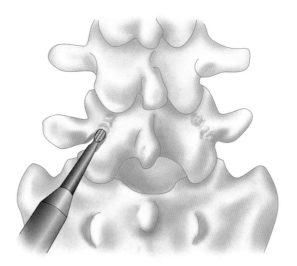

FIGURE 3

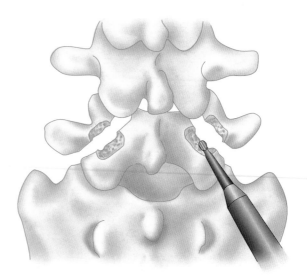

FIGURE 4

STEP 2

- A pedicle screw with a hole through its post is inserted using standard techniques.
- A cable is threaded through the hole in the pedicle screw post and around the spinous process (Fig. 5A and 5B).

Instrumentation/Implantion

• Pedicle screw insertion

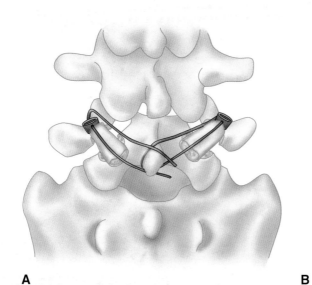
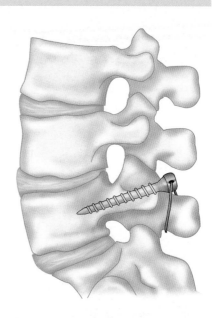

FIGURE 5A-B **A** **B**

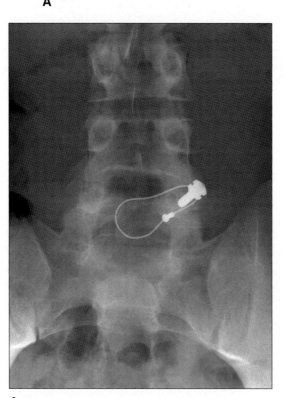
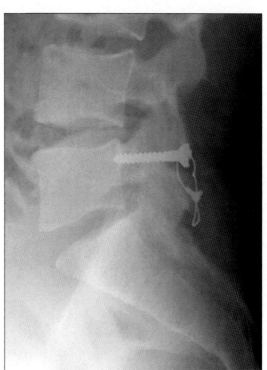

FIGURE 6A-B **A** **B**

Instrumentation/ Implantation

- Pedicle screw insertion
- Sublaminar hook insertion

STEP 3

- An alternative technique uses a hook/rod construct (Fig. 7).
- A pedicle screw with a hole through its post is inserted using standard techniques
- A sublaminar hook is placed, connected to the pedicle screw with a rod, and secured after compression force is applied.

STEP 4

- Standard would closure

Postoperative Care and Expected Outcomes

- Camp brace is used for 6 weeks.

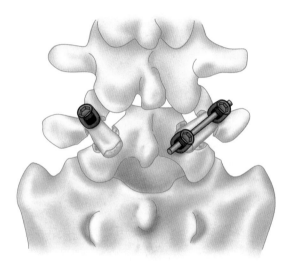

FIGURE 7

Evidence

Buck JE. Direct repair of the defect in spondylolisthesis: preliminary report. J Bone Joint Surg Br. 1970;52:432-7.

Grade-B description of a direct screw fixation technique across the pars defect.

Morscher E, Gerber B, Fasel J. Surgical treatment of spondylolisthesis by bone grafting and direct stabilization of spondylolysis by means of a hook screw. Arch Orthop Trauma Surg. 1988;103:178-88.

Grade-B description of a hook screw fixation technique in 12 patients, 10 of whom had an excellent or good outcome.

Nichol RO, Scott JHS. Lytic spondylolysis repair by wiring. Spine. 1986;11:1027-30.

Grade-C retrospective review of a wiring technique.

Songer MN, Rovin R. Repair of the pars interarticularis defect with a cable-screw construct: a preliminary report. Spine. 1998;23:263-9.

Grade-B report with an excellent description of the technique. The outcomes of seven patients are retrospectively reviewed.

Tokuhasi Y, Matsuzaki H. Repair of defects in spondylolysis by segmental pedicular screw hook fixation: a preliminary report. Spine. 1996;21:2041-5.

Grade-B report of six patients treated with a screw-hook technique.

Reduction of High-Grade Spondylolisthesis

Rachana Tyagi and David H. Clements

Controversies

• Diskography is performed by some surgeons to elucidate the contribution of the disk as a pain generator.

Treatment Options

• Bracing
• Selective nerve root blocks
• Facet blocks (if pain is mechanical)
• Physical therapy
• Nonsteroidal anti-inflammatory drugs

Indications

■ Intractable pain (may be back pain, radiculopathy, or neurogenic claudication)
■ Neurologic deficit
■ Spinal instability

Examination/Imaging

PHYSICAL EXAMINATION

■ May note stepoff of spinous processes (Fig. 1A).
■ Heart-shaped buttocks with spondyloptosis may be noted.
■ Symptoms are reproduced with lumbar extension.
■ Examine entire spine in upright and flexed positions for scoliosis.
■ Patients often stand with hips and knees flexed to bring sacrum more parallel with the floor, and have a large popliteal angle with tight hamstrings.
■ Document careful neurologic examination for baseline deficits, including cystometrics.
■ If hyperreflexia is present, evaluate for concomitant cervical spine disease.

IMAGING

■ Plain films with anteroposterior, lateral, and oblique views to assess degree of slip, angulation, pars abnormality, and scoliosis (Fig. 1B)

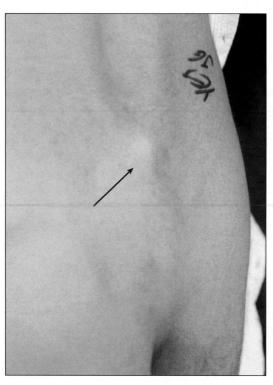

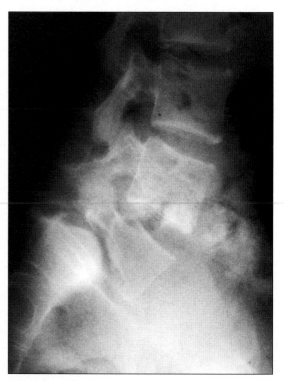

A **B**

FIGURE 1A-B

- Flexion/extension films to evaluate stability
- Examine films closely for possible spina bifida occulta.
- Magnetic resonance imaging to evaluate the degree of central and foraminal stenosis (Fig. 1C and 1D)
- Computed tomography (Fig. 1E–1G)

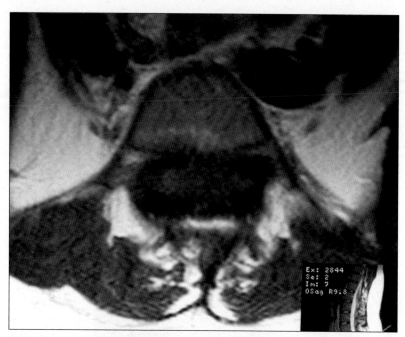

C

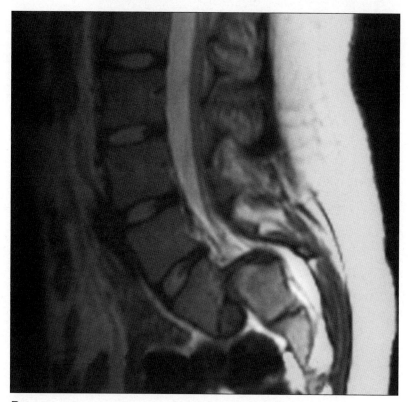

D

FIGURE 1C-D *Continued*

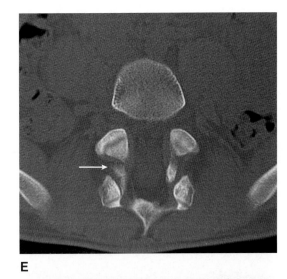

E

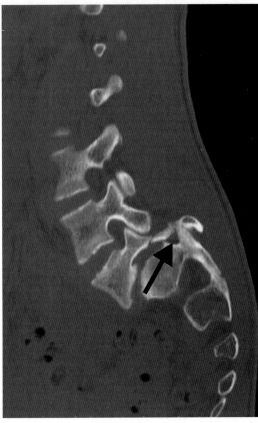

F

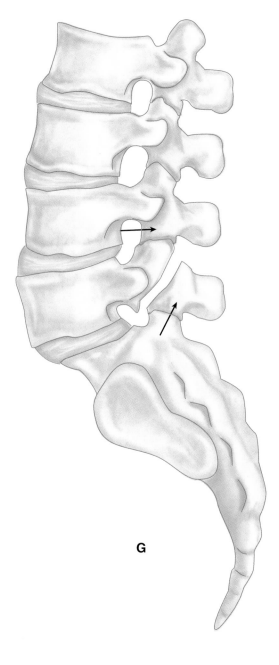

G

FIGURE 1E-G *Continued*

Surgical Anatomy

- Anterior
  - Iliac and segmental vessels
  - Sympathetic chain/lumbar plexus
- Posterior
  - Lamina/pars/facets (Fig. 2)
  - Ligamentum flavum
  - Nerve roots/thecal sac
  - Pedicles/transverse processes
  - Sacral alae/iliac crests

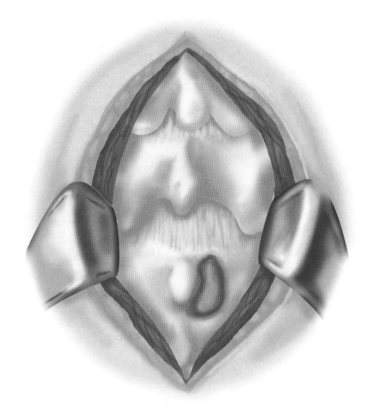

FIGURE 2

PEARLS

- *Confirm good fluoroscopic imaging prior to draping (Fig. 3B).*

- *Obtain baseline electromyogram (EMG) after positioning.*

PITFALLS

- *Stretched nerve roots due to poor positioning can cause a neurologic deficit.*

Positioning

- Position with lumbar lordosis and hip flexion (Fig. 3A).
- Pad pressure points at shoulder/axilla (brachial plexus), elbow (ulnar nerve), breast (nipple), iliac crest, genitals, knees, and toes.

Equipment

- Gel rolls
- Sliding tabletop bed (to allow for C-arm fluoroscope)
- C-arm fluoroscope
- Blankets and/or padding for head, elbows, knees, and feet
- Neurologic monitoring equipment

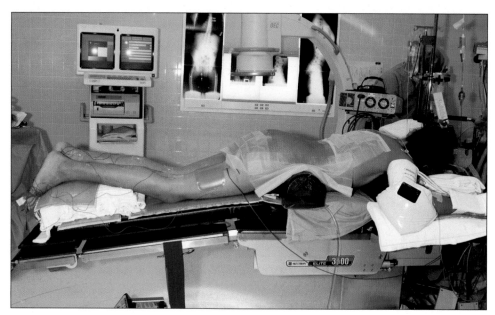

A

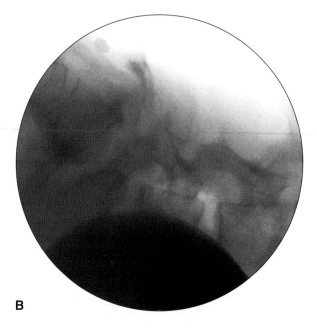

FIGURE 3A-B

B

Portals/Exposures

- Expose at least from S2 to the inferior portion of the L3 lamina.
- Expose the sacral alae and the transverse processes of L4 and L5 (Fig. 4).

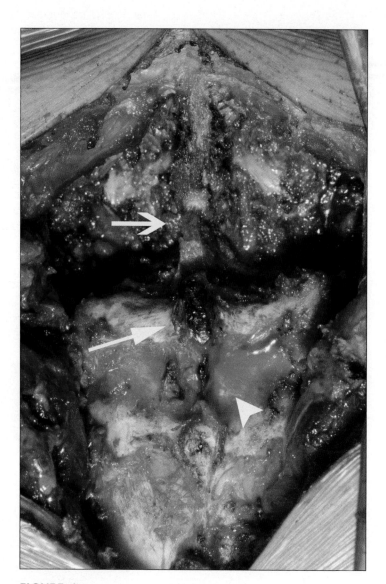

FIGURE 4

Procedure

STEP 1

- Perform a Gill laminectomy, detaching the lamina and inferior facets of L5 from S1 and the dysplastic/ fractured pars (Fig. 5A and 5B).
- Remove the remaining fragments of the pars, making sure the L5 roots are well decompressed.
- Perform a partial facetectomy of the inferior facet of L4 to completely open the foramen.
- Identify the L4, L5, and S1 pedicles and roots.

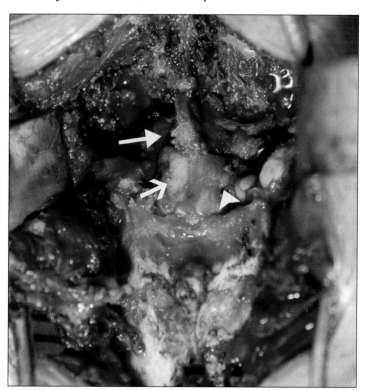

A

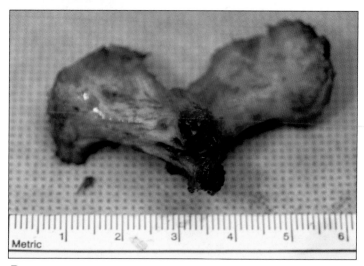

B

FIGURE 5A-B

PEARLS

• *Use fluoroscopic guidance—the L5 pedicles will likely be at an extreme lordotic angle.*

• *Use the largest diameter screws possible at S1, and place them bicortically.*

STEP 2

■ Place pedicle screws at L4 and S1 (Fig. 6A and 6B).
■ Place reduction screws at L5.

PITFALLS

• *Do not place the S1 screws into the superior end plate, as this will compromise the diskectomy and cage placement.*

Instrumentation/Implantion

• Four regular pedicle screws
• Two reduction pedicle screws
• C-arm fluoroscope

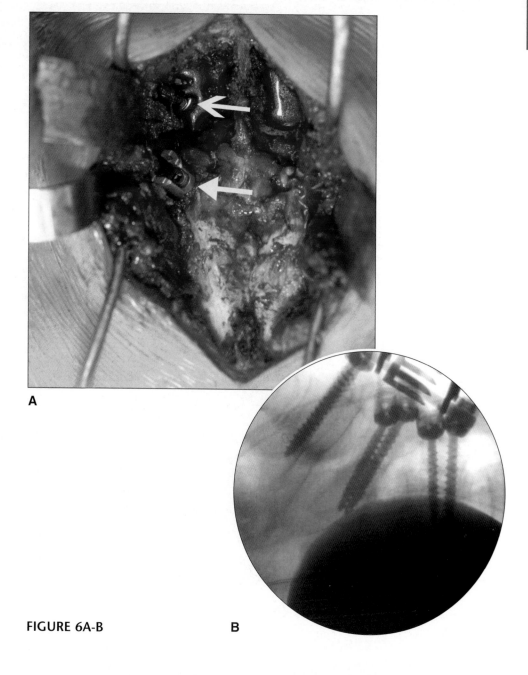

A

B

FIGURE 6A-B

STEP 3

- Secure the L4 and S1 screws to the temporary rods, distracting between L4 and S1 to help reduce L5 and open the disk space (Fig. 7A and 7B).
- Retract the S1 root/thecal sac medially, being careful not to place too much tension on it.
- Make an annulotomy and remove as much of the disk as possible.
- Repeat the procedure on the opposite side.
- Under fluoroscopic guidance, use an osteotome to resect the dome of S1 (Fig. 7C).

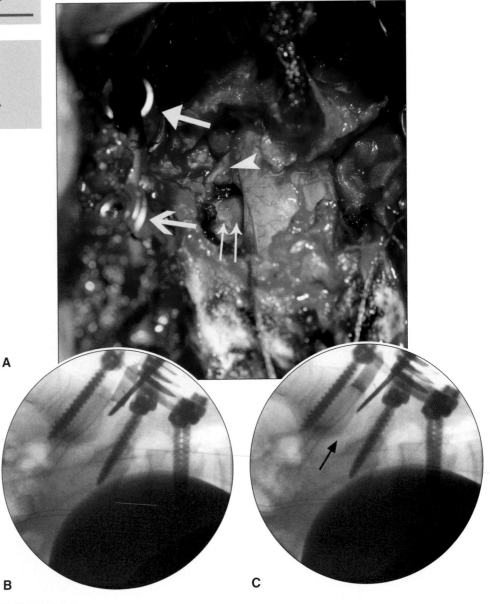

A

B

C

FIGURE 7A-C

Instrumentation/ Implantation

- Two ring clamps, guides, and inner screwdrivers
- C-arm fluroscope

STEP 4

- Place ring clamps on the reduction screws (Fig. 8A).
- Slowly advance caps down the reduction screws with guide and screwdriver, at a symmetric rate, pausing to allow the soft tissues to relax (Fig. 8B).
- When the caps are fully tightened, remove the ring clamps and break off the reduction guide tabs (Fig. 8C).
- Monitor reduction using Garm fluoroscope (Fig. 8D).
- An interdiscal trial may help facilitate reduction (Fig. 8E).

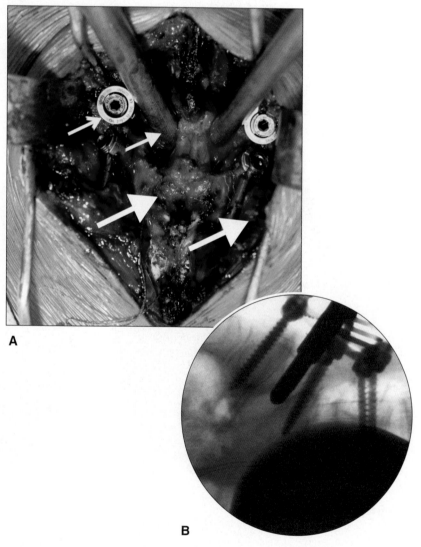

A

B

FIGURE 8A-B *Continued*

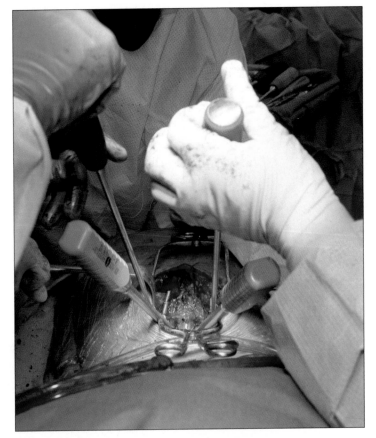

C

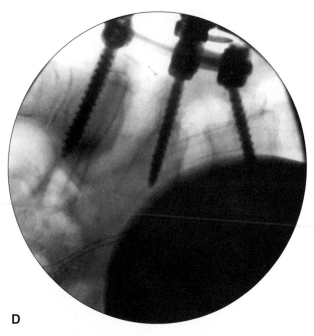

D

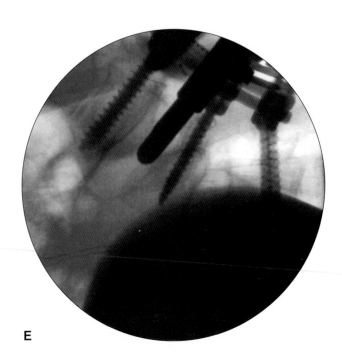

E

FIGURE 8C-E *Continued*

Instrumentation/ Implantation

- Interbody cages
- Graft supplements
- Iliac bolts/connectors
- C-arm fluoroscope

Controversies

- Fusion to L4 may not be necessary if the L4/5 disk is normal. In this case, the L4 screws may be removed and the fusion done only to L5-S1/ pelvis.

STEP 5

- Rasp/curette the end plates to bleeding bone.
- Use trials to measure disk space for appropriate cage size.
- Pack cage with autograft and any additional materials to aid fusion.
- Place cages into disk space after reduction under fluoroscopic guidance (Fig. 9A and 9B).
- Place iliac bolts under fluoroscopic guidance (Fig. 9C).
- Replace one temporary rod at a time with the final rod, compressing across the L5/S1 disk space.
- Place grafting material in lateral gutters.
- Use a large drain and waterproof closure.

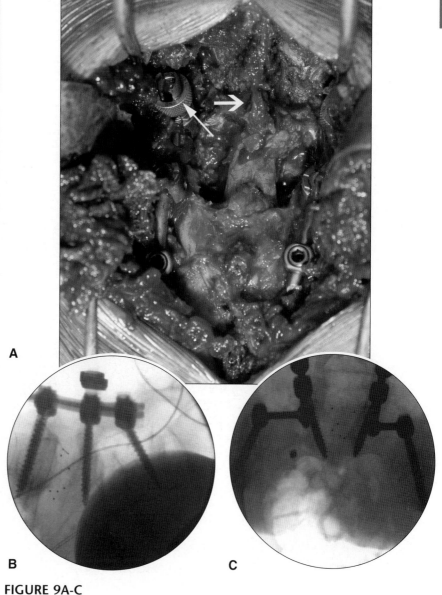

A

B

C

FIGURE 9A-C

PEARLS

- *Monitor for 48 hours with frequent neurologic checks to watch for L4, L5, or S1 root traction injuries.*

- *The most common root injury is to L5 (Fig. 10D and 10E).*

PITFALLS

- *Traction injuries are common, and should be managed with supportive care and physical therapy.*

- *A root injury may not be noticed until 1 or 2 days postoperatively, when the patient is mobilized.*

Postoperative Care and Expected Outcomes (Fig. 10A–10C)

- Position patients with the hips and knees flexed at all times to reduce stretch on the femoral nerve for the first few days (very often patients have a temporary neuropathy that improves with time and therapy).
- Avoid hypotension/anemia.
- Use patient-controlled analgesia for pain relief.
- Monitor in the intensive care unit for at least overnight with hourly neurologic checks.

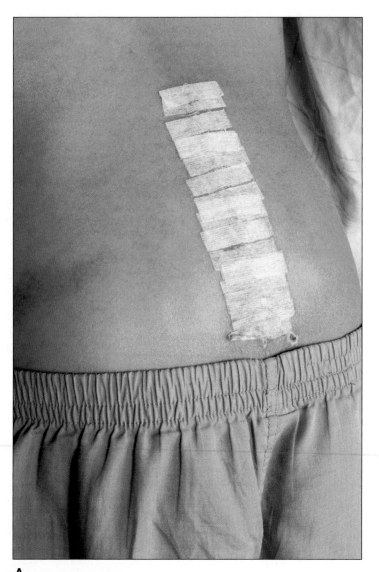

A

FIGURE 10A

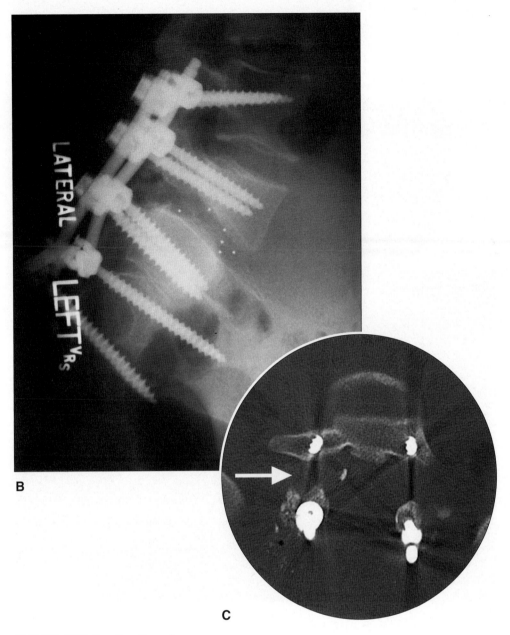

B

C

FIGURE 10B-C *Continued*

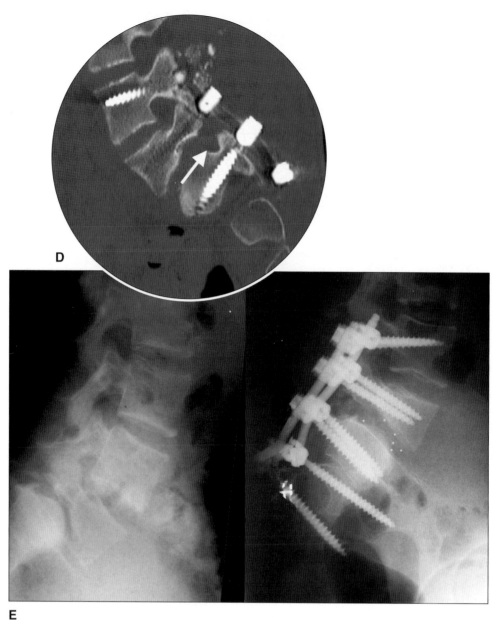

D

E

FIGURE 10D-E *Continued*

Evidence

DeWald CJ, Vartabedian JE, Rodts MF, Hammerberg KW. Evaluation and management of high-grade spondylolisthesis in adults. Spine. 2005;30(6 Suppl):S49-59.

Reviews 21 adult patients with surgical treatment of symptomatic high-grade spondylolisthesis. Patients who had a reduction maneuver were provided with anterior column support. There were no pseudarthroses. Many patients developed at least temporary neurologic deficits, even if no reduction was performed. Surgery in adults is more challenging due to the stiffer deformity.

Kumar R, Niall D, Walsh A, Khalikullah K, McCormack D. Spina bifida occulta in isthmic spondylolisthesis: a surgical trap. Eur Spine J. 2002;11:159-61.

A case report on the presence of a significant bony defect of S1 noted during an in situ fusion of a grade II dysplastic spondylolisthesis. Highlights the risks of injury to the thecal sac/nerves during the dissection.

McAfee PC, DeVine JG, Chaput CD, Prybis BG, Fedder IL, Cunningham BW, Farrell DJ, Hess SJ, Vigna FE. The indications for interbody fusion cages in the treatment of spondylolisthesis. Spine 2005;30(6 Suppl):S60-5.

Retrospectively evaluates the results of a unilateral transforaminal lumbar interbody fusion (TLIF) procedure performed in 120 patients with spondylolisthesis of various causes. Had excellent results with 98% fusion success despite many revision surgeries, increase in disk height, and 23% slip reduction (not a primary goal of surgery). Lists indications for TLIF, including slip angle greater than 40°, limited fusion mass available in posterolateral gutter, revision cases, dysplastic etiology, and three-column injury.

Molinari RW, Bridwell KH, Lenke LG, Baldus C. Anterior column support in surgery for high-grade, isthmic spondylolisthesis. Clin Orthop Relat Res. 2002;394:109-20.

A review of patients with various fusion techniques, analyzed by whether anterior column support was used or not (from a posterior lumbar interbody fusion/TLIF approach). Describes a much higher pseudarthrosis rate if no anterior column support was used, but these patients did go on to fusion when revised with an anterior interbody graft.

Molinari RW, Bridwell KH, Lenke LG, Ungacta FF, Riew KD. Complications in the surgical treatment of pediatric high-grade, isthmic dysplastic spondylolisthesis: a comparison of three surgical approaches. Spine. 1999;24:1701-11.

A review of patients with in situ fusion, simple decompression and instrumented fusion, or reduction and circumferential fusion. Reports high rates of pseudarthrosis with in situ fusion, and excellent results of reduction with circumferential fusion with low complication rate long-term. Also recommends the use of bicortical sacral screws and long iliac bolts to reduce instrumentation failure.

Ogilvie JW. Complications in spondylolisthesis surgery. Spine. 2005;30(6 Suppl):S97-101.

Review of the most common complications during and subsequent to isthmic spondylolisthesis surgery. Pseudarthrosis has historically been the most common complication, but is less so with modern instrumentation and anterior column fusion. The rate of neurologic injury is somewhat increased over the last few years in patients undergoing a reduction, although the etiology is unclear. Transition syndromes with postoperative degeneration or spondylolisthesis aquisita at adjacent levels are discussed, including techniques to reduce these complications.

Petraco DM, Spivak JM, Cappadona JG, Kummer FJ, Neuwirth MG. An anatomic evaluation of L5 nerve stretch in spondylolisthesis reduction. Spine. 1996; 21:1133-38; discussion 1139.

Anatomic study evaluating factors and quantifying stretch on the L5 root during spondylolisthesis reduction, including slip angle, sagittal translation, and disk height. Recommends reduction of the slip angle, but emphasizes increased risk of root injury if sagittal translation is completely reduced.

Ruf M, Koch H, Melcher RP, Harms J. Anatomic reduction and monosegmental fusion in high-grade developmental spondylolisthesis. Spine. 2006;31:269-74.

A retrospective review assessing radiographic and clinical outcomes of single-segment fusion for L5/S1 high-grade spondylolisthesis. Discusses technique of temporary fixation of L4 only for surgery, then removal of screws to preserve the L4-5 motion segment. Most patients did very well, but 4 of 23 had decompensation at L4-5.

Transfeldt EE, Dendrinos GK, Bradford DS. Paresis of proximal lumbar roots after reduction of L5-S1 spondylolisthesis. Spine. 1989;14:884-7.

A case report of a patient who developed paresis in the L2, L3, and L4 roots after reduction of a grade 5 spondylolisthesis that was not detected intraoperatively secondary to inadequate monitoring and wake-up test. Proximal roots must also be assessed for a stretch injury during the procedure.

Interspinous Process Motion-Sparing Implant

Ralph J. Mobbs and Charles Fisher

Controversies

- Interspinous process motion-sparing devices continue to be evaluated in clinical trials. Early results suggest a possible role in the management of degenerative disorders of the lumbar spine.

Treatment Options

- Would be dependent on underlying pathology:
  - Conservative management for degenerative disk disease
  - Laminectomy and spinal fusion for canal stenosis with spondylolisthesis
  - Disk replacement

Indications

- Diskectomy for massive herniated disk leading to substantial loss of disk material
- Second diskectomy for recurrence of herniated disk
- Neurogenic claudication: placing the stenotic segment in slight flexion and preventing extension
- Degenerative disk disease at a level adjacent to a previous fusion, or at the time of a fusion procedure.

Examination/Imaging

- Plain standing lateral radiograph of the lumbar spine to assess antero- or retrolisthesis (Fig. 1).
- Magnetic resonance imaging scan to assess disk Modic changes, disk herniation, canal stenosis, and facet joint degeneration (Fig. 2).

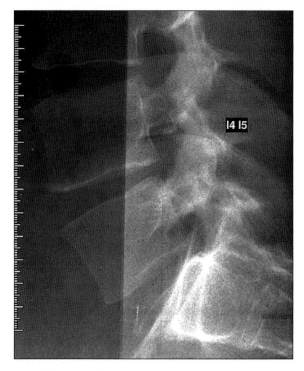

FIGURE 1

Surgical Anatomy

- Radiograph prior to incision to limit exposure
- Midline lumbar incision
- Bilateral exposure to reveal the inferior and superior aspect of the spinous process adjacent to the interspinous segment being treated

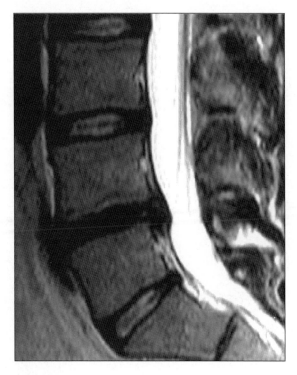

FIGURE 2

■ The supraspinous ligament MUST be kept intact so that the device does not dislodge posteriorly (Fig. 3).

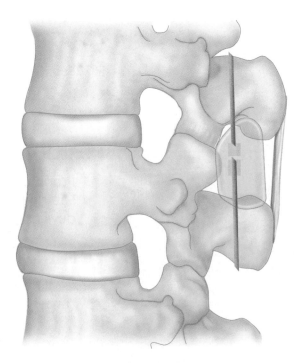

FIGURE 3

- Most interspinous devices will require a bilateral exposure of the interspinous space for safe insertion of the device (Fig. 4).
- Facet joint anatomy should not be disrupted, as the facets are structures the device is attempting to support.

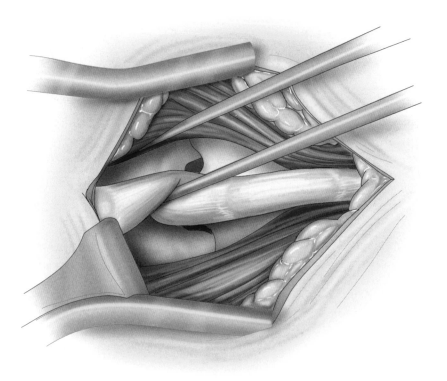

FIGURE 4

Positioning

- Prone position: Jackson or 90/90 table *or*
- Lateral position with local anesthesia for specific devices (X-stop)

Portals/Exposures

- Midline approach as for standard lumbar spine surgery

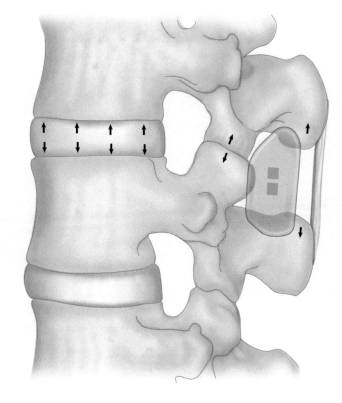

FIGURE 5

Procedure

STEP 1

- Local **or** general anesthesia. General anesthesia is usually required if the device is being used in combination with a decompressive laminotomy or a diskectomy procedure.

STEP 2

- Midline lumbar incision over the spinous processes being treated with the interspinous process motion-sparing device (Fig. 5). For an L4-5 procedure, expose the superior aspect of the L5 spinous process and the inferior aspect of the L4 spinous process.

STEP 3

- The method of implantation of the interspinous device varies among designs. The goal is to limit terminal extension at the implanted level.
- All designs, however, require a "spacer" or cushioning component between the spinous processes that is inserted in combination with distraction between the spinous processes (see Fig. 5).

Instrumentation/Implantation

- When distracting the interspinous space, be careful not to aggressively overdistract as fracture of a spinous process is a common initial surgeon mistake.

Controversies

- If the surgeon overdistracts between the spinous processes and inserts too large a device, the result may be over-kyphosis of the motion segment.

- Distract the interspace until the supraspinous ligament is just taut but not overstretched (Fig. 6).
- Choose the correct implant size based on distraction.
- With each design, the spacer is supported by a unique fixation method.

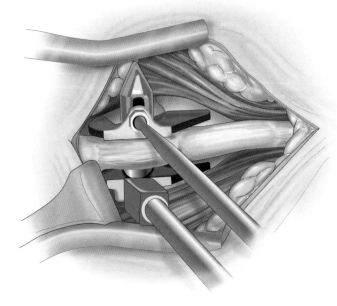

FIGURE 6

Postoperative Care and Expected Outcomes

- With adequate analgesia, the patient can be mobilized postoperatively and be discharged either the same day or on postoperative day 1 depending on surgeon preference.

Evidence

Christie S, Song J, Fessler R. Dynamic interspinous process technology. Spine. 2005;30(16 Suppl):S73-8.

Siddiqui M, Nicol M, Karadimas E, et al. The positional magnetic resonance imaging changes in the lumbar spine following insertion of a novel interspinous process distraction device. Spine. 2005;30:2677-82.

Weiner BK. Interspinous process decompression system device affords superior outcomes and equal safety to nonoperative therapy. Spine. 2005;30:2846-7.

Zucherman JF, Hsu KY, Hartjen CA, et al. A prospective randomized multi-center study for the treatment of lumbar spinal stenosis with the X STOP interspinous implant: 1-year results. Eur Spine J. 2004;13:22-31.

Anterior Lumbar Interbody Fusion

Michael D. Daubs

Controversies

• Males have a 2-5% risk for retrograde ejaculation with the anterior lumbar approach.

Treatment Options

• Posterior intertransverse fusion
• Posterior lumbar interbody fusion
• Lateral retroperitoneal lumbar interbody fusion

Indications

■ Lumbar degenerative disk disease
■ Anterior column support in long fusion constructs
■ Restoring lumbar lordosis
■ Pseudarthrosis following posterior lumbar fusion
■ Lumbar fusions at high risk for nonunion
■ Tumor and trauma

Examination/Imaging

■ Magnetic resonance imaging to assess degree of disk degeneration (Fig. 1)
■ Standing lateral radiograph of the lumbar spine to assess whether sacral slope and L5-S1 disk are at an angle that can be accessed through the anterior approach. (Fig. 2). If sacral slope is severe (L5/S1 spondylolisthesis), access to the disk can be very difficult.

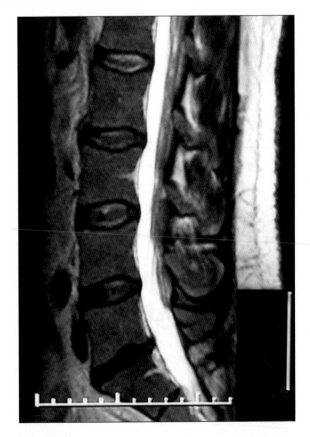

FIGURE 1

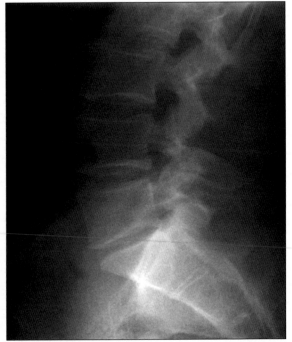

FIGURE 2

Surgical Anatomy

- Aorta, vena cava, iliac veins and arteries (Figs. 3 and 4)
- Ureter
- Sympathetic nerves
- Hypogastric plexus

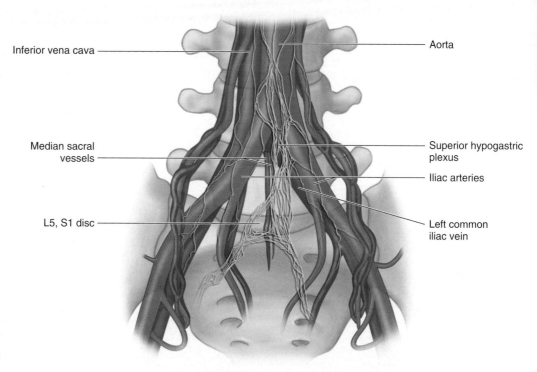

Inferior vena cava —
Aorta

Median sacral vessels —
Superior hypogastric plexus

Iliac arteries

L5, S1 disc —
Left common iliac vein

FIGURE 3

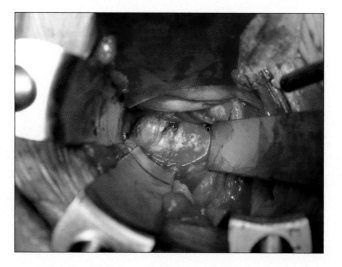

FIGURE 4

PEARLS

- *A bolster can be used in the lumbar region to accentuate lordosis as needed.*

PITFALLS

- *If using fluoroscopy, obtain images preoperatively to ensure that all views are obtainable without obstruction from the table or the patient's extremities.*

Equipment

- An operating room table that can rotate side to side can be helpful for visualization during the approach.

PEARLS

- *If the L5/S1 disk lies low in the pelvis and is at an acute angle, the incision will need to be lower on the abdomen to allow the proper trajectory for disk excision and graft placement.*

- *Always confirm the disk level with fluoroscopy or radiographs to avoid wrong-level surgery.*

PITFALLS

- *Improper incision placement can make the disk excision and instrumentation very difficult to perform, and may compromise implant insertion.*

- *Be aware of the correct disk level to be addressed in cases in which there is transitional lumbosacral anatomy.*

- *Avoidance of electrocautery may reduce the incidence of retrograde ejaculation. Bipolar cautery or other means to achieve hemostasis is recommended.*

Positioning

- The patient is positioned supine on a radiolucent operating room table.
- The patient's arms are positioned at the sides in an abducted position on rests to allow for lateral imaging (Fig. 5).

Portals/Exposures

- A lateral fluoroscopic image is used to mark the level of incision.
- A radiopaque rod or pin is used to mark the angle of the disk and the corresponding trajectory to the abdominal wall. The incision site is adjusted to give optimum access to the disk to be operated upon.
- A transverse or longitudinal incision is made a few centimeters lateral to midline at the corresponding disk level in line with the angle of the disk space. Figure 6A shows the more vertical approach to L4-L5 and a higher incision level, and Figure 6B displays the trajectory to the L5/S1 disk. If both levels are being addressed, the incision should be between the levels, or a longitudinal incision can be used.
- The anterior rectus sheath is incised transversely while avoiding the underlying rectus muscle.
- The transversalis fascia is gently incised with a no. 15 scalpel, and the interval between the peritoneum and fascia is developed.
- The retroperitoneal cavity is dissected bluntly toward the midline (left to right), and the peritoneal contents are retracted to expose the anterior spine.
- Blunt dissection is performed down to the anterior disk space.

Instrumentation

- Smooth-edged retractors are important to avoid inadvertent vessel injuries.
- Proper illumination into the abdominal cavity is key. A head light or direct fiberoptic lighting is helpful.

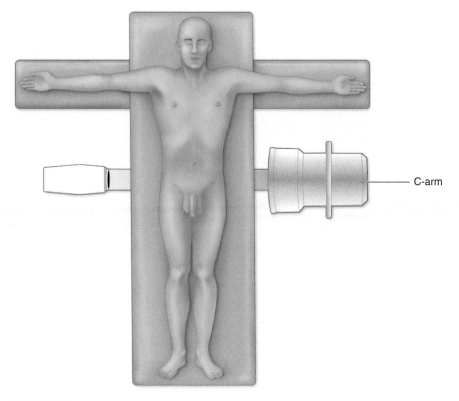

FIGURE 5

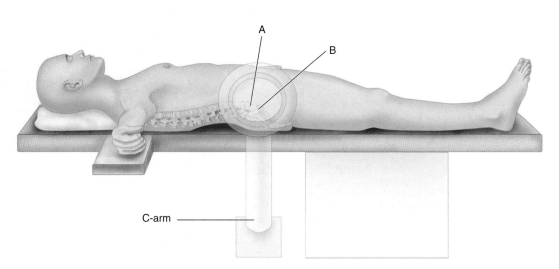

FIGURE 6

Controversies

- The use of a co-surgeon (general or vascular surgeon) during the anterior lumbar approach is dependent upon the individual surgeon's training and expertise.

PEARLS

- *Properly developing the interval between the subchondral bone and the cartilaginous end plate with a disk elevator is crucial for efficient and complete disk excision.*

- *If the end plates are sclerotic, a bone hook can be used to perforate the subchondral bone in several areas to expose bleeding bone.*

PITFALLS

- *When incising the disk margins, the sharp edge of the blade should always point away from the vascular structures.*

- *When exiting and entering the disk space during excision, maintain an awareness of the location of the vascular structures. Veins can easily slip beneath the edges of retractors.*

- *Be aware of the orientation of the end plates when excising the disk to avoid disruption of the subchondral bone.*

- Retractors are placed appropriately depending on the disk space being addressed. At L4/L5, the aorta and inferior vena cava are retracted left to right. At L5/S1 the middle sacral artery and vein are ligated (see Fig. 4) and the iliac veins are retracted laterally.

Procedure

STEP 1

- The anterior disk is incised with a long-handled no. 10 scalpel.
- An end plate elevator is used to develop the interval between the subchondral bone and the cartilaginous end plate (Fig. 7).
- Disk rongeurs are used to remove large disk fragments (Fig. 8).
- Long-handled curettes are utilized to gently scrape the end plates of any remaining pieces of cartilage and to expose bleeding bone.

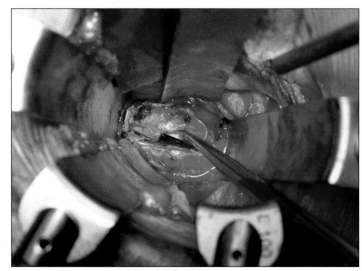

FIGURE 7

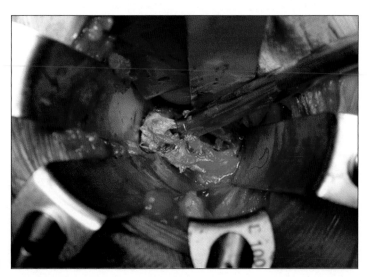

FIGURE 8

Instrumentation/Implantion

• Various anterior lumbar interbody implants are available, including allograft, titanium, polyether ether ketone (PEEK), and absorbable. They come in many shapes and sizes.

Controversies

• The use of an anterior plate for interspace fixation or buttressing of the implant is surgeon dependent.
• Many surgeons believe anterior implants alone are not stable enough to obtain a successful fusion. However, recent studies using bone morphogenic protein (BMP) in conjunction with stand-alone devices have reported a fusion rate of up to 99%.

STEP 2

■ Distraction is applied to the disk space to restore proper disk space height.
■ A trial implant or sizing device is used to determine the appropriate-sized graft or cage.
■ An implant is selected that corresponds to the correct trial implant.
■ The implant is packed with bone graft material and inserted into the disk space in an anterior-posterior direction (Figs. 9 and 10). The insertion

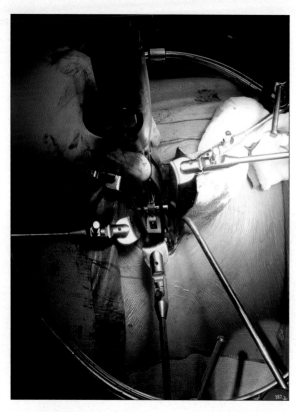

FIGURE 9

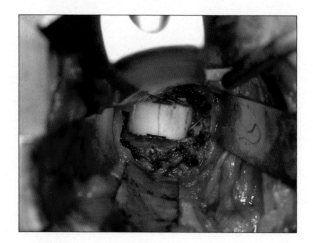

FIGURE 10

device distracts the disk space as the implant is inserted.

■ Fluoroscopic imaging is used to ensure correct positioning of the implant.

■ If utilized, anterior instrumentation is applied across the disk space (Figs. 11, 12, and 13).

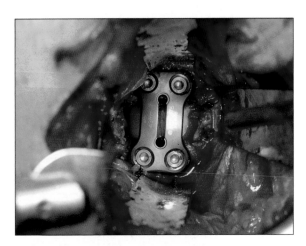

FIGURE 11

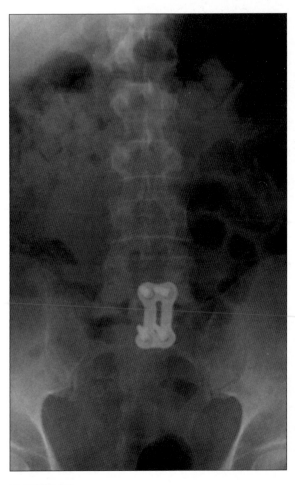

FIGURE 12

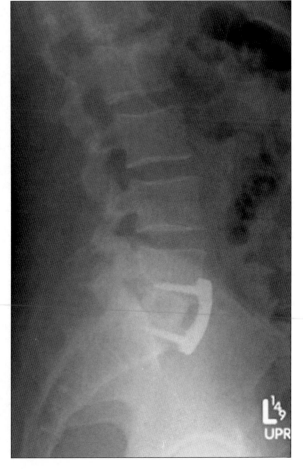

FIGURE 13

Postoperative Care and Expected Outcomes

- Patients are started on clear liquids and their diets are advanced as tolerated.
- Patients are mobilized on postoperative day 1 and encouraged to ambulate as tolerated.
- A simple lumbar corsette brace is used for 6 weeks postoperatively.
- If the procedure is a stand-alone anterior lumbar interbody fusion, patients are typically discharged on postoperative day 2 or 3.
- A successful fusion rate in the 90% range can be expected with an anterior lumbar interbody fusion when combined with a posterior stabilizing procedure or when BMP is used in conjunction with an implant stabilized anteriorly.

Evidence

Brau SA. Mini-open approach to the spine for anterior lumbar interbody fusion: description of the procedure, results and complications. Spine J. 2002;2:216-23.

A review of the complications of the anterior lumbar approach using a mini-open technique. (Level IV evidence)

Burkus JK, Sandhu HS, Gornet MF, Longley MC. Use of rhBMP-2 in combination with structural cortical allografts: clinical and radiographic outcomes in anterior lumbar spinal surgery. J Bone Joint Surg Am. 2005;87:1205-12.

A prospective Investigational Device Exemption study evaluating the use of BMP in anterior lumbar fusion with cortical allograft dowels. The fusion rate was 99%. (Level I evidence)

Burkus JK, Transfeldt EE, Kitchel SH, et al. Clinical and radiographic outcomes of anterior lumbar interbody fusion using recombinant human bone morphogenic protein-2. Spine. 2002;27:2396-408.

A 94% fusion rate was achieved with tapered titanium cylinder cages and rh-BMP2. (Level II evidence)

Sasso RC, Kitchel SH, Dawson EG. A prospective randomized controlled clinical trial of anterior lumbar interbody fusion using a titanium cylindrical threaded fusion device. Spine. 2004;29:113-22.

Titanium cylinder cages had better results when used alone than did femoral allograft implants. (Level II evidence)

Transforaminal Lumbar Interbody Fusion

Jacob M. Buchowski and Michael D. Daubs

Controversies

- Multilevel (>3 levels) degenerative disk disease
- Disk disease causing radicular pain without mechanical symptoms or instability
- Revision posterior surgery (epidural scarring)

Treatment Options

- Anterior lumbar interbody fusion
- Posterior lumbar interbody fusion

Equipment

- A radiolucent table and the use of fluoroscopy are helpful in properly positioning the interbody device.

Indications

- Spondylolisthesis (ideally grades 1 and 2)
- Symptomatic degenerative disk disease
- Recurrent disk herniation associated with mechanical back pain
- Postdiskectomy disk space collapse with foraminal stenosis/radiculopathy
- Distal end of a long posterior fusion (scoliosis)

Examination/Imaging

- A plain lateral radiograph (Fig. 1) or fluoroscopic image after the patient is positioned prone on the operating table is helpful to evaluate overall alignment, angle of end plates and approach to the disk interspace, and proper angles of insertion for pedicle screw instrumentation. After positioning on the table, the spondylolisthesis often reduces with the patient in the prone, hips extended position.
- The most symptomatic side (left or right) or the side with the most pathology (i.e., recurrent lumbar disk herniation) should be noted on magnetic resonance imaging (Fig. 2) and/or computed tomography myelography images.

Surgical Anatomy

- The working zone for the transforaminal lumbar interbody fusion (TLIF) approach (Fig. 3) is bounded by the traversing nerve root and thecal sac medially, the exiting nerve root and pedicle of the vertebra above the disk of interest cranially, and the pedicle of the vertebra below the disk of interest caudally.

Positioning

- The patient should be positioned in prone with the abdomen free of any compression.

Portals/Exposures

- With an open approach, the spine is exposed to the tips of the transverse processes via a standard midline lumbar incision (Fig. 4). If no central decompression is being performed, the midline posterior ligamentous and osseous structures are preserved.
- A paramedian, muscle-splitting, or Wiltse-type approach can also be used if no central decompression is planned.

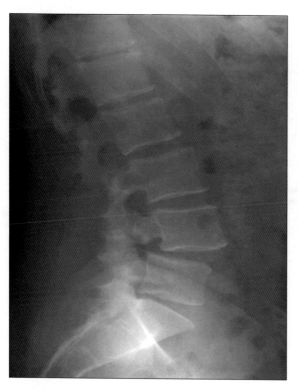

FIGURE 1

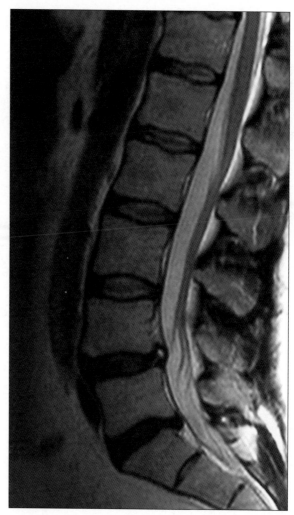

FIGURE 2

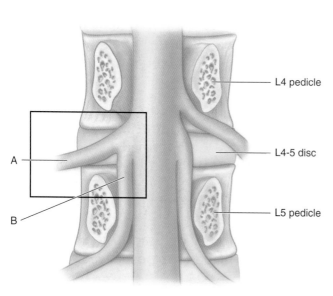

L4 pedicle

L4-5 disc

L5 pedicle

A

B

FIGURE 3

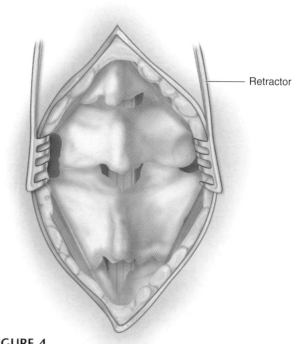

Retractor

FIGURE 4

Instrumentation

• Standard posterior lumbar spine retractors are used most often with an open approach.

Procedure

STEP 1

■ Pedicle screw instrumentation is placed.
■ The inferior facet and a portion of the pars above the level of the disk is removed from the cephalad level (Fig. 5).

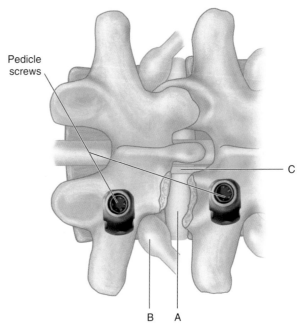

Pedicle screws

C

B   A

FIGURE 5

■ The superior facet of the caudad level is resected flush with the pedicle.
■ The lateral aspect of the lamina and the ligamentum are resected as needed to perform a decompression and to visualize the nerve roots.
■ Bipolar cautery is used to obtain hemostasis.

STEP 2

■ The pedicle screws contralateral to the facetectomy are connected to a rod, and distraction across the intervertebral disk space is performed.
■ The disk space is incised with a no. 10 or no. 15 scalpel.
■ Various disk ronguers are used to remove disk material (Fig. 6).
■ Standard and ring curettes are used to scrape the end plates free of cartilage to expose bleeding subchondral bone.

Instrumentation/ Implantion

- Slightly curved curettes and up-biting ronguers are useful in removing disk material from the contralateral side (see Fig. 6).

Controversies

- Some surgeons recommend using an osteotome to decorticate the most anterior aspect of the end plates when preparing the interspace for fusion.

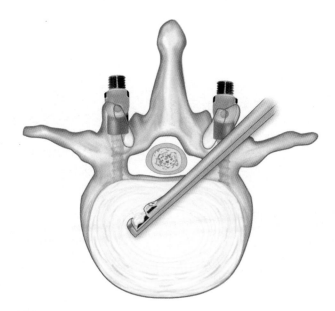

FIGURE 6

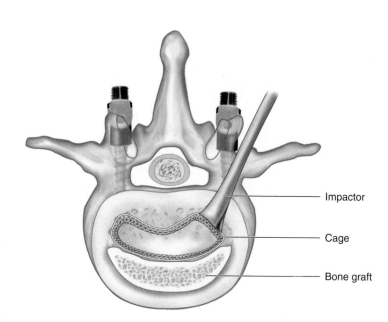

Impactor

Cage

Bone graft

FIGURE 7

STEP 3

- Interbody spacers can be used to further distract across the disk space (Fig. 8). The contralateral rod is loosened and retightened.
- Cancellous autograft is packed into the anterior aspect of the disk space.
- If utilized, a collagen sponge soaked with an osteoinductive protein (bone morphogenic protein [BMP]) is inserted anteriorly with the autograft.
- A trial implant is used to size the interspace.

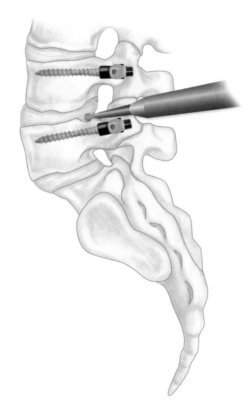

FIGURE 8

- A curvilinear implant is inserted and tapped into position.
- More autograft is packed posterior to the implant.
- Distraction is let down, and pedicle screws are retightened and the ipsilateral rod is placed.
- Radiographs confirm proper position of the implant.
- A posterolateral intertransverse fusion may be added. It is typically performed on the contralateral side of the TLIF to avoid bone graft fragments falling into the zone of decompression onto the nerve roots and epidural space (Fig. 9).

PEARLS

- *Removing the posterior osteophytes or concave ridge of the posterior vertebral body will help in placing the proper-size implant.*

- *Tap the implant to the contralateral side of the disk space prior to impacting it completely anteriorly.*

PITFALLS

- *Breeching the anulus and inserting the implant anterior to the disk space into the retroperitoneal space*

- *Inserting an oversized implant can disrupt the end plate and lead to settling and loss of sagittal alignment.*

- *Inserting the implant at an incorrect angle (unparallel to the end plates) will disrupt the subchondral bone and lead to settling.*

- *Impinging on a nerve root while inserting the implant*

Controversies

- The use of BMP for TLIFs is controversial and is considered an off-label application of BMP. Overgrowth of bone into the epidural space has been reported. Using a fibrin glue sealant along the posterior disk and keeping the collagen sponge contained in the implant and anteriorly in the interspace may prevent this complication.

Instrumentation/ Implantation

- Intervertebral distractors are helpful in achieving further distraction of the disk space and reducing the strain on the pedicle screws.
- Choose an implant that gives maximal surface area of contact.
- Overdistracting through the pedicle screws can cause loosening at the bone-screw interface. Check the screws for loosening and insert a larger diameter screw if possible if they are loose.
- Options for structural interbody spacers include machined allograft, shaped autograft, titanium cages, polyether ether ketone (PEEK), and resorbable cages, with titanium or PEEK cages used most commonly.

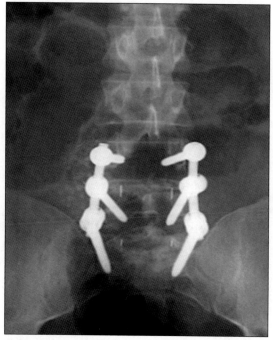

A

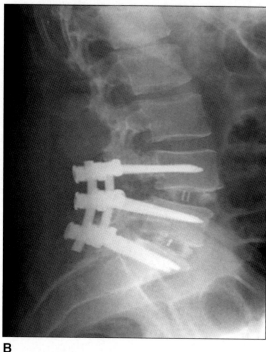

B

FIGURE 9A-B

Postoperative Care And Expected Outcomes

- Postoperatively, patients are mobilized the same day of surgery or the following morning.
  - Physical therapy is started on the day of surgery or on the first postoperative day.

Controversies

• The use of externally worn bone graft stimulators is advocated by some surgeons in patients at high risk for nonhealing (tobacco users).

- Walking is encouraged.
- Low-impact activities and swimming are usually allowed 8-12 weeks following surgery.
- Repetitive bending is restricted until the fusion is solid.

■ Successful fusion can be expected in approximately 90% of patients, and typically a majority of patients will report improvement in functional outcome.

Evidence

Hackenberg L, Halm H, Bullmann V, Vieth V, Schneider M, Liljenqvist U. Transforaminal lumbar interbody fusion: a safe technique with satisfactory three to five year results. Eur Spine J. 2005;14:551-8.

The authors of this Level IV study found that TLIF performed in 52 patients was associated with an 89% radiographic fusion rate. The authors found that pain (as measured by the Visual Analogue Scale[VAS]) and Oswestry Disability Index improved significantly following surgery.

Lowe TG, Tahernia AD. Unilateral transforaminal posterior lumbar interbody fusion. Clin Orthop Rel Res. 2002;394:64-72.

The authors of this Level IV study found that TLIF performed in 40 patients was associated with a 90% radiographic fusion rate. The authors found that 85% of patients had excellent or good clinical outcomes and there were few complications.

Lowe TG, Tahernia AD, O'Brien MF, Smith DAB. Unilateral transforaminal posterior lumbar interbody fusion (TLIF): indications, technique, and 2-year results. J Spinal Disord Tech. 2002;14:31-8.

The authors of this Level IV study found that TLIF performed in 40 patients was associated with a 90% radiographic fusion rate. The authors found that 79% of patients had excellent or good clinical outcomes and there were few complications.

Potter BK, Freedman BA, Verwiebe EG, Hall JM, Polly DW Jr, Kuklo TR. Transforaminal lumbar interbody fusion: clinical and radiographic results and complications in 100 consecutive patients. J Spinal Disord Tech. 2005;18:337-46.

The authors of this Level IV study found that TLIF is a safe and effective method of achieving lumbar fusion with a 93% radiographic fusion rate. Although 81% of patients reported greater than 50% decrease in their symptoms and 76% would choose to have the procedure again, only 29% were entirely pain free. Complications from the procedure were found to be uncommon and generally minor and transient.

Salehi SA, Tawk R, Ganju A, LaMarca F, Liu JC, Ondra SL. Transforaminal lumbar interbody fusion: surgical technique and results in 24 patients. Neurosurgery 2004;54:368-74.

The authors of this Level IV study found that TLIF performed in 24 patients was associated with a 87.5% radiographic fusion rate and a 83.5% patient satisfaction rate with 71% of patients choosing to have the same surgery again. Complications were found to be uncommon.

Schwender JD, Holly LT, Rouben DP, Foley KT. Minimally invasive transforaminal lumbar interbody fusion (TLIF): technical feasibility and initial results. J Spinal Disord Tech. 2005;18(Suppl 1):S1-6.

The authors of this Level IV study found that minimally invasive TLIF performed in 49 patients was safe and effective, resulting in a 100% radiographic fusion rate. The authors found that pain (as measured by the VAS) and Oswestry Disability Index improved significantly following surgery.

Lumbar Spine Arthroplasty: Charité Total Disk Replacement

Kern Singh, Demian M. Yakel, Bart Wojewnik, Donna D. Ohnmeiss, Alexander R Vaccaro, and Scott L. Blumenthal

PITFALLS

- *Conditions compromising the structural integrity of the vertebral end plates and bodies*

  - *Osteoporosis*

  - *Osteomalacia*

  - *Acute fracture*

  - *Intraspinal neoplasm*

- *Conditions prohibiting safe anterior spinal access*

  - *Previous major abdominal surgery or irradiation*

- *Conditions affecting the stability of the implant*

  - *Scoliosis*

  - *Spondylolysis*

  - *Spondylolisthesis*

  - *Previous destabilizing posterior surgery*

- *Conditions not addressed by disk replacement*

  - *Disk herniation with predominantly radicular symptoms or signs of cauda equina syndrome*

  - *Substantial (grade III or IV) facet arthrosis*

  - *Central or lateral recess stenosis*

- *Miscellaneous*

  - *Pregnancy*

  - *Active infection (of the spine or elsewhere)*

  - *Severe obesity*

Indications

- Age 18-60 years (optimally below 50 years)
- Symptomatic degenerative disk disease or lumbar spondylosis with objective evidence of degenerative disk disease by computed tomography or magnetic resonance imaging (MRI)
  - Specific radiographic findings include vacuum disk sign, high-intensity zone signal, and Modic changes
  - Provocative diskography is helpful to confirm the diagnosis
- Only single- or two-level intervertebral disk disease
- Nonradicular leg pain or back pain in the absence of nerve root compression
- Postdiskectomy syndrome
- Failure of at least 6 months of conservative, nonoperative treatment

Examination/Imaging

- MRI to evaluate the intervertebral disks, spinal canal, and neural foramen (Fig. 1)
  - One must be cautious in assuming that every degenerated "black disk" found on MRI is a source of pain.
  - Assessment of facet arthrosis in combination with computed tomography
- Anteroposterior and lateral and flexion/extension radiographs (Fig. 2)

Controversies

- The presence of radicular pain in addition to axial pain is acceptable if there is no severe canal stenosis and it is thought that the radicular pain is mostly from foraminal stenosis secondary to loss of disk height at that level.

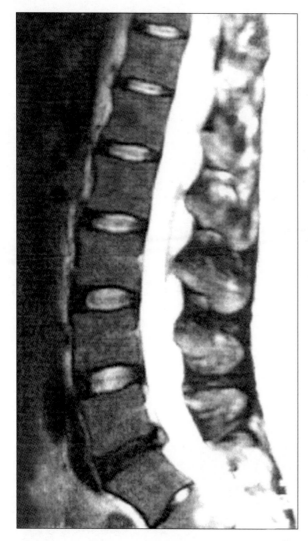

FIGURE 1

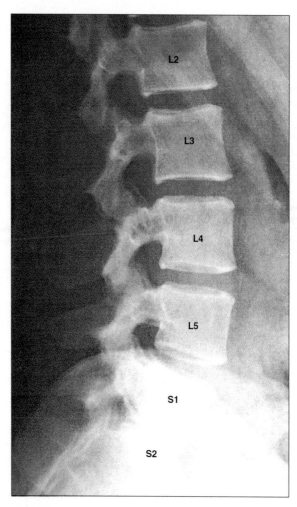

L2

L3

L4

L5

S1

S2

FIGURE 2

Treatment Options

- Anterior lumbar interbody fusion
- Posterior lumbar arthrodesis
  - Posterolateral instrumented fusion
  - Transforaminal lumbar interbody fusion
  - Posterolateral lumbar interbody fusion
- Intradiscal electrothermal therapy (IDET)
- Spinal cord stimulation
- Posterior motion-sparing stabilization (pedicle screw or intraspinous process device)

- Discography: discogram should demonstrate concordant pain reproduction with at least one control level that is not painful and does not reproduce the patient's symptoms (Figs. 3 and 4).

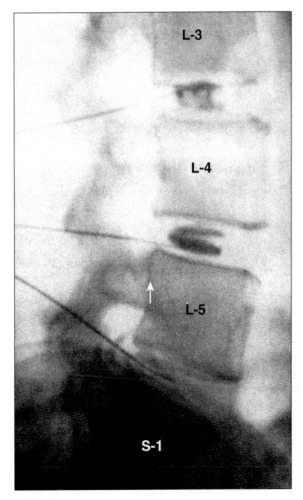

FIGURE 3

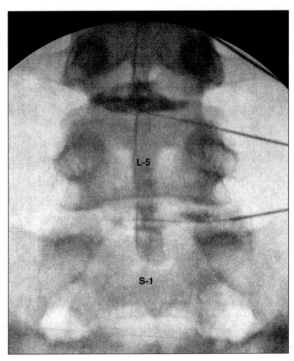

FIGURE 4

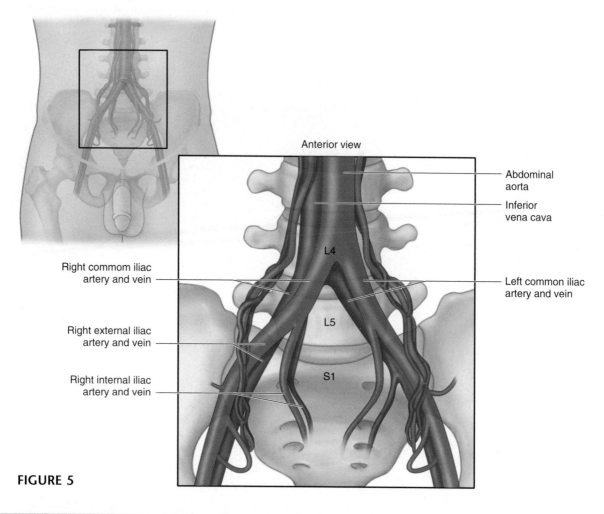

Anterior view

Abdominal aorta

Inferior vena cava

L4

Right commom iliac artery and vein

Left common iliac artery and vein

L5

Right external iliac artery and vein

S1

Right internal iliac artery and vein

FIGURE 5

Surgical Anatomy

RETROPERITONEAL APPROACH (FIG. 5)

- The approach for this procedure is typically left sided because the aorta lies to the left of the vena cava.
  - The aorta is relatively resilient and easy to mobilize as compared to the vena cava.
  - An exception is in male patients at L5/S1, where a right-sided approach may be preferable to reduce the risk of injury to the superior hypogastric plexus, resulting in retrograde ejaculation.
    - Anatomically, the hypogastric plexus sits to the left side and anastamoses with the left perivascular sympathetic plexus.
- The ureter is swept medially with the peritoneum.
- The iliac vessels are identified and protected.
  - At L5/S1, the ureter typically crosses the iliac vessels and marks the cephalad region of the disk space.
  - For an L3/4 or L4/5 disk replacement, the vessels are mobilized from the left to the right.

Equipment

• Radiolucent operating room table
• C-arm fluoroscope

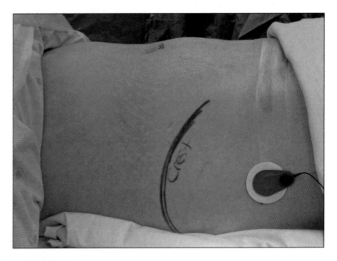

FIGURE 6

Positioning

■ The patient is positioned in supine on a radiolucent table.
■ Prior to preparation, the surgeon verifies that clear anteroposterior and lateral fluoroscopic images of the index level can be achieved.

Portals/Exposures

■ A horizontal incision is preferred for a one level replacement and a vertical incision for multi-level procedures (Fig. 7).
  • A retroperitoneal approach is preferred, but a transperitoneal approach may also be used at L5/S1.

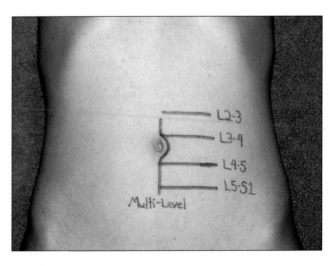

FIGURE 7

- *A lateral fluoroscopic image can be used to ensure that the skin incision is centered over the index level.*

- *Care must be taken to preserve sympathetic and parasympathetic nerves to avoid erectile dysfunction and retrograde ejaculation in the male patient.*

■ The retroperitoneal space lies deep to the rectus sheath.

- The retroperitoneal space is entered by pushing the peritoneum posteriorly at the edge of the fascial incision (Fig. 8).
- Blunt dissection with sponge sticks is used to dissect within the retroperitoneal plane leading to the lateral edge of the psoas.
- The ureter is typically swept medially with the peritoneum.

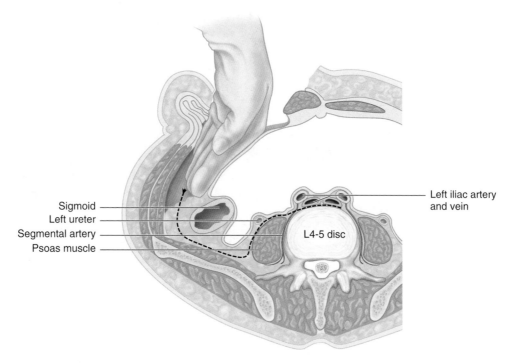

Sigmoid
Left ureter
Segmental artery
Psoas muscle

L4-5 disc

Left iliac artery and vein

FIGURE 8

Controversies

- The transperitoneal approach may be used in patients who have had previous open abdominal surgery, obese patients, and patients who have had revision anterior retroperitoneal surgery.

■ Vascular structures provide the biggest obstace to adequate access to the disk space.
  - Elevation of vascular structures is necessary for exposure of the anterior spine. The retractor blades should not pass posterior to the anterior 50% of the vertebral body, in order to protect the ventral nerve root (Figs. 9 and 10).

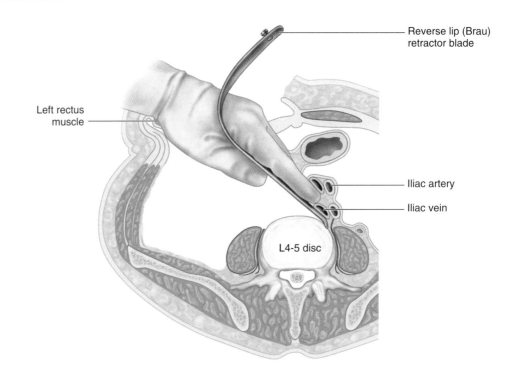

Reverse lip (Brau) retractor blade

Left rectus muscle

Iliac artery

Iliac vein

L4-5 disc

FIGURE 9

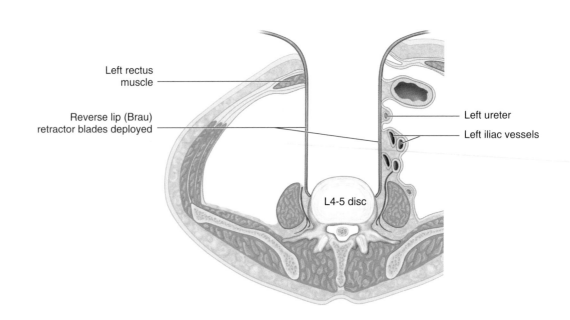

Left rectus muscle

Reverse lip (Brau) retractor blades deployed

Left ureter

Left iliac vessels

L4-5 disc

FIGURE 10

• At L5/S1, the disk space is situated caudad to the aortic bifurcation. The left iliac vein typically covers a portion of the left side of the disk and must be mobilized (Fig. 11).

• At L4/5, the iliolumbar vein must be ligated in order to allow safe retraction of the left iliac vein.

Procedure

STEP 1: DISK SPACE PREPARATION

■ The appropriate disk level and midline are determined using a marking screw and fluoroscopic images (Figs. 12, 13, and 14), and the midline

■ *If the posterior part of the disk does not distract, it is necessary to release the posterior longitudinal ligament and osteophytes.*

■ *Mobilization allows appropriate posterior placement of the implant and increases the range of motion.*

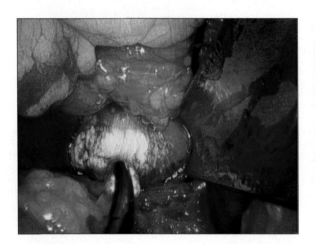

FIGURE 11

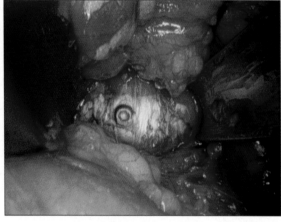

FIGURE 12

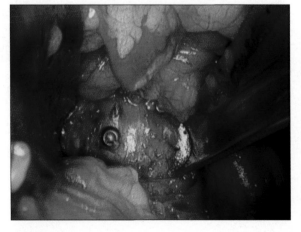

FIGURE 13

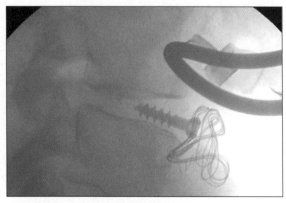

FIGURE 14

reference point is marked on the superior vereberal body (Fig. 15).

- An anterior anulotomy is performed with a scalpel or cautery (Fig. 16).
- A large Cobb elevator is used to separate the cartilaginous end plate from the osseous end plate.
- The disk is subtotally resected, leaving the lateral aspect of the anulus intact (Fig. 17).

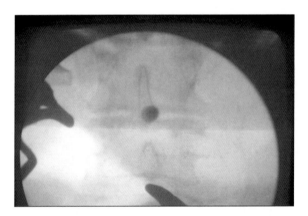

FIGURE 15

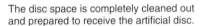
The disc space is completely cleaned out and prepared to receive the artificial disc.

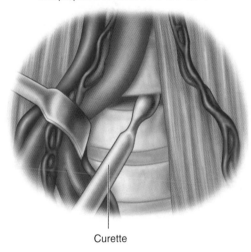

Curette

FIGURE 16

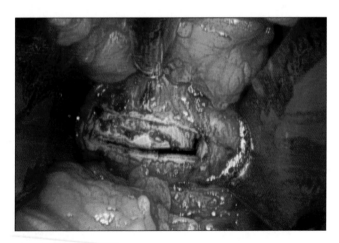

FIGURE 17

Instrumentation/ Implantion

• End plate sizing guide

STEP 2: END PLATE SIZING

■ Using visual landmarks, insert the end plate sizing gauge in the midline (Fig. 18A).
■ Verify that the gauge maximally covers the end plate using lateral fluoroscopy (Fig. 18B).
■ Verify the ability to place the implant posteriorly.

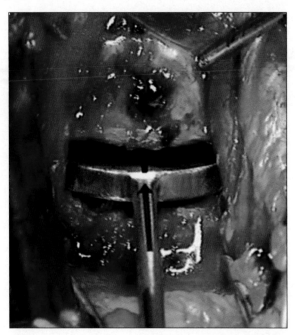

A

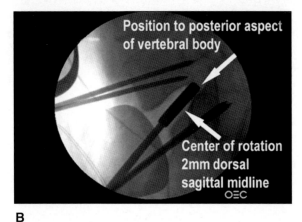

Position to posterior aspect of vertebral body

Center of rotation 2mm dorsal sagittal midline

OEC

B

FIGURE 18A-B

Instrumentation/ Implantation

• Trial insertion instrument
• Trial guide

STEP 3: TRIAL INSERTION

■ Based on the patient's anatomy and preoperative assessment, select the appropriate radiolucent trial (size and lordotic angle) and insert into the trial insertion instrument.

■ Insert the trial insertion instrument through the insertion guide, allowing the trial channels to track along the insertion guide rails (Fig. 19A).

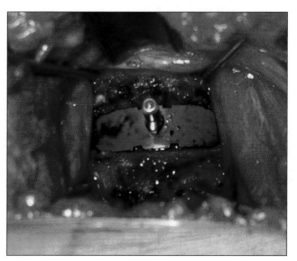

A

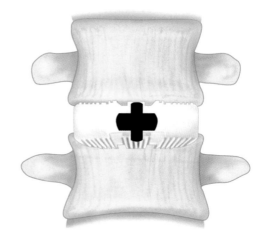

B

FIGURE 19A-B

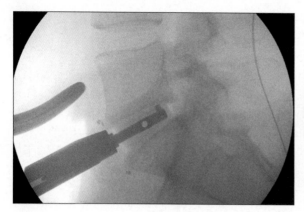

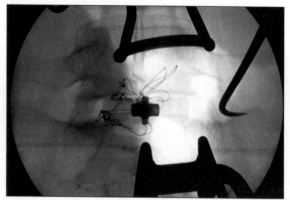

A

B

FIGURE 20A-B

STEP 4: PILOT DRIVER INSERTION

- Select the appropriate-size pilot driver.
- Align the center tooth with the midline marker to verify a perpendicular trajectory.
- Carefully impact the pilot driver to verify the ability to accurately place the end plates into the proper position (Fig. 21A).
- The center of the pilot driver should be 2 mm dorsal to the lateral midline (Fig. 21B).
- Use the slap hammer to safely remove the pilot driver from the disk space.

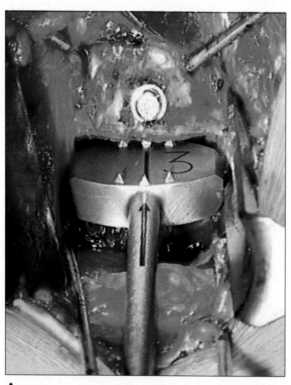

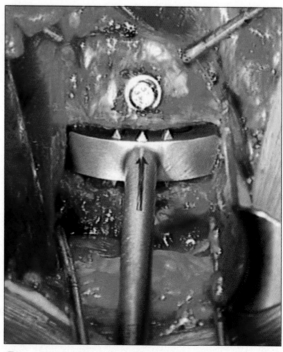

A

B

FIGURE 21A-B

Instrumentation

- Charité disk replacement prosthesis

STEP 5: IMPLANT INSERTION

- Insert the end plate insertion tips into the spreading and insertion instrument (Fig. 22A).
- Once the proper end plates have been selected, load into the end plate insertion instrument.
- Insert the end plates into the disk space (Fig. 22B).
  - Insert into the disk space with the guided impactor, with care not to fracture the end plate (Fig. 22C).

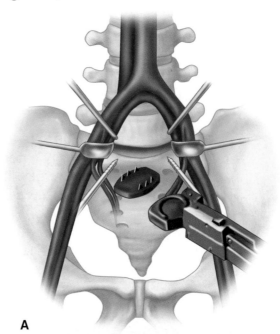

FIGURE 22A-C   A

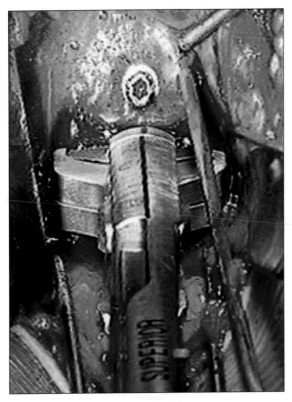

B

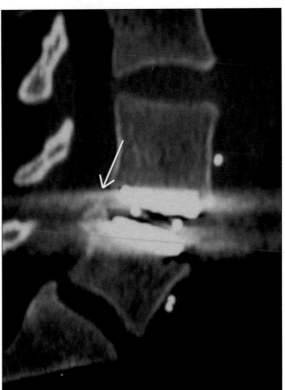

C

- During insertion, there is subtle disengagement of the S1 end plate via a caudal "walking" technique (Fig. 23A). With subtle cephalad tilting of the guide impactor, S1 is engaged and L5 is disengaged to further "walk" the prosthesis posteriorly (Fig. 23B).
- Verify posterior positioning with a lateral radiograph.

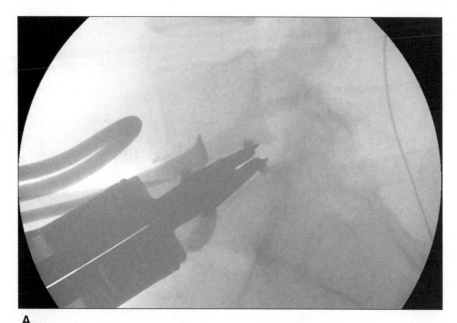

A

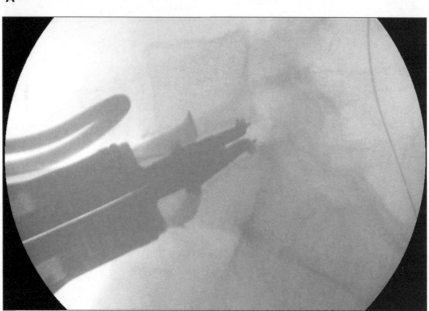

B

FIGURE 23A-B

Instrumentation

- Disk space distractor
- Polyethylene core

STEP 6: POLYETHYLENE CORE INSERTION

- Sequentially distract the disk space using the distraction spacers and modular T-handle corresponding to the core heights (Fig. 24A and 24B).
  - Care must be taken to avoid contact between the distraction spacer and the articulating surface of the end plates.
- Core insertion (Fig. 24C)
  - Confirm sliding core height by placing the core trial between the distracted end plates. Fluoroscopic images can be used to demonstrate that the sliding core has been placed to restore height to Mc Nab's line (Fig. 24D and Fig. 25A and 25B).

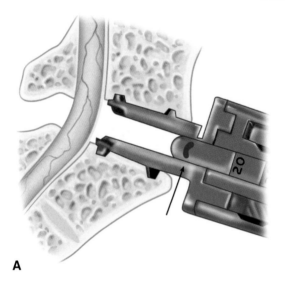

A

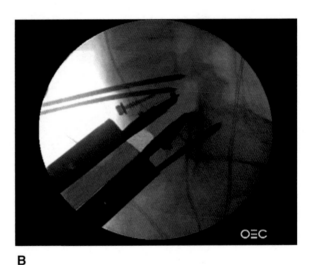

B

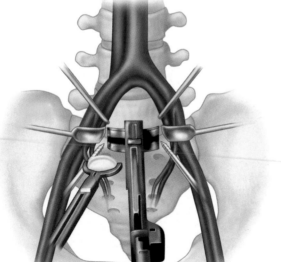

C

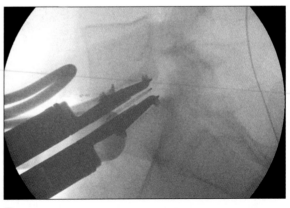

D

FIGURE 24A-D

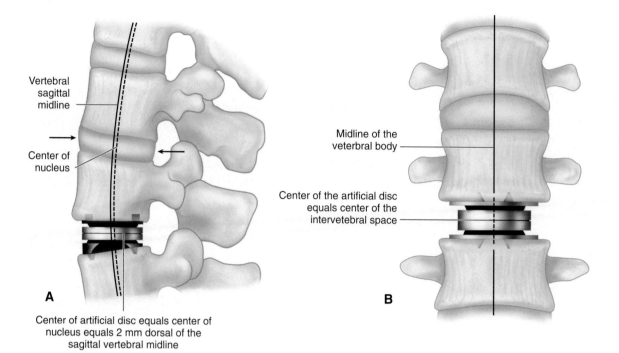

Vertebral sagittal midline

Center of nucleus

A

Center of artificial disc equals center of nucleus equals 2 mm dorsal of the sagittal vertebral midline

Midline of the veterbral body

Center of the artificial disc equals center of the intervetebral space

B

FIGURE 25A-B

- Never impact the core trial.
- Lateral fluoroscopic images may be taken to show the restoration of both the disk height and the lordosis (Fig. 26).

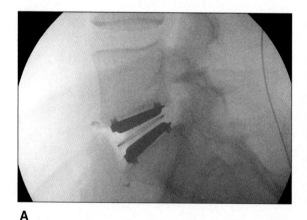

A

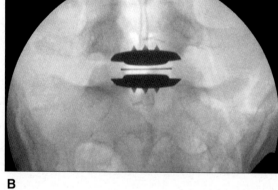

B

FIGURE 26A-B

PITFALLS

- *Potential complications of disk replacement*

  - *Subsidence*

  - *Device dislocation and migration*

  - *Radicular pain, weakness, dysesthesia*

  - *Infection*

  - *Polyethylene wear, osteolysis, and loosening*

  - *Metal debris and oncogenic potential (no clinical cases identified)*

  - *Acceleration of facet joint arthrosis*

  - *Instability (too thin of a spacer)*

  - *Postoperative scoliosis (poor device positioning)*

Controversies

- Revision options include avoiding the entire anterior implantation area completely and performing a posterior fusion.
- If removal of the device is indicated, it may be replaced with a new TDR, or an anterior fusion may be performed with or without a supplemental posterior construct.
- The approach for removing the primary TDR prosthesis may be done through a repeat direct anterior approach or through a lateral approach, avoiding the area of scar tissue.

Postoperative Care And Expected Outcomes

- All patients may be weight bearing immediately after surgery.
- Standing radiographs are obtained the morning after surgery to document position and to rule out migration in the weight-bearing position.
- Patients are advised to avoid extension, stooping, excessive twisting, or any heavy lifting for the first 6 weeks postsurgery.
- After 6 weeks, unrestricted activities are allowed in a progressive fashion. Participation in extreme or contact sports is not encouraged.

RESULTS OF THE CHARITÉ ARTIFICIAL DISK

- Recently, results of the multicenter Food and Drug Administration–regulated trial conducted to assess the safety and effectiveness of the Charité Artificial Disk were published.
  - The study involved 304 patients and included 24-month follow-up. Patients were randomized to total disk replacement (TDR) or anterior interbody fusion using cages. While patients in both groups improved, the TDR group experienced improvement more quickly and were significantly more satisfied.
  - Complications in the two groups were similar.
- Long-term follow-up of TDR patients has been published from Europe, where TDR has been performed since the mid-1980s.
  - A study with a minimum 10-year follow-up for 100 patients found that 62% of patients had an excellent outcome, with an additional 28% indicating a good outcome. The return-to-work rate was 91%. Five patients (5%) required a secondary posterior fusion.
  - There was no indication of significant problems with the durability of the devices long term.

FUTURE DESIGN MODIFICATIONS AND GOALS

- The goals of spinal arthroplasty are to maintain motion, relieve pain, preserve disk space height, maintain neural foraminal height, and preserve the facet joints.
- It is important to have longevity of any implant through millions of cycles and to aim for avoidance of revision surgery. This requires excellent wear

characteristics of any spacer, excellent shock-absorbing capacity, and a solid interface between the device and the host bone without sacrificing revision options. As we look toward the future in design concepts, we must bear these goals in mind and make careful modifications based on carefully collected data from current designs over a mid- to long-term duration.

Evidence

Lemaire JP, Carrier H, Sariali el-H, Skalli W, Lavaste F. Clinical and radiological outcomes with the Charité artificial disc: a 10-year minimum follow-up. J Spinal Disord Tech. 2005;18:353-9.

With a minimum follow-up of 10 years, the Charité artificial disk demonstrated excellent flexion/extension and lateral range of motion with no significant complications in 107 patients.

Regan JJ. Clinical results of Charité lumbar total disc replacement. Orthop Clin North Am. 2005;36:323-40.

Kyphoplasty

Daniel Shedid and Isador H. Lieberman

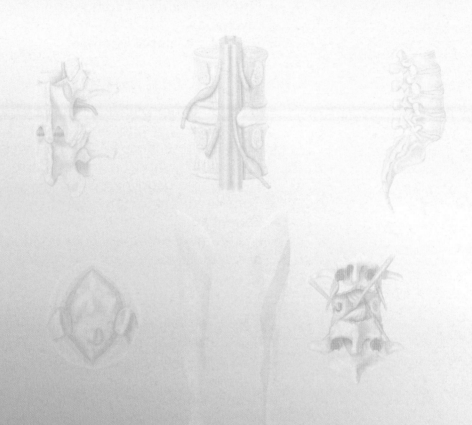

Controversies

- Progressive kyphotic deformity secondary to osteoporotic fracture

Treatment Options

- Bed rest
- Brace
- Narcotic analgesics
- Vertebroplasty
- Open surgical procedure

INDICATIONS

- Progressive, painful osteoporotic vertebral wedge compression fractures in the absence of neurologic signs
- Osteolytic vertebral compression fractures (multiple myeloma)
- Sagittal spinal malalignment

Examination/Imaging

- Plain radiographs, including 36-inch cassette scoliosis films (anteroposterior and lateral)
- Magnetic resonance imaging (T_1-weighted, T_2-weighted, short time inversion recovery [STIR], T_1-weighted gadolinium)
- Computed tomography scan
- Bone scan
- Prothrombin time/partial thromboplastin time and platelet count

Surgical Anatomy

- Define the pedicular rings (waist of the pedicle): to define the starting point
- Define the spinous process: to gauge vertebral body rotation
- Define end plates: to plan the trajectory anterior to posterior and superior to inferior
- Define cortical margins: to avoid anterior margin of the spinal canal, the great vessels, and the lungs

Positioning

- General or local anesthesia
- Patient prone on a Jackson table or other radiolucent table with appropriate padding for spine surgery
- Biplanar fluoroscopy

Portals/Exposures

- The approach to the vertebral body is percutaneously via the transpedicular or extrapedicular approach with a Jamshidi needle.

- *The spinous processes should be equidistant between vertebral body pedicles.*

- *On lateral fluoroscopic images, the pedicles should be superimposed.*

Equipment

- Biplanar fluoroscopy

Procedure

STEP 1

- Using biplanar fluoroscopy, identify the entry point and the skin incision.
- After injecting local anesthetic, a 3-mm paramedian skin incision is created over the entry site to the fractured bone.
- Use a Jamshidi needle to locate the entry point to the pedicle and to feel the bony landmarks.
- The Jamshidi needle is advanced through the bone of the pedicle using a tapping mallet.
- The Jamshidi needle should be positioned at the junction of the pedicle and the vertebral body.
- After removing the trocar, place a guidewire in the hollow core of the needle.
- Advance the guidewire until it is slightly posterior to the anterior cortex of the vertebral body.
- Remove the Jamshidi needle.
- A cannulated blunt dissector is passed over the guidewire into the vertebral body.
- The working cannula is passed over the blunt dissector, and becomes seated just anterior to the posterior cortex (Fig. 1).
- Remove the blunt dissector.
- A drill or solid stylet is used to create a channel in the vertebral body to accommodate the inflatable bone tamp. A vertebral body biopsy with the appropriate trephine may be obtained at this time.
- The procedure is repeated on the contralateral side.

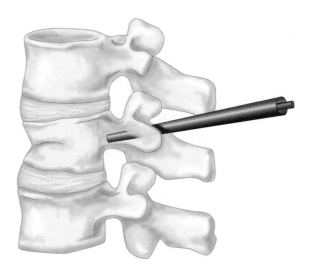

FIGURE 1

STEP 2

- The deflated balloon tamp is passed down the working cannula under fluoroscopic control.
- The radiographic markers within the balloon tamp are used for proper positioning.
- Once the balloon is properly positioned (Fig. 2), start gradually inflating it with frequent AP and lateral imaging.
- The balloon is inflated with sterile saline and radiocontrast dye to monitor the position of the balloon. The liquid is delivered via a flexible cannula connected to a twist syringe with a pressure transducer to monitor the volume and inflation pressure.
- A reduction of the fracture after inflating the balloon is a satisfactory result (Fig. 3).
- The procedure is repeated on the contralateral side.

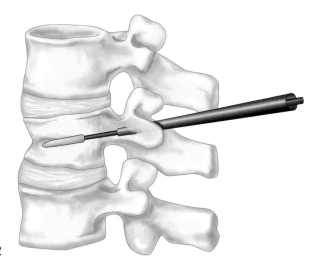

FIGURE 2

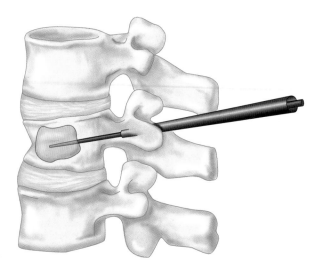

FIGURE 3

Instrumentation/ Implantation

- Local anesthetic
- Jamshidi needle
- Mallet
- Guidewire
- Blunt dissector
- Working cannula

Instrumentation/ Implantion

- Balloon tamps
- Curette
- Biopsy forceps

PEARLS

- *Care is taken not to pierce the anterior cortex.*

- *During balloon inflation, care must be taken not to pierce the lateral cortex of the vertebral body.*

- *During balloon inflation, rigorously monitor the inflation pressure. Do not inflate above 300 psi.*

- *If the balloon is not inflated enough and high inflation pressures have been reached, one could remove the ballon and use a curette that can be angled inside the vertebral body in order to create a partial cavity for the balloon (Fig. 4A).*

- *If a biopsy is needed, a forceps can be used through the working cannula prior to the balloon tamps (Fig. 4B).*

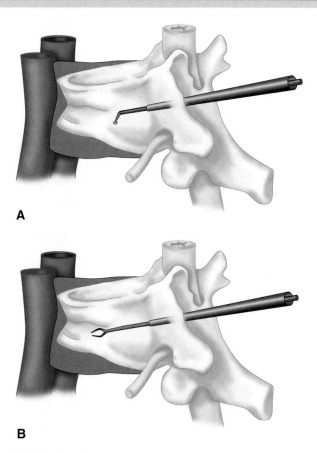

A

B

FIGURE 4A-B

STEP 3

- After inflating the balloon tamps bilaterally and obtaining a satisfactory reduction of the fracture, the balloons are deflated and removed (Fig. 5). A void is left inside the vertebral bodies.
- The PMMA bone cement is mixed and the cement applicators are filled. Before the cement hardens,

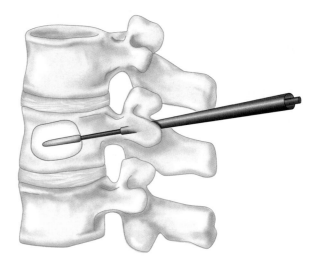

FIGURE 5

it is extruded from the cement applicators via the working cannula into the defect in the vertebral body.

■ Bone cement is slowly deposited under low pressure, filling the deepest area first, then withdrawing the needle slightly to fill upper areas (Fig. 6). The pressure and amount of cement extruded are closely monitored to avoid unwanted leakage into nearby areas, such as through the upper or lower end plates or the posterior and anterior cortices.

■ The volume of cement that can safely be deposited is usually the same as the volume to which the balloon tamps had been inflated.

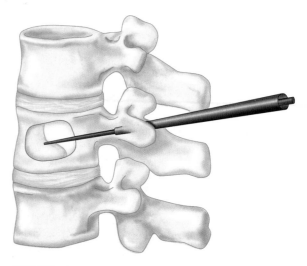

FIGURE 6

Instrumentation/ Implantation

- PMMA
- Cement applicator

- Cement injection is stopped when it approaches the end plates or lateral wall or the posterior cortex, or if leakage is seen.
- The cement applicator is left in place until the cement fully cures to prevent cement from expanding up the working cannula.
- The procedure is repeated in the contralateral side.
- The working cannula is removed (Fig. 7) and the skin incision is closed with a resorbable suture.

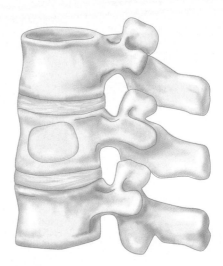

FIGURE 7

Postoperative Care and Expected Outcomes

- No bracing is required.
- Most patients can be released home the same day if a neurologic examination is normal.
- Pain is managed for a limited period with narcotic medication.
- Potential complications include cement leakage, adjacent vertebral compression fracture, and epidural hematoma.

Evidence

Garfin SR, Reilley MA. Minimally invasive treatment of osteoporotic vertebral body compression fractures. Spine J. 2002;2:76-80.

In this prospective multicenter series, there were six major complications among 600 cases, with 0.75% neurologic complications.

Ledlie JT, Renfro M. Balloon kyphoplasty: one-year outcomes in vertebral body height restoration, chronic pain, and activity levels. J Neurosurg. 2003;98(1 Suppl):36-42.

Ninety percent of patients were ambulating without assistance post-kyphoplasty. No device- or procedure-related complications were noted; 9% had asymptomatic cement leaks.

Lieberman IH, Dudeney S, Reinhardt MK, Bell G. Initial outcome and efficacy of "kyphoplasty" in the treatment of painful osteoporotic vertebral compression fractures. Spine. 2001;26:1631-8.

Seventy percent of the vertebral bodies achieved hight restoration.

Majd ME, Farley S, Holt RT. Preliminary outcomes and efficacy of the first 360 consecutive kyphoplasties for the treatment of painful osteoporotic vertebral compression fractures. Spine J. 2005;5:244-55.

Immediate pain relief was achieved in 89% of patients. More than 20% had restoration of height loss in 69% of the fractures. Cement leaks occurred in 10% of patients, and 12% had adjacent-level or remote fractures.

Phillips FM, Ho E, Campbell-Hupp M, McNally T, Todd Wetzel F, Gupta P. Early radiographic and clinical results of balloon kyphoplasty for the treatment of osteoporotic vertebral compression fractures. Spine. 2003;28:2260-5; discussion 2265-7.

Mean correction of kyphosis was 14.2°. No device- or procedure-related complications were noted; 9.8% of patients had asymptomatic cement leaks and 9% had remote or adjacent-level fractures.

Balloon-Assisted End Plate Reduction (BAER) Techniques

F.C. Öner and J.J. Verlaan

Controversies

• Many burst fractures, especially with intact posterior ligamentary complex (PLC) and without neurologic involvement, can be managed nonoperatively.

Treatment Options

• Anterior corpectomy and reconstruction with iliac crest bone graft, allograft strut, or cage.

Indications

■ Burst type fractures of thoracic and lumbar spine of:
  • Traumatic origin
  • Osteoporotic origin
  • Pathologic origin

Examination/Imaging

■ Thin-slice computed tomography with sagittal reconstructions (Fig. 1)
■ T_1- and T_2-weighted sagittal magnetic resonance imaging (MRI) (Fig. 2)

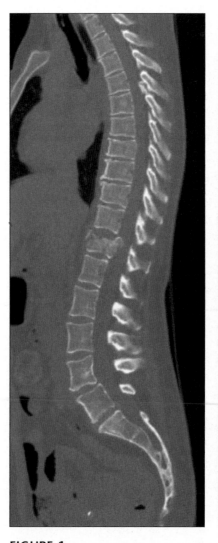
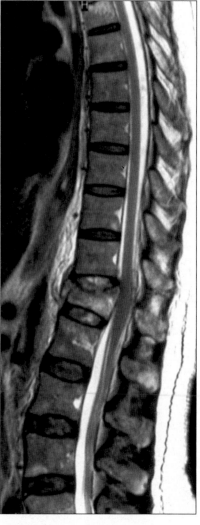

FIGURE 1   **FIGURE 2**

Surgical Anatomy

- Standard posterior transpedicular approach through midline incision

Positioning

- Place the patient in the prone position with chest and pelvic support.
- Assure that the abdomen is free and uncompressed.

Portals/Exposures

- Midline incision allowing access to the pedicle entry points of the fractured vertebra and the adjacent levels (Fig. 3)

Procedure

STEP 1

- Insert the optimal-sized pedicle screws into the vertebrae cranial and caudal to the fractured vertebra (Fig. 4).

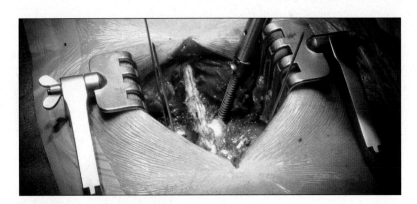

FIGURE 3

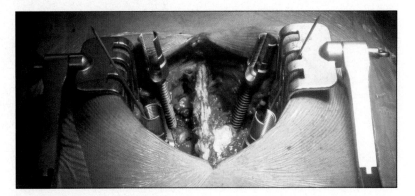

FIGURE 4

440

Instrumentation/ Implantion

• Not every pedicle screw instrumentation is suitable for fracture reduction.
• Check whether you can carry out different reduction maneuvers independently with the available implants.

STEP 2

■ Depending on the type of instrumentation used, attempt initially to correct the posttraumatic kyphosis (Fig. 5), followed by fracture distraction (Fig. 6).
■ Correct scoliotic deformity by asymmetric distraction.
■ Check correction with posteroanterior and lateral fluoroscopy and lock the screws.

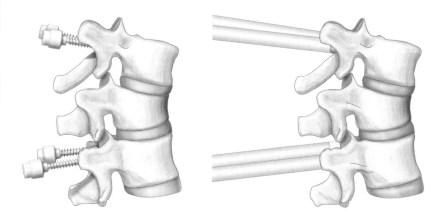

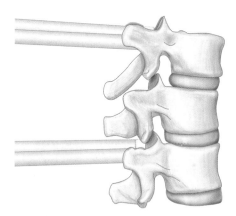

FIGURE 5

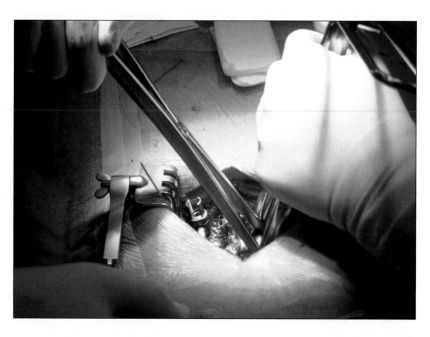

FIGURE 6

Instrumentation/ Implantation

- KyphX inflatable bone tamps
- BoneSource or other CaP cement

STEP 3

- Probe the pedicles of the fractured vertebra carefully.
- Insert the cannulas of the KyphX set (Fig. 7).
- Under fluoroscopic control, insert the drill of the set. Try to get the drill under the most depressed portion of the end plate.
- Fill the KyphX bone tamps with contrast fluid as instructed by the company.
- Insert balloons and check their position under the end plate using AP and lateral fluoroscopy (Fig. 8).
- Make sure that the balloons are placed under the central end plate depression (Fig. 9)

Controversies

- PMMA cement can be used for osteoporotic or pathologic fractures. The advantages of CaP cements in trauma patients are theoretical and not proven in comparative studies.
- In young trauma patients, a posterolateral fusion is recommended, although there is no evidence as of yet for this practice.

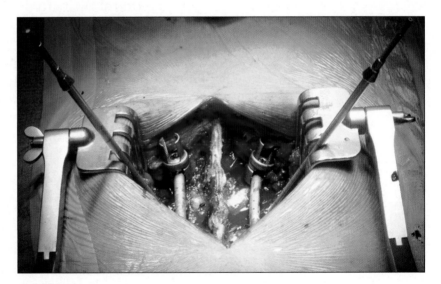

FIGURE 7

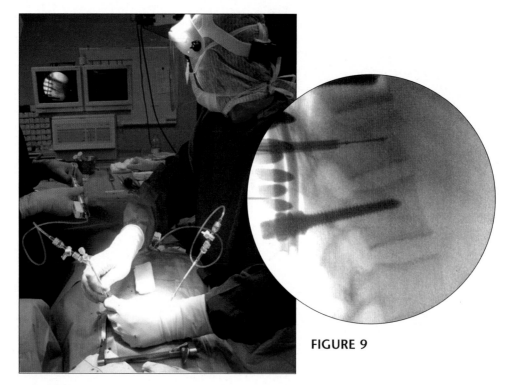

FIGURE 9

FIGURE 8

- Reduce the end plate under lateral fluoroscopic control by incremental inflation of the balloons (Fig. 10).
- Remove the balloons and inject saline into one cannula with a syringe, making sure that it comes out of the contralateral cannula unimpeded.
- Inject the cement from only one side to avoid high-pressure buildup within the cement mass. Injection should be monitored fluoroscopically (Fig. 11).

Postoperative Care and Expected Outcomes

- Obtain standing AP and lateral radiographs. In cases of neurologic impairment, obtain postoperative MRI to confirm canal clearance.
- A thoracolumbar orthosis is recommended for 4-6 weeks.

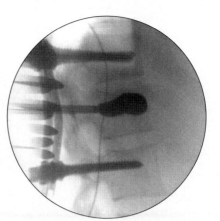

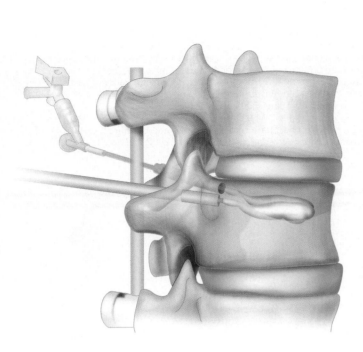

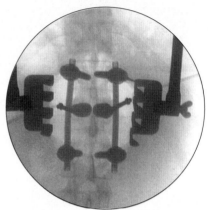

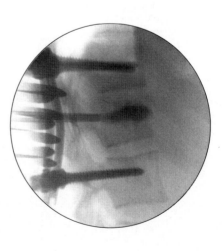

FIGURE 10

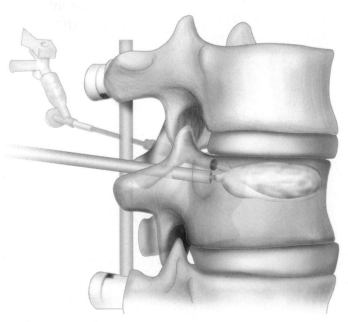

FIGURE 11

Evidence

Öner FC, Dhert WJ, Verlaan JJ. Less invasive anterior column reconstruction in thoracolumbar fractures. Injury. 2005;36(Suppl 2):B82-9.

Öner FC, Verlaan JJ, Verbout AJ, Dhert WJ: Cement augmentation techniques in traumatic thoracolumbar spine fractures. Spine. 2006;31(11 Suppl):S89-95.

Verlaan JJ, Dhert WJA, Verbout AJ, Oner FC: Balloon vertebroplasty in combination with pedicle screw instrumentation: a novel technique to treat thoracic and lumbar burst fractures. Spine. 2005;30:E73-9.

Verlaan JJ, van Helden WH, Oner FC, Verbout AJ, Dhert WJA. Balloon vertebroplasty with calcium phosphate cement augmentation for direct restoration of traumatic thoracolumbar vertebral fractures. Spine. 2002;27:543-554

Minimally Invasive Exposure Techniques of the Lumbar Spine

Kornelis A. Poelstra, Chadi Tannoury, Swetha Srinivisan, and D. Greg Anderson

---

PITFALLS

- *Any diagnosis making adequate fluoroscopic imaging difficult or impossible, such as:*

  - *Severe osteopenia*

  - *Intra-abdominal contrast*

- *Severe obesity, wherein a tubular retractor system is unable to reach bony anatomy*

Controversies

- Revision decompression due to scarring of neural elements

Treatment Options

- The alternative to any MISS procedure for the lumbar spine is traditional open surgery to achieve proper decompression of neural elements and fusion of the bony spine. With experience, MISS can be applied to most degenerative conditions; however, since certain clinical situations are not amenable to a minimally invasive approach, the surgeon should always prepare a MISS surgical candidate for the possibility of conversion to a larger exposure to adequately address all spinal pathology.

Indications

- Lumbar diskectomy/decompression
- Posterior lumbar fusion
  - Posterolateral (onlay)
  - Posterior interbody fusions
    - Posterior lumbar interbody fusion (PLIF)
    - Transforaminal lumbar interbody fusion (TLIF)
- Anterior lumbar interbody fusion (ALIF)

Examination/Imaging

- Although it might be difficult to define the exact boundaries of a percutaneous, mini-open, or traditional "open" surgery, the applications of less invasive spinal surgery principles are much more important than the length of the skin incision (Jaikumar et al., 2002; Lehman et al., 2005).

- As with an open procedure, evaluation of the problem should always begin with careful analysis of all pertinent imaging studies (magnetic resonance imaging [MRI], computed tomography [CT], and plain radiographs) to define the exact location of spinal pathology. This is critical because all relevant anatomic regions of the spine must be visualized and be treatable during the less invasive procedure, just as with a traditional open operation. For example, the typical lumbar degeneration with grade 1 spondylolisthesis (L4/5) and two-level disk herniations with lateral recess stenosis (L4/5 and L5/S1) requires vast minimally invasive spine surgery (MISS) experience prior to addressing these problems using minimal access surgery (Fig. 1). Knowing one's individual limitations can aid in proficiency rather than result in disappointment when starting to use MISS.

- Patients with severe osteopenia, obesity, or intra-abdominal contrast may be challenging to image using a C-arm because their bony anatomy may be obscured or difficult to visualize. If adequate fluoroscopic images cannot be obtained, an alternative surgical strategy should be employed.

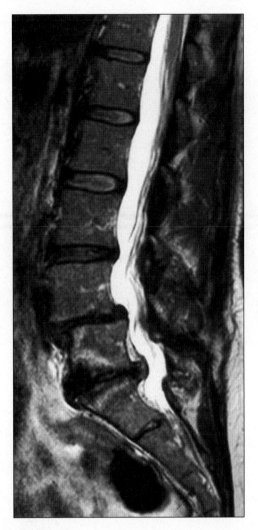

FIGURE 1

Surgical Anatomy

■ To perform a decompression and fusion in any part of the spinal column through a small opening, it is crucial to localize the precise site for all skin incisions using fluoroscopy in order to ensure successful exposure of all underlying spinal pathology (Seldomridge and Phillips, 2005).

  • After the skin and fascial incisions are made, serial dilation allows for parting of the paraspinal muscles, while minimal cutting during exposure prevents blood loss and optimizes visualization of the structures ahead. Depending on the retractor system used, some type of serial dilation and "docking" of a final, fixed retractor onto bony landmarks of the spine secures the area of interest inside the field of view (Fig. 2A and 2B). Fluoroscopic confirmation of the location is paramount.

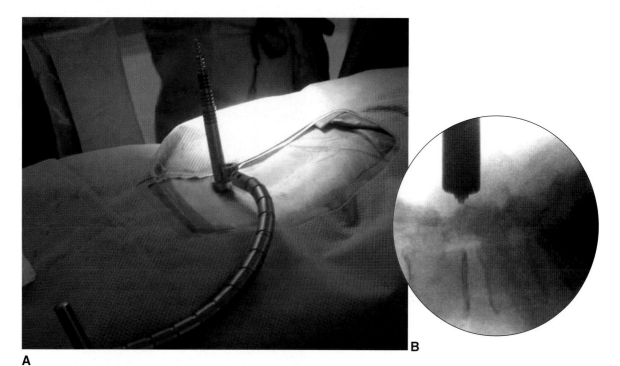

A

B

FIGURE 2A-B

- To facilitate easy placement of a tubular retractor system and prior to dilation of the paraspinal muscles, a narrow Cobb retractor placed through the initial skin incision and delivered to the level of interest on the bony anatomy can aid in removing some of the smaller attached musculature.
- Use of an operative microscope provides the best visualization for most cases, especially where decompression procedures are planned.

■ The advent of expandable tubular retractor systems has allowed for a significant increase in visualization. Once it is securely docked against the spine, soft tissue creep from underneath the outer edges of the retractor, obscuring visibility, can usually be prevented (Khoo et al., 2002; Tafazal and Sell, 2004).

- It is important to realize that the length of a narrow tubular retractor dictates the angular freedom of the surgical tools placed down inside of it. Therefore, the final retractor should have just the correct length to reach from the skin just down to the bony elements, where it can be safely docked, after which it needs to be checked on a lateral fluoroscopic image. Small adjustments in retractor position can be easily made after this, and only if a significant amount of soft tissue remains at the bottom of the retractor should it be replaced.

- With the bony elements of the spine clearly exposed and correctly identified, the surgical procedure may begin.
- Although the instruments used for MISS procedures are similar to those used with traditional open procedures, longer, bayoneted instruments are useful to ensure that visualization is not obscured by the surgeon's hands.
  - The most ergonomic approach involves using a narrow suction tool in one hand and a working instrument (e.g., Kerrison rongeur or curette) in the other, dominant, hand (Fig. 3), allowing optimal visualization at the tip of the working instrument (Seldomridge and Phillips, 2005).
  - In most cases, only minimal assistance is required from a surgical assistant during the decompression portion of a MISS case.
- "Wanding" is an important technique that allows for access outside of the small initial area exposed at the end of the tubular retractor.
  - It is usually performed by first loosening the attachment of the retractor to the operating table. Then, the tubular retractor can be shifted or angled through the soft tissues to the new position, while gently holding the retractor against the spine to minimize soft tissue creep (Fig. 4).

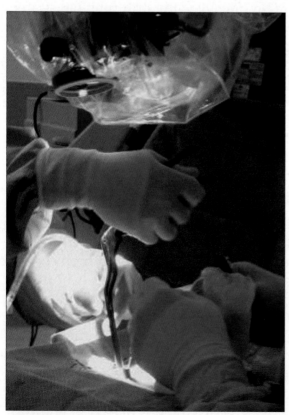

FIGURE 3

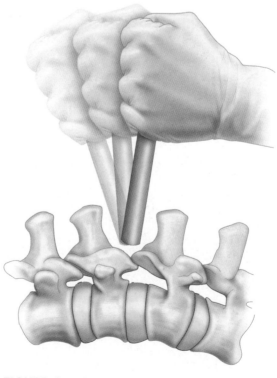

FIGURE 4

- Migration of the tip over small distances through the soft tissues is generally also possible, enabling an increased field of view without further need for dissection.
- The best way to manipulate the final retractor is to place the largest dilator back into the tubular retractor to act as a joystick for manipulating the tip position of the tubular retractor. Using this technique, it is usually possible to reach both sides of the spine canal during a spinal decompressive procedure or two adjacent vertebral levels on the ipsilateral side of the spine.

■ In addition to direct visualization through the retractor, tactile feedback is almost as important to perform MISS safely and effectively. The surgeon should learn to "feel" the spine and neural elements during the MISS case. Care must be taken when decompressing the spinal canal in a region along the edge of the tubular retractor, where soft tissue encroachment may obscure visualization. A useful technique is to gently twist the Kerrison rongeur after a decompressive bite, while watching the dura, prior to pulling away to see if the dura is entrapped. This careful technique can avoid most accidental dural tears.

■ In the unfortunate event of a dural laceration, proper repair may be difficult. Although multiple strategies for managing dural tears are available, the authors believe that direct repair of a significant dural laceration is optimal (Bosacco et al., 2001). This may require extension of the incision to gain adequate access, and it is important to discuss this with the patient prior to surgical intervention as well as to include the need for traditional open access in the preoperative consent form.

Positioning

■ After the patient has been placed on a radiolucent table or frame, the position of surgical incisions should be localized in the operating room prior to the beginning of the procedure. This is normally done using C-arm fluoroscopy and is particularly important because the surgeon must ensure that the skin incisions will allow access to the relevant region of the spinal column (Lehman et al., 2005; Seldomridge and Phillips, 2005).

- Often, incisions are not made immediately over palpable anatomy, but placed in line with

PEARLS

- *It is mandatory to obtain adequate AP and lateral fluoroscopic images and localize the incisions on the skin of the patient prior to draping and the start of the case.*

PITFALLS

- *In order to gain proper access, the incisions for percutaneous pedicle screw placement need to be approximately 1 cm lateral to the lateral border of the pedicle on an adequate AP fluoroscopic image, parallel to the superior end plate of the vertebral body involved.*

- *The incision for a percutaneous TLIF procedure needs to be 2-2.5 inches lateral to the midline in order to be able to angulate medially and perform an effective diskectomy on the contralateral side of the spine.*

Equipment

- When neuromonitoring is used, ensure that no wires are taped underneath the patient that can obscure the surgeon's view of the bony anatomy.

anticipated linear access to the spinal structures of interest. Ideally, MISS allows less extensive manipulation of surrounding tissues than a conventional open procedure while accomplishing the same goals and objectives at the target structure.

- Since MISS is more dependent on fluoroscopy than traditional open surgery, it is paramount that good fluoroscopic images of the spinal region of interest are obtained prior to the skin incision.

■ The vertebrae should be aligned so that, on an AP image, the spinous process is centered between the pedicles and the superior end plate is parallel to the fluoroscopy beam (Fig. 5). On the lateral image, the pedicles should be superimposed and only a single posterior cortex of the vertebral body should be seen (Fig. 6, arrow). The superior end plates of the vertebral bodies appear as a single straight line also. Incorrect images can cause malpositioning of the screws and possible neural element compromise.

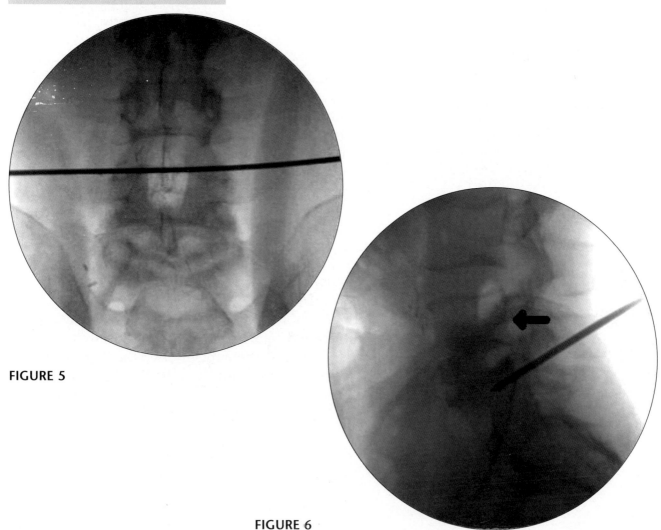

FIGURE 5

FIGURE 6

PEARLS

- *When starting with limited-access spinal surgery, simple diskectomies are appropriate after adequate MISS experience has been gained using cadaver courses.*

PITFALLS

- *When performing a decompression of the neural elements at the perimeter of the tubular retractor, a useful technique is to gently twist the Kerrison rongeur while watching the dura prior to pulling away to see if the dura is entrapped. Careful technique can avoid most accidental dural tears.*

Controversies

- Never hesitate to increase the size of an incision to perform your procedure adequately. Minimally invasive should not equate to minimally effective, and patients selected to undergo a MISS procedure need to be told that traditional open surgery may be required to adequately address their pathology or deal with an intraoperative complication (e.g., accidental dural laceration).

Procedure

STEP 1: DECOMPRESSION TECHNIQUES

- MISS is an excellent option for localized cases of spinal canal stenosis or herniated lumbar disks. Simple decompressive surgery is generally straightforward and is an appropriate starting point for the novice MISS surgeon after adequate training has been gained through cadaver courses. It is important to remember that, although MISS decompressions are done through a smaller skin incision, the same adequate decompression must be achieved to have a good clinical outcome. Minimally invasive should not equate to minimally effective.

- In the case of a disk herniation, any free fragments should be localized on preoperative imaging studies (recent MRI preferred) relative to the pedicles and the disk space. A simple laminotomy over the disk fragment will allow the surgeon to remove the fragment and decompress the compromised neural elements.

- With spinal stenosis, the location of the obstruction within the spinal canal should be clearly defined to reduce the risk of residual neural element compression postoperatively.

- In addition to a laminectomy, a "laminoplasty" technique can be used to address bilateral stenosis through a single unilateral portal. With the laminoplasty technique, a wide hemilaminectomy is performed first, after which a medial facet resection can be done to decompress the ipsilateral side of the spine. Then, the tube is angled (utilizing the wanding technique outlined previously) underneath the lamina while the ligamentum flavum remains intact. The decompression can be completed using a long, thin, high-speed burr to perform undercutting of the lamina on the contralateral side (Fig. 7).

- During drilling across the midline of the spine canal on the contralateral side, the ligamentum flavum should be left intact to protect the underlying dura from the drill. At the conclusion of laminectomy, the ligamentum flavum should be resected so the dura can be fully visualized and the surgeon can be assured that an adequate decompression was performed.

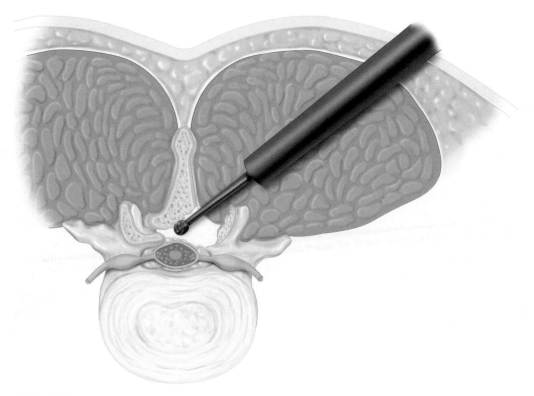

FIGURE 7

STEP 2: SPINAL FUSION

- In addition to anterior interbody fusion (traditional ALIF or lateral ALIF), posterolateral (onlay) fusion and posterior interbody fusion (PLIF or TLIF) also can be successfully performed using MISS surgery.
- Posterolateral (Onlay) Fusion
  - Posterolateral fusion between the transverse processes of two adjacent levels is achieved by serial dilation of the paraspinal muscles to allow docking of a tubular retractor against the transverse process of one of the levels to be fused. An expandable retractor system can facilitate the exposure of both the superior and inferior transverse process at the fusion level simultaneously.
  - It is important to localize the correct anatomic levels prior to making the skin incisions. Using a Steinmann pin or its equivalent, the lateral margins of the pedicles and superior end plates of the vertebral elements can be easily identified using AP and lateral fluoroscopy. Both the superior end plates and the lateral margins of the pedicles need

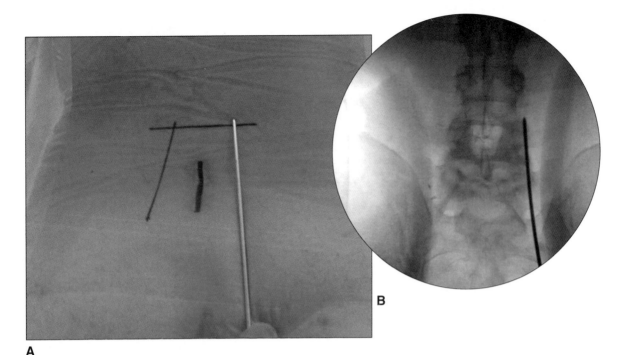

A

B

FIGURE 8A-B

Instrumentation/Implantion

- Implantation of a cage or allograft bone into a collapsed disk space can be difficult, and care must be taken not to cause misdirection of the graft into the softer cancellous bone of either vertebral body.
- Additional bone graft can be placed behind the PLIF/TLIF cage to improve the rate of arthrodesis.

to be drawn on the skin (Fig. 8A and 8B). An incision 1 cm lateral to this margin gives excellent exposure of the transverse processes in line with the fluoroscopic beam (Fig. 9). Keep in mind that the dissection and pedicle screw placement has to be directed slightly medially.

- After reaching the correct level, the soft tissues can be cleared from the intertransverse space and decortication of the transverse process, pars interarticularis, and facet joints can be achieved, followed by grafting with a suitable bone graft substance. It is important not to violate the intertransverse membrane since continuous bloody oozing can obscure the field of view, putting the nerve roots located directly anterior to this membrane at risk.

- Posterior Interbody Fusion
  - Although more technically challenging, posterior interbody fusion using either a PLIF or TLIF approach can also be achieved (German and Foley, 2005; Khoo et al., 2002; Lehman et al., 2005). As we learned from traditional open fusion procedures, the placement of an interbody device provides a more favorable fusion environment (compression) and allows the surgeon to reconstruct a collapsed disk space. The skills necessary to perform this type of surgery can be gained as the surgeon becomes familiar with spinal canal decompression through a tubular retractor.

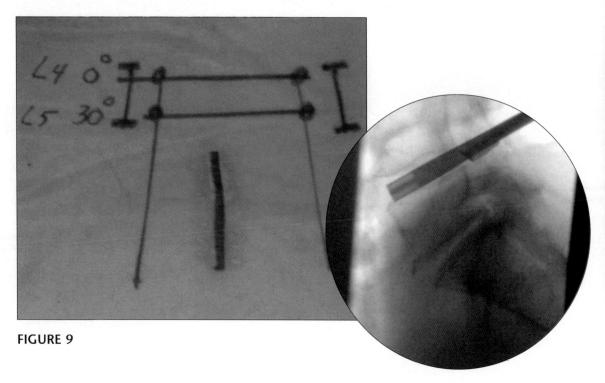

FIGURE 9

FIGURE 10

Controversies

- When prone patients are placed in lordosis on a radiolucent frame, their posterior disk space often collapses, and insertion of intravertebral body dilators can sometimes be difficult. Distraction using a rod seated inside percutaneously placed pedicle screws opposite to the PLIF/TLIF side can safely aid in opening the disk space. However, when larger dilators or further distraction is required, the rod may need to be loosened and retightened to prevent subsequent dilators from digging into the softer cancellous bone of the vertebral end plates.

- To reach the disk space, a partial or complete removal of the facet joint is required to obtain optimal access through the foramen. The surgeon should remove enough facet so that minimal retraction of the dural sac is required to place the interbody cage.
- Using a side-to-side technique rather than an up-and-down scraping technique with various sizes of curettes, the exposed disk space can be cleared of all disk material and cartilaginous end plate in preparation for fusion. Lateral fluoroscopy can also be used to prevent anterior perforation of the anulus while clearing remaining material out of the disk space.
- It is imperative to select an appropriate-sized interbody graft that fits optimally inside the disk space to support the vertebral bodies (Fig. 10). The end plates should not be violated in order to prevent graft subsidence, and the interbody spacer (whether made from titanium, polyether ether ketone [PEEK], or bone allograft) should be placed far enough anterior to minimize the risk of dural impingement. In addition to the cage, the remainder of the disk space should be filled with an adequate volume of graft material

to achieve an optimal fusion environment. The fusion is then supplemented with adjunctive spinal instrumentation (e.g., pedicle screws).

- When performing a minimally invasive TLIF, the skin incision should be placed 2-2.5 inches lateral to the midline in order to attain proper access to the contralateral disk space through angulation of the retractor to remove disk material and achieve equal amounts of distraction.

■ ALIF can be performed as a laparoscopic or mini-open procedure. ALIF provides an excellent reconstruction of the disk space and eliminates the need to operate alongside the dural sac posteriorly, thereby decreasing the risk of neural injury or epidural scarring. After ALIF, percutaneous pedicle screws can be placed to achieve a posterior tension band construct and provide circumferential stability of the spine.

■ The lateral transpsoas approach is gaining popularity for fusion of the L2/3, L3/4, and/or L4/5 disk spaces. The advantages of this approach are that no vascular mobilization is required and the risk of damage to the hypogastric plexus or postoperative ileus is minimized (Seldomridge and Phillips, 2005).

STEP 3: INSTRUMENTATION

■ Minimally invasive spinal instrumentation has been greatly simplified with the advent of percutaneous cannulated pedicle screw systems. Surgeons should familiarize themselves with the specific system to be used prior to the procedure.

■ Using AP fluoroscopic guidance, the location and trajectory of the pedicles can easily be determined (see Fig. 9) (Lehman et al., 2005; Seldomridge and Phillips, 2005).

■ The skin incisions for percutaneous pedicle screws should be positioned at least 1 cm lateral (or farther lateral in an obese patient) to the lateral wall of the pedicles on the true AP image.

■ A large Jamshidi needle (used for bone marrow biopsies) can then be introduced through the skin incision. With gentle mallet taps (Fig. 11A), the needle is slowly advanced into the lateral part of the pedicle. The Jamshidi needle must be "docked" on the spine with the tip directly over the lateral border of the pedicle image on the AP view. Once docked just inside of the cortex of the bone, fluoroscopic confirmation of the location needs to be obtained prior to advancing it any deeper (Fig. 11B). Marking the needle at this point approximately 20 mm from

PEARLS

- *Obtaining a true AP fluoroscopic image, parallel to the superior end plate of the vertebral body where pedicle fixation is desired, is paramount for the success of percutaneous screw placement.*

PITFALLS

- *Guidewires need to be held in place when the Jamshidi needle or the tap is removed from the bone to prevent accidental pullout of the wire prior to screw placement.*

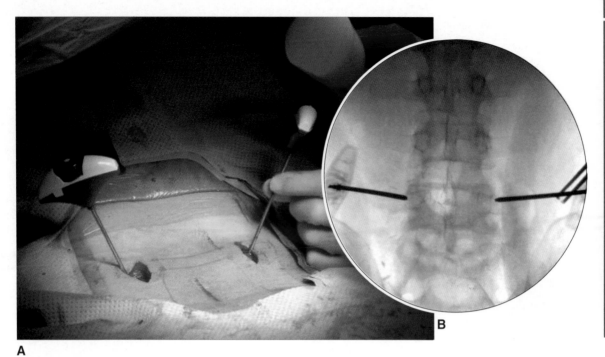

A

B

FIGURE 11A-B

Instrumentation/ Implantation

- Percutaneous pedicle screws placed over narrow guidewires can be redirected (while followed on lateral fluoroscopy) once the tip of the screw has reached the posterior margin of the vertebral body inside of the pedicle and the wire has been removed.
- Redirection prior to this can result in penetration of the outer pedicle cortex, or breaking of the guidewire!

the skin surface serves as a reminder as to the depth of the needle within the vertebral body.

■ On an AP fluoroscopic image, the tip of the needle will appear to move medially across the pedicle as the needle moves deeper into the pedicle. When the tip of the needle is at the level of the posterior cortex of the vertebral body on a lateral view, it should appear no more than two thirds the distance across the pedicle on an AP view (Fig. 12). Placement of the needle traversing the lateral pedicle by approximately two thirds and approximately 20 mm from the bony starting point (in depth) will ensure safe placement of the guidewire into the vertebral body.

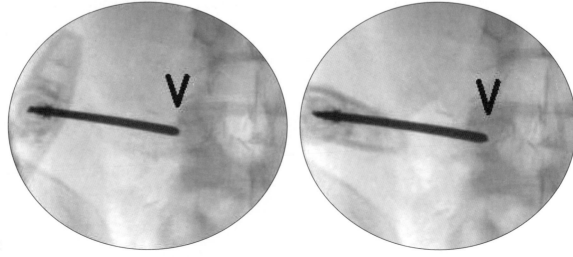

FIGURE 12

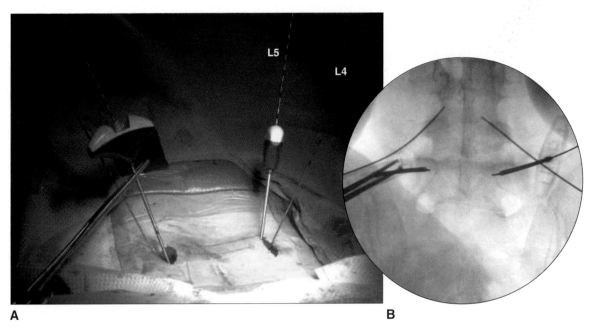

A   B

FIGURE 13A-B

- When the Jamshidi needle properly traverses the pedicle, the obturator can be removed and a guidewire is advanced into the vertebral body (Fig. 13A and 13B).
- The guidewire is then used to guide a cannulated tap and subsequently to place the cannulated pedicle screws. If desired, the screw trajectory can be tested for pedicle breach by electromyography using the tap (Fig. 14).
- As soon as the guide wires are advanced into the pedicles and vertebral bodies, lateral fluoroscopy needs to be obtained to check wire depth and direction parallel to the superior end plates. After the wires are tapped, cannulated screws can be placed (Fig. 15). When the tip of the screw reaches the posterior cortex of the vertebral body (just through the pedicle), the guidewire can be pulled out, and directional changes (especially in the superior-inferior direction) can be made to the screw.
- After all the screws are placed, the rods can be introduced according to the manufacturer's specifications and end caps can be placed into the tulip heads of the pedicle screws (Fig. 16).
- Once the screws and rods are connected, manually holding the screw extensions attached to the screw heads allows one to exert a counterforce during final tightening of the screw caps using a torque-limiting screwdriver (Fig. 17).

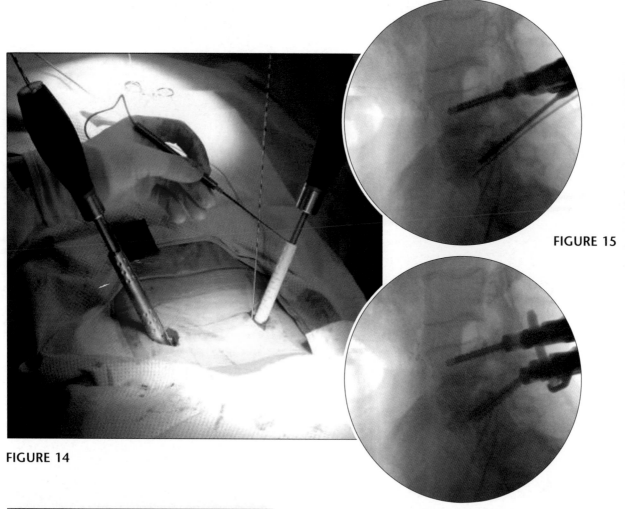

FIGURE 14

FIGURE 15

FIGURE 16

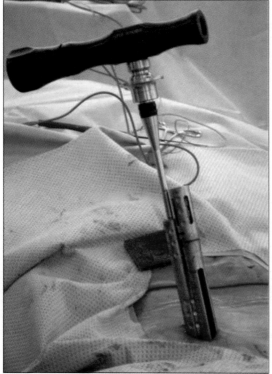

FIGURE 17

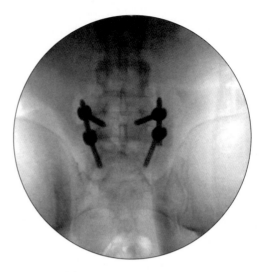

FIGURE 18

- Final AP fluoroscopy (Fig. 18) should show appropriate pedicular fixation of this revision AP fusion without the need for violation of the initial midline incision.
- The authors prefer to use subcuticular resorbable sutures to close the wound, resulting in a desirable cosmetic result (Fig. 19).

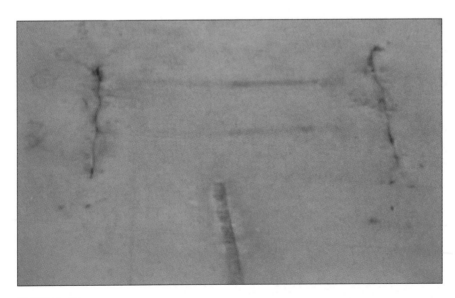

FIGURE 19

Postoperative Care and Expected Outcomes

- Postoperative care is similar to that after traditional open lumbar spinal decompression and/or fusion. The most significant difference is that the patient usually experiences less local incisional pain, and can be mobilized earlier in the postoperative period. Often the authors prefer to encourage patients to sit in a chair and ambulate to the restroom on the same afternoon of their surgery.
- Blood loss is typically less during and after the procedure, so patients feel stronger when getting up for physical therapy and require no Hemovac drainage. Aggressive rehabilitation can begin the next day after MISS intervention since risks for incisional breakdown are minimal.
- Potential perioperative complications include accidental dural laceration, unrecognized bleeding, and postoperative infection. Inadequate neural decompression is a potential complication, especially early in the learning curve. Meticulous scrutiny of preoperative CT, myelographic, and MRI images to adequately localize compressive pathology is therefore paramount when embarking on MISS decompression.

Evidence

Bosacco SJ, Gardner MJ, Guille JT. Evaluation and treatment of dural tears in lumbar spine surgery: a review. Clin Orthop Relat Res. 2001;389:238-47.

Dural lacerations are fortunately not a very common misadventure during spinal surgery, but neglect can lead to significant complications. This review addresses their prevalence and treatment options.

German JW, Foley KT. Minimal access surgical techniques in the management of the painful lumbar motion segment. Spine. 2005;30(Suppl):S52-9.

This paper reports good results following minimally invasive spinal fusion procedures. Although the preliminary data appear promising, long-term studies are required for critical review.

Jaikumar S, Kim DH, Kam AC. History of minimally invasive spine surgery. Neurosurgery. 2002;51(Suppl):S1-14.

MISS appeals to patients due to early recovery and the cosmetic benefits. Advances in this field are influenced by the evolving technologies in lasers, endoscopy, and image guidance. Reviewing the history of MISS is helpful in understanding this emerging technique in spine surgery.

Khoo LT, Palmer S, Laich DT, Fessler AG. Minimally invasive percutaneous posterior lumbar interbody fusion. Neurosurgery. 2002;51(Suppl):S166-71.

With minimally invasive techniques, a complete posterior lumbar interbody fusion can be achieved safely with good results. However, the efficacy of these procedures remains to be validated by further studies.

Lehman RA, Vacarro AR, Bartagnoli R, Kuklo TR. Standard and minimally invasive approaches to the spine. Orthop Clin North Am. 2005;36:281-92.

Minimal-access retractors and specialized instruments are being designed to access and treat different spinal pathologies with minimal access surgery. These minimally invasive procedures are safe and effective, and avoid the surgical morbidities and disadvantages associated with standard open techniques.

Seldomridge JA, Phillips FM. Minimally invasive spine surgery. Am J Orthop. 2005;34:224-32.

This paper reviews the rationale of MISS, highlighting its benefits and describing common MISS procedures.

Tafazal SI, Sell PJ. Incidental durotomy in lumbar spine surgery: incidence and management. Eur Spine J. 2004;14:287-90.

This paper describes the incidence and sequelae of an accidental dural laceration as well as the preferred treatment method once a dural tear has been diagnosed.

Hemivertebrae Resection

Matías G. Petracchi and Oheneba Boachie-Adjei

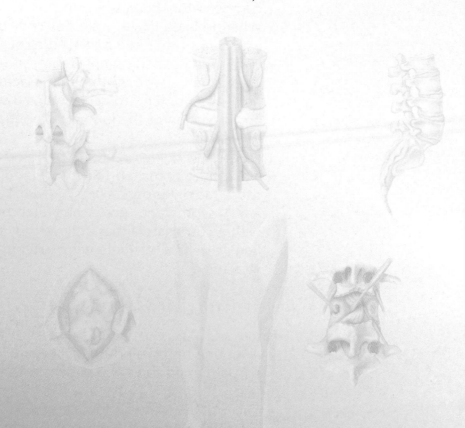

Indications

- To resect an isolated hemivertebra causing a progressive congenital deformity. Recommended in patients more than 2 years old, preferably before compensatory curves become structural.
- When isolated in situ fusion or convex epiphysiodesis would not result in a balanced spine.
- When the isolated hemivertebra causes marked coronal imbalance. In the lumbosacral area, the hemivertebra tend to cause marked pelvic obliquity and deviation of the lumbar spine, generating spinal imbalance.
- Progressive curve greater than 40°.
- If it can be predicted that the type of anomaly can cause rapidly progression. The worst situation is a fully segmented, nonincarcerated hemivertebra with a contralateral bar, followed by two unilateral hemivertebrae, a single hemivertebra, and wedge vertebra.

Examination/Imaging

HISTORY AND PHYSICAL

- A routine history and physical examination should be performed as in any patient with spinal deformity (Fig. 1).
- Rule out associated anomalies (62%)
  - VATER syndrome (vertebral anomalies, anorectal atresia, tracheoesophageal fistula, and renal and vascular anomalies)
  - VACTERL syndrome (VATER + cardiac and limb defects)
  - Genitourinary tract anomalies (20%)
  - Cardiac defects (26%)
  - Intraspinal anomalies (18%)
  - Other musculoskeletal problems
    - Other spinal anomalies
    - Clubfoot
    - Development dysplasia of the hip
    - Limb hypoplasia
    - Sprengel's deformity

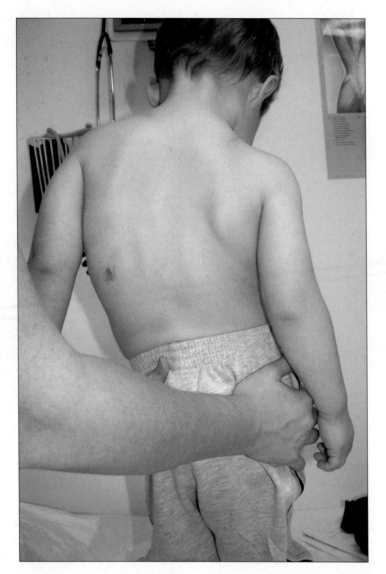

FIGURE 1

Radiographs

- Rule out other vertebral abnormalities
- Panoramic anteroposterior and lateral radiographs of the complete spine (Fig. 2A and 2B)
- Focal radiographs in the area of the anomaly (Fig. 2C)
- Dynamic evaluation to understand the compensatory curves adjacent to the hemivertebra: left (Fig. 3A) and right (Fig. 3B) bending and traction films

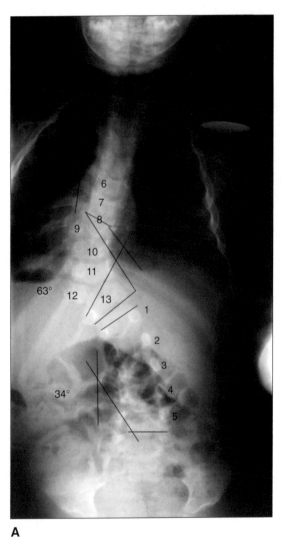

A

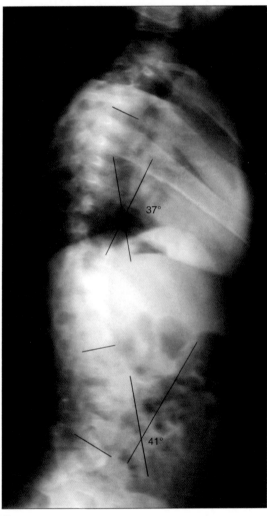

B

FIGURE 2A-B

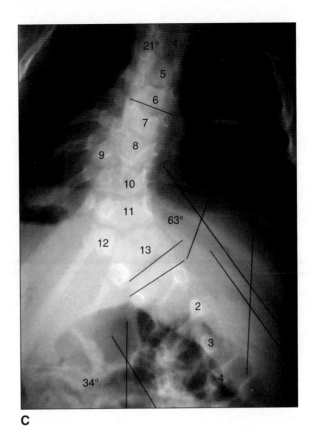

C

FIGURE 2C *Continued*

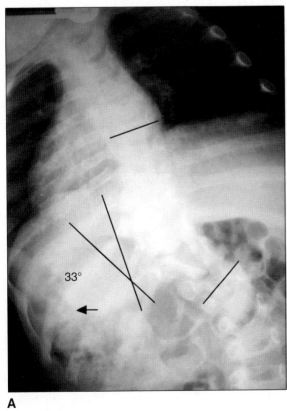

A

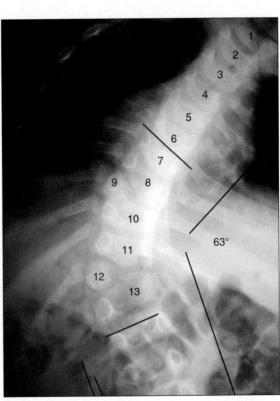

B

FIGURE 3A-B

Treatment Options

- In situ posterior fusion
  - When progression is documented and no major deformity is present
  - Usually in patients younger than 5 years
  - The fusion is one level proximal and distal to the hemivertebra
  - The addition of instrumentation helps to avoid or decrease the cast time.
  - An anterior procedure can be combined with posterior fusion to avoid a crankshaft phenomenon.
- Convex-side growth arrest (unilateral epiphysiodesis)
  - Best results in patients less than 5 years old with single lumbar hemivertebra and in curves not greater than 50-60°
  - Results are uncertain because the growth potential of the concave side is variable and unpredicted.
  - The procedure must be done along the entire curve.
- Convex-side growth arrest combined with concave distraction: for unpredicted growth on the concave side
- Hemivertebra excision
  - Potential benefit of better correction (60-70% of the curve), permits good control of the trunk shift and the kyphosis, decreases the likelihood of pseudarthrosis, and prevents crankshaft phenomenon
  - Combined anterior and posterior approach, either simultaneous or sequential (same day or two stages separated by 10 days)
  - Alternative isolated posterior procedure: one-approach, one-stage procedure that is technically more demanding, with a theoretically increased risk for neurologic injury

COMPUTED TOMOGRAPHY

- Coronal, sagittal, and three-dimensional reconstructions
- Facilitates visualization of complex anatomic structures
- Helps to define the vertebral anomaly, especially the associated posterior anomalies (bifid or fused posterior elements)

MAGNETIC RESONANCE IMAGING (MRI)

- Complete spine evaluation to rule out intracanal abnormalities (14-18%) such as Arnold-Chiari malformation, syringomyelia, diastematomyelia, diplomyelia, or a tethered cord
- To evaluate the anatomy of the anomaly (e.g., disk, end plates, bar) (Fig. 4A and 4B)
- To study the segmentation of the hemivertebra and the growth plate
- Size, shape, and location of the kidneys

TESTING TO RULE OUT OTHER ABNORMALITIES

- Genitourinary abnormalities (29%): ultrasound, intravenous pyelography, MRI
- Cardiac abnormalities: echocardiogram

Surgical Anatomy

- Associated vascular anomalies could be present. Try to preserve the adjacent segmental vessels.
- Expose the convex and anterior side of the hemivertebra.
- Complete removal of the disk. Avoid residual disk during the anterior resection because it can displace toward the spinal canal during the correcting maneuvers.
- Try to resect the most of the pedicles during the anterior approach.
- Be prepared with a wide range of instrumentation to adapt to the size and anatomy of the patient; low-profile systems are preferable.

Positioning

- Lateral decubitus with convex side up
  - For the anterior approach or simultaneous anterior and posterior approaches
  - A roll under the level of the deformity and/or a table that can be flexed will facilitate the exposure.

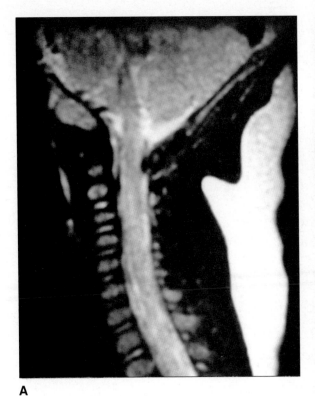

A

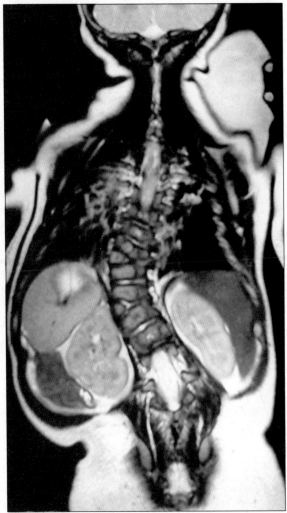

B

FIGURE 4A-B

- The approach depends on the level of the anomaly.
  - ◆ Thoracic (usually above T10): one or two levels above the area of the hemivertebra
  - ◆ Thoracoabdominal: usually the 10th rib is resected.
  - ◆ Retroperitoneal lumbar (below L2-3 space)
- ■ Prone position
  - For sequential anterior-posterior or single posterior approach
  - Position the patient in a four-poster frame, rolls, or another frame that allows the abdomen to hang free.

Portals/Exposures

- Anterior
  - The approach is centered in the area of the vertebral resection.
  - For a thoracic or a thoracolumbar approach, the rib to be removed is that which is one or two levels above the anomaly.
- Posterior
  - The posterior elements of the hemivertebra are removed.
  - The hemivertebra can be resected by this approach, avoiding the anterior exposure.

Procedure: Hemivertebra Resection and Fusion: Anterior and Posterior Approach

Anterior Approach

- Expose the vertebra from the approach side toward the opposite site. Retract the soft tissue off the spine (pleura, psoas muscle).
- Remove the adjacent disks and cartilage from the end plates utilizing a scalpel, rongeurs, curettes, Cobb retractors, and burr. A hinge consisting of a small portion of the anulus is preserved on the concave side to avoid lateral translation of the adjacent structures.
- Resect the vertebral body
  - Special attention should be paid to resecting the posterior wall and part of the pedicle.
  - Avoid damaging the dura and the nerve root exiting below the pedicle.
  - If profuse bleeding occurs from epidural veins, utilize bipolar cautery if possible and/or apply hemostatic agents (Gelfoam soaked with thrombin [Pharmacia Corp., Peapak, NJ], Tisseel) combined with focal pressure.
- Morselized bone graft, structural bone graft, or cages combined with morselized bone graft can be inserted in the gap. Usually the structural interbody devices help to correct the associated kyphosis.
- Some surgeons perform the instrumentation during this part of the procedure and supplement it with a posterior fusion. This can be done when the bone stock is adequate.

PEARLS

- *Consider Cell Saver utilization.*

- *In thoracic and thoracolumbar levels, consider spinal cord monitoring.*

  - *Somatosensory and motor evoked potentials during the procedure*

  - *Wake-up test after reducing maneuvers and stabilization if the intraoperative monitoring is not reliable*

- *Free-running electromyographic potentials may be used.*

- *After resecting the body of the hemivertebra, a structural interbody device helps to correct the deformity.,*

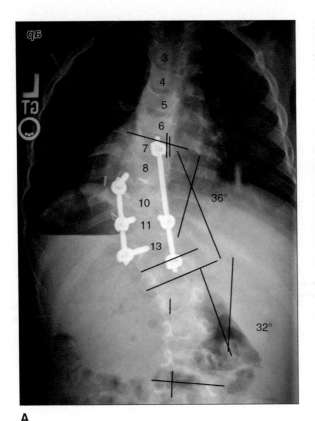

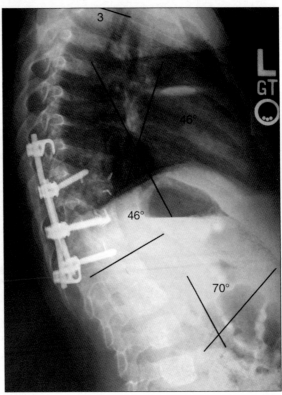

A   **B**

FIGURE 5A-B

Posterior Approach

■ Remove the posterior elements.
  • Excise the adjacent soft tissue attached to the lamina (ligaments and capsules).
  • Excise the lamina, facets, transverse process, and the remaining pedicle if it was partially resected from the anterior approach.
■ The stabilization can be performed with casting.
  • Pantaloon spica cast
  • Cast molded with the patient bent toward the convexity and avoiding kyphosis in the area of the vertebral resection
■ Alternatively, the stabilization can be performed with instrumentation adapted to the size of the patient.
  • A wide range of instrumentation should be available in the operating room, including screws (pedicle, iliac), hooks, and cables or wires (Fig. 5A and 5B).
  • Part of the instrumentation can be done before beginning with the posterior element resection, and temporary stabilization may be done to avoid instability and translation of the adjacent vertebrae.
  • Definitive stabilization is done compressing on the convex side to avoid kyphosis.

Procedure: Isolated Posterior Hemivertebra Resection and Fusion

- The hemivertebra can be resected by a single posterior approach, avoiding the anterior exposure.
- The posterior elements of the hemivertebra are removed, including the posterior parts of the pedicle. Expose and protect the adjacent nerve roots. The dural sac usually has deviated to the concave side.
- In thoracic hemivertebra, the attached rib head is excised.
- The lateral and anterior parts of the hemivertebra are exposed.
- The disks adjacent to the hemivertebra are cut, and the rest of the hemivertebra is resected with osteotomes, curettes, rongeurs, or Kerrison punches depending on the personal choice of the surgeon. It can be done like an eggshell procedure.
- The remaining disk and end plates adjacent to the hemivertebra have to be removed.
- Morselized bone graft, structural bone graft, or cages combined with morselized bone graft can be inserted in the gap. Anterior column support with structural interbody devices helps to correct the associated kyphosis.
- Part of the instrumentation can be done before beginning with the posterior element resection, and temporary stabilization may be done to avoid instability and translation of the adjacent vertebrae.
- Definitive stabilization is done by compressing on the convex side to avoid kyphosis.
- Short segmental fusions can be done in cases of a single hemivertebra without bars, rib synostosis, or other major structural changes.

Postoperative Care and Expected Outcomes

- Place the patient in a brace or cast for 3 months.

Evidence

Benli IT, Aydin E, Alanay A, Uzumcugil O, Buyukgullu O, Kis M. Results of complete hemivertebra excision followed by circumferential fusion and anterior or posterior instrumentation in patients with type-IA formation defect. Eur Spine J. 2006;16: 1-11.

Bollini G, Docquier PL, Viehweger E, Launay F, Jouve JL. Lumbar hemivertebra resection. J Bone Joint Surg Am. 2006;88:1043-52.

Bollini G, Docquier PL, Viehweger E, Launay F, Jouve JL. Thoracolumbar hemivertebrae resection by double approach in a single procedure: long-term follow-up. Spine. 2006;31:1745-57.

Bradford DS, Boachie-Adjei O. One-stage anterior and posterior hemivertebral resection and arthrodesis for congenital scoliosis. J Bone Joint Surg Am. 1990;72:536-40.

Hedequist D, Emans J. Congenital scoliosis. J Am Acad Orthop Surg. 2004;12:266-75.

Hedequist DJ, Emans JB. The correlation of preoperative three-dimensional computed tomography reconstructions with operative findings in congenital scoliosis. Spine. 2003;28:2531-4.

Hedequist DJ, Hall JE, Emans JB. Hemivertebra excision in children via simultaneous anterior and posterior exposures. J Pediatr Orthop. 2005;25:60-3.

Holte DC, Winter RB, Lonstein JE, Denis F. Excision of hemivertebrae and wedge resection in the treatment of congenital scoliosis. J Bone Joint Surg Am. 1995;77:159-71.

Lazar RD, Hall JE. Simultaneous anterior and posterior hemivertebra excision. Clin Orthop Relat Res. 1999;364:76-84.

McMaster MJ, Ohtsuka K. The natural history of congenital scoliosis: a study of two hundred and fifty-one patients. J Bone Joint Surg Am. 1982;64:1128-47.

Nasca RJ, Stilling FH 3rd, Stell HH. Progression of congenital scoliosis due to hemivertebrae and hemivertebrae with bars. J Bone Joint Surg Am. 1975;57):456-66.

Ruf M, Harms J. Posterior hemivertebra resection with transpedicular instrumentation: early correction in children aged 1 to 6 years. Spine. 2003;28:2132-8.

Shono Y, Abumi K, Kaneda K. One-stage posterior hemivertebra resection and correction using segmental posterior instrumentation. Spine. 2001;26:752-7.

Slabaugh PB, Winter RB, Lonstein JE, Moe JH. Lumbosacral hemivertebrae: a review of twenty-four patients, with excision in eight. Spine. 1980;5:234-44.

Suh SW, Sarwark JF, Vora A, Huang BK. Evaluating congenital spine deformities for intraspinal anomalies with magnetic resonance imaging. J Pediatr Orthop. 2001;21:525-31.

INDEX

Note: Page numbers followed by f refer to figures; page numbers followed by t refer to tables.